# TOTAL HEALTH
# TURNAROUND

## THE **ALL-NATURAL PLAN** TO REVERSE ADRENAL FATIGUE, LOSE WEIGHT, AND **FEEL BETTER FAST**

# DR. TRICIA PINGEL
### NATUROPATHIC PHYSICIAN

RODALE

© 2014 by Tricia Pingel, NMD

Printed in the United States of America

Rodale Inc. makes every effort to use acid-free ∞, recycled paper ♲.

Photo page 82: courtesy of Steve Gladys; photo page 111: courtesy of Erin Mulkins; photo page 280: © Misty Moffitt Photography

Book design by Joanna Williams

Library of Congress Cataloging-in-Publication Data is on file with the publisher.

ISBN 978–1–62336–200–3

4   6   8   10   9   7   5   3      hardcover

We inspire and enable people to improve their lives and the world around them.
rodalebooks.com

To those who have inspired me and given me
the support and direction I needed to find my path:

Mr. Moppet, whose unfortunate passing
inspired me to become a doctor.

Birdie, who continues to amaze me every day and has
shown me how impactful natural medicine can be on your health.

Audie and Doe, who taught me to be strong, pursue my dreams,
and made your love for me abundantly clear.

My patients, who have amazed me with their dedication,
devotion, and support. You have enriched my life.

# CONTENTS

Preface                                          vii
Acknowledgments                                   xi

## PART I:
## UNDERSTANDING ADRENAL FATIGUE

1 Do You Have Adrenal Fatigue?                     3
2 The Adrenal-Diabetes Connection                 31
3 Adrenal Fatigue and Your Hormones               52
4 Fighting the Battle Within                       69
5 Take Adrenal Fatigue to Heart                   83
6 Adrenal Fatigue and Your Thyroid                95
7 Stress and Your Digestive System               112
8 Is Adrenal Fatigue Keeping You Awake?          132
9 Adrenal Fatigue: The Nutrient Thief            145
10 Is Your Medication Keeping You Sick?          175

## PART II:
## THE ADRENAL RESTORATION PLAN

11 The Total Health Nutritional Plan             203
12 Healing with Nature's Pharmacy                224
13 Your Adrenal Exercise Prescription            240
14 The Mind-Body Connection                      281

## PART III:
## RECIPES FOR ADRENAL RESTORATION

Breakfasts                                       303
Lunches                                          315
Dinners                                          325
Snacks                                           335
Desserts                                         339

Endnotes                                         347
Index                                            362

# PREFACE

I was sitting in a coffee shop working on research when I found myself distracted by a woman at the next table. She was obese, sitting by herself, and seemed to be in deep thought. She looked sad, depressed, and worried. She also looked lonely. In front of her sat a plate of waffles with butter, syrup, and powdered sugar. Next to it, there was a second plate with a double serving of bacon. She drank a very large, iced coffee drink that appeared to be made with cream. While she ate fairly slowly, she stared off into the air, obviously distracted. I began to wonder what—or who—she was thinking about.

As I looked around the rest of the coffee shop, I noticed that it was filled with people chatting. They were smiling, laughing, and enjoying their company. I highly doubt they were even thinking about how healthy the food was that they were consuming. Meanwhile, this woman took out a bottle of medication, swallowed three different pills, and sipped her coffee. She pulled out something to read, but then she put it away and continued to stare off. As I looked around the room, my eyes caught hers, and she quickly looked away.

Suddenly, I was reminded of a patient I had seen the day before; she weighed about 300 pounds and had come to me for a wellness consultation. She was nervous, shaking at the thought of seeing a doctor. Having not seen a doctor in 20 years out of fear of what one might say to her, she stated that her husband had left her a few years before because she was "fat." She shared that she did not used to be fat, but when the state of her marriage became stressful, she turned to food. Now she couldn't seem to leave it; she was addicted.

I could see the pain in her eyes. I wanted to hold her, but I couldn't. She agreed to a blood sample, which I suspected would show significant issues with her cardiovascular system, thyroid, and blood sugar. How would I tell her that her obesity has led to diseases that could kill her if she doesn't get them under control—that her grandchildren may never know her? Who am I to tell someone what is wrong with them? Everyone else in her life has left her due to her obesity. What will she say to me when I confront her with the damage that has been done? Will I be the "bad guy" who depresses her even further?

Everyone has felt this way at some point, regardless of his or her weight. Everyone feels insecure at some time, feels unloved, feels lost. What is the difference between the women who recover and those who continue down this path? Why do they let food harm their bodies? Do they consciously know what they are doing to themselves?

How does a doctor motivate someone in this state to believe in herself and reverse her disease? I know it's possible. I know it can be done, if you love yourself enough. Society is adapting to people who are overweight or obese by telling them to be happy with their weight, to cherish who they are. Although I agree that self-esteem needs to be improved and the focus on dieting until you are rail thin is inappropriate, it is this practice of teaching that it is okay to emotionally eat that enables people to eat foods that have no nutritional value. It is not okay for people to eat themselves into diet-related disease. It is not okay to live a life of pain, disease, and depression. Where is the balance? How do we help these people love themselves and reverse disease development?

## I'VE BEEN WHERE YOU ARE NOW

When the woman from the coffee shop stood up to leave, I noticed that she was having difficulty moving her body. As she walked out the door with her head down, my heart felt for her pain, her disease, her state of health. I pray that someone or something gives her the strength to see her own value. In that moment, she reminded me of why I became a doctor. I am a teacher, a motivator, a support team for health. I am not a god, I am not omniscient, and I am not a lecturer. I am a voice of reason, and I realize that everyone needs support in order to grow. It is not my responsibility to make you well, but it is my responsibility to teach you how to make yourself well; to inspire you to want to improve; to let you know that you are not alone—that there is hope. This is why I became a doctor. And this is also why I am writing this book.

Like you, I wear a lot of hats. I am a wife, a mother, and a doctor. I am also a house cleaner, an errand runner, and a peacemaker. I am the boss of my practice, I am human resources, I am a trainer and a confidant. In addition, I am responsible for healing my patients. Needless to say, I take on a lot and I, just like you, face numerous daily demands. Odds are, you stretch yourself too thin—so much so that you think you do not have the time to commit to healing yourself. But you do. The problem is that you probably put yourself last on your own list. I hope that, after reading this book, you will move yourself up higher on your list and make your health a priority, as you do all of your other tasks.

## THERE IS HOPE

In my quest to heal my own adrenal fatigue, I have been faced with numerous health issues: menstrual cycle abnormalities, acne, hair loss, skin dryness, moodiness, lack of libido, mental fogginess, gastrointestinal disturbances, insomnia, and extreme fatigue. At times, as I worked through each of these symptoms, I would find myself frustrated or overwhelmed. I had to become more positive and remind myself that I was ill and needed to allow my body to heal, which it did. I will likely always have some form of adrenal fatigue due to the massive impact of the stress I choose to take on, but by following a four-pronged approach to healing—eating the right foods, taking the time to exercise, supplementing the nutrients depleted by adrenal fatigue, and practicing calming mind-body techniques—I am asymptomatic. And by following this same approach, as outlined in this book, you can be, too!

This book will serve as a guide to wellness, giving you the tools to heal your body. You have the power to be well. Realize that you will feel lost at times, perhaps even overwhelmed, and that you may want to give up—but don't. Never give up hope, because you *can* do this. You can start on the path to achieving total health today!

# ACKNOWLEDGMENTS

This book could not have surfaced without the input and support of the following people:

To the three men in my life, Spud, Munchie, and Bucky: You hold my heart, and I could never have made it this far without your continued love and support. You are my world.

To Dr. Gorgeous: Your contributions as a friend and colleague have been invaluable to me. Thank you.

To everyone at Rodale and to my agent, Trina Becksted: Thank you for the confidence and support I needed to complete this book.

To everyone reading this book: Your support is what drives me to continue down the path I began. I thank you for your commitment to health.

# PART I

# UNDERSTANDING ADRENAL FATIGUE

# 1

# DO YOU HAVE ADRENAL FATIGUE?

Are you tired all the time, despite the amount of sleep you get each night? When you lie down in bed, do you toss and turn, worrying about minute details? Are you snappy or irritable toward your loved ones for no real reason? If so, you may have an underlying condition that's causing these issues. In the conventional medicine community, this condition is known as burnout syndrome, hypothalamic pituitary dysfunction, adrenal exhaustion, or hypocortisolism. But in naturopathic medicine, this condition is simply known as adrenal fatigue. And the simple truth of the matter is that you may very well have it.

When describing how someone who is in the throes of adrenal fatigue might feel, the best word to accurately convey it is "overwhelmed." You may feel that the demands placed on you by your daily responsibilities are great, but your ability to handle it all has diminished. If you're someone who used to get everything done with a smile, you may suddenly find yourself struggling to gather the energy to simply get up in the morning. This feeling is depressing. After all, you used to be fun! You used to enjoy every aspect of your life, and now you just feel stuck, like you're running in a hamster wheel with no positive change in your mood, weight, or overall health.

Have you experienced a trip to your doctor's office where you spilled out all of your symptoms only to be told that you are healthy and this is simply a part of aging? Or perhaps you were just handed a prescription for a medication designed to suppress the symptoms you described. Even worse, you may have been given a referral for a psychological consult. It's frustrating! You know you don't feel well, yet no one seems to know why. As a result, you spend time on the Internet and find many other people who feel just like you do. You begin to suspect that maybe your thyroid is the problem, or that perhaps you are experiencing low hormone levels. Yet your doctor says these symptoms are age appropriate and don't warrant treatment.

But that simply isn't true. In 1969, John Tintera, MD, who specialized in treating people with low-functioning adrenal glands, estimated that approximately 16 percent of the public could be classified as having severe adrenal fatigue. However, he added that if all indications of low cortisol were included, it would be closer to 66 percent. And with our lives becoming ever more demanding, this number continues to grow. In 2001, James L. Wilson, ND, reported that approximately 80 percent of Americans have suffered from adrenal fatigue at some point in their lives.[1] But even though it's such a common syndrome, it remains one of the most underdiagnosed conditions in our country, as proven in a 2010 study. Scientists performed a cross-sectional study and found that less than 30 percent of women and 50 percent of men with adrenal insufficiency (AI, also known as late-stage adrenal fatigue) were diagnosed within the first 6 months after onset of symptoms. And 20 percent of patients suffered for more than 5 years before being diagnosed. In addition, the researchers found that almost 70 percent of the patients had consulted at least three different physicians, and 68 percent of those patients were given a false diagnosis. These inaccurate diagnoses proved to have a substantial impact on the patients' health, as those who were diagnosed correctly within 3 months of onset of symptoms were in much better health than those who were diagnosed later. The researchers concluded that, "Because of the unspecific symptoms, diagnosis is often delayed, not recognized by physicians, or diagnosed falsely. An early diagnosis is necessary and might positively influence overall health status in patients with AI."[2]

If you have had any of these experiences, this book is intended for you. This book is written for those who have been told that they are healthy when they know that they are not. For those who have been prescribed medications to suppress a symptom that is likely related to the body's response to stress. For those whose symptoms are typically the result of adrenal fatigue. Because this condition can be treated with natural therapies, you can feel like you again!

## WHAT IS ADRENAL FATIGUE?

So you know how you're feeling, but what exactly is adrenal fatigue and where does it come from? Adrenal fatigue is a syndrome, or a collection of signs and symptoms, that appears when your adrenal glands are doing a poor job managing hormones in response to chronic stress. It results in a fatigue that is not improved with sleep and is accompanied by a variety of other hormone-mediated symptoms, such as insomnia, menstrual cycle changes, lack of libido, hair loss, poor thyroid function, depression, anxiety, pain, and poor immune health.

Adrenal fatigue is at the root of most disease development because your adrenal glands control your entire body. Think of your adrenal glands as your body's control center; their function is connected to almost every one of your organs. They regulate digestion, cardiovascular health, neurological balance, inflammatory response, sleep and wake cycles, production of sex hormones, electrolyte balance, and blood sugar usage, and they give you the energy to adapt and respond to acute stress quickly. After all, we are creatures of adaptation. This means that when your body has been exposed to chronic stress, it will have an impact on all of these biological functions, ultimately resulting in progressing symptoms and disease development. This adaptation to stress is controlled solely by your adrenal glands and results in changes to your biochemistry. These changes in chemistry cause symptoms that can range from a mild headache to the development of a severe cancer (see "Common Symptoms of Adrenal Fatigue" below).

# THE CONSTANT STATE OF FIGHT-OR-FLIGHT

Imagine that you're sitting in the woods, relaxing and enjoying nature. You hear a sound and turn. Your heart starts to beat a little faster, and your hearing is heightened. Suddenly, you hear another sound and focus

## COMMON SYMPTOMS OF ADRENAL FATIGUE

Take a look at some of the most common symptoms of adrenal fatigue. Are you currently experiencing any of these?

- Morning fatigue (difficulty waking up)
- Afternoon lows (feeling sleepy or "foggy" from 2 p.m. to 4 p.m.)
- Surges of energy at 6 p.m.
- Insomnia
- Cravings for foods high in salt and fat
- Increased PMS or menopausal symptoms
- Mild depression
- Lack of energy
- Decreased ability to handle stress
- Muscular weakness
- Increased allergies
- Lightheadedness upon standing
- Decreased sex drive
- Frequent sighing
- Hot flashes
- IBS/digestive issues
- Commonly feeling overwhelmed or exhausted
- Frequent headaches
- Sugar cravings
- Inability to lose weight
- Frequent sickness— coughs, sore throats, colds, and flu

your eyes on the bushes to try and identify where the sound is coming from. That's when you spot a bear. He is much taller than you and growls to reveal his massive teeth. He stands about 25 feet away, staring you down. You experience panic, and your first instinct is to run. Your mind races as you decide in a split second in which direction to head, after taking a quick inventory of your surroundings. It's do-or-die: Your life depends on the decision you make.

In primal times, the bear would have been avoided, or killed, and life would have returned to a calm state. A significant amount of time would likely pass before the next threat. Unfortunately, in today's society, there is always another bear. Regardless of what you do with the first one, whether you run away, or kill it, the minute you "get away," there is another new rustle in the bushes that keeps you on high alert.

We are all surrounded by "bears." We have our jobs to do, spouses to support, children to care for, and social status to maintain. We worry about the impact of our culture, attacks on our land, our leaders, our legacies. Constantly surrounded by the beeping of our text messages, phones calls, and e-mails, we shove food into our mouths while we drive to and from work to save time during the day just so we can get more done. We are in a constant state of fight-or-flight, wondering where to run and how to get there as fast as possible, with the goal of completing every task on our never-ending to-do lists. This fight-or-flight reaction is a normal physiological response to increased stress, but because today's stresses never seem to let up, this continual response now leads to the development of disease. We have become an incredibly ill nation, spending billions of dollars every year on health care while we continue to live with constant fatigue, insomnia, obesity, and disease.

Due to this physiological phenomenon, medical science has begun investigating the effects of chronic stress on society. In fact, a 2012 study showed that when workers were exposed to repeated stress or perceived themselves to be under stress for extended periods of time at the workplace, they were found to be suffering from burnout syndrome and were the clinical pictures of adrenal fatigue.[3] Once considered an area of psychiatric medicine, treatment of the physiological response to stress is now moving into mainstream medicine, as more people develop heart disease, cancer, gastrointestinal disease, mental disturbances, and diabetes. In fact, studies have shown that adrenal responses to stress occur in a way that reflects activation of the adrenal system, called the hypothalamic–pituitary–adrenocortical (HPA) axis. In emergencies such as fight-or-flight situations, your sympathetic nervous system (the excitatory, acute reaction to stress) remains stable, protecting you from disease, but if the stress response is excessive or prolonged, then your body becomes vulnerable and any of a variety of clinical disorders can arise.[4]

## Your Body's Reaction to the "Bear"

While running from a bear, your body changes its entire biochemistry. How? Your adrenal glands release the hormones epinephrine, norepinephrine, and cortisol in response to actual or anticipated stress. Epinephrine and norepinephrine are part of your sympathetic nervous system and give you the feeling of an adrenaline rush. Just the simple release of these hormones begins a cascade of biochemical events.

When released, these hormones cause an increase in your heart rate and help your eyes focus on the target as your body anticipates running. As a result of this anticipation, your body has to begin raising your blood sugar by converting stored energy into glucose (sugar) so you can run. Your liver is called upon to help with this conversion, so it puts aside its daily chore of detoxifying your body to help with the acute threat. The norepinephrine raises your blood pressure by constricting your blood vessels so that blood can easily get to your muscles and you can run. Your gastrointestinal system slows in response to this stimulatory effect, and you are so focused on your target that you ignore your peripheral vision. In fact, by the time you stop running, you cannot remember how you got to where you are. You can't remember if you ran to the left or right, or whether you saw a lake, flower, or tree stump. You simply forget. Sound familiar?

I often hear stories like this from my patients. How many times have you made it home from work, but you don't remember the drive home? Or you walk into the laundry room and cannot remember why you went in there? In medicine, this is described as "mental fogginess" and it's commonly dismissed as a symptom of aging. However, it is incredibly common at all ages.

Another very common concern is a lack of sexual desire for a loved one. Many of my patients are just "too tired." They cannot understand why they do not want to engage in sexual activity with someone they find attractive. This is not a separate symptom, but rather another result of adrenal fatigue. Consider how you feel when you're running from your bear. Do you stop to engage in sexual activity? Or do you pass on it, admitting that you are "too tired" or "do not have time" to stop?

This makes sense if you think about it from a primal perspective: If a threat is high, your body does not find the need to reproduce. We are evolving creatures, and only the strongest of us survive. Mental fogginess, a lack of libido, an inability to maintain weight due to poor gastrointestinal and liver function, and a sense of living in a constant state of worry are likely to lead to feelings of depression and anxiety. You lie awake at night worrying about your future. You are exhausted, but you cannot sleep. Your limbs hurt. Why? Because all we do is run. We binge eat to keep up with the demands of stress and then restrict calories to compensate for our bingeing. We yo-yo diet, causing further stress on our bodies by providing an unpredictable pattern of fuel—fuel we need in order to run from that bear.

Consider this: What if you hired someone to answer your phones, but some days she showed up and some days she didn't? What if some days she worked extra hard and some days she surfed the Internet all day? How would that make you feel? Would you consider hiring additional people as backup for the days when she did not do her job? This need for backup is why, when you do not provide your adrenally fatigued body with a constant, predictable supply of food (fuel), you get fat deposits in your abdomen and your weight loss is limited despite "dieting." Going without meals, eating very small meals, or eating very large meals in an unpredictable pattern when your adrenal glands are under stress will reduce your weight-loss success. Often, this pattern and the failure to achieve weight-loss goals results in depression, as your self-esteem takes a hit due to weight gain. You get stuck in a cycle that prevents your body from doing its job, which is to keep you well.

## The Ins and Outs of Your Adrenal Glands

The source of all of this chaos is your adrenal glands, which are located on top of your kidneys and are responsible for regulating hormones in your endocrine system. Your body runs its endocrine system via signaled responses. This is similar to a sophisticated reception telephone. A call comes in, it is directed to the appropriate party, and then the call is disconnected. This results in either another phone call (signal) or completion of the task. Your endocrine system works the same way: Your body takes the call, sends the call to your brain, and your brain decides whether that call needs to be sent to another department or handled locally. This system is run by a negative feedback loop, meaning that if there is enough of any particular hormone, your body will stop making it.

So if your thyroid function is slowing down, your brain will increase the signal, asking for more. Once the levels are perfect (and it's an intricate process, achieving "normal" for any given person), the call will be disconnected. It is a very sophisticated business and is run very precisely. When one signal is off, it will affect all the other signals and hormones being released. Any stress, whether it is simply a cell phone ringing or something more extreme, like a divorce, will signal a response, or call, from the adrenal glands to the brain for an answer.

I know you may not be excited by the idea of learning biochemistry, but for the purposes of further discussion it is important that you know which hormones are controlled by your adrenal glands so that you can determine which adaptations are occurring in your body, as each body is different. While the primary hormones released from these glands are norepinephrine, epinephrine, cortisol, aldosterone, and dopamine, the adrenal glands are also responsible for the production of the sex hormones progesterone, testosterone, and DHEA. Each gland is divided into two parts, the cortex (the outer portion of the adrenal gland) and the medulla (the inner portion of the gland). Each part releases different hormones designed to keep your body in balance. The cortex releases cortisol, aldosterone, and the androgens (sex hormones) and is responsible for regulating inflammatory response and immune function. The cortex will modify its production based on long-term responses, not simply an occasional stress. This means that low stress levels over a longer period of time will cause adaptation to the hormones released from the cortex. The medulla releases our adrenaline hormones, norepinephrine and epinephrine, and is responsible for the acute response to stress, as discussed in the "running from a bear" example above. The adaptations that occur due to chronic stress are rooted in the adrenal cortex, so let's spend some time discussing the impact of those changes.

## Cortisol

Cortisol is a hormone released from your adrenal glands during times of stress, and it has a significant impact on how your body converts fats, proteins, and carbohydrates into energy. It also regulates blood pressure and cardiovascular function. But its main job is to regulate your sleep-wake cycle. The release of cortisol is what wakes you up in the morning and what tires you out at night. It is intended to be highest in the morning and slowly decrease throughout the day, eventually rising right before you wake from sleep. It is responsible for assisting you when you need energy from glucose, and it affects your use of insulin, which is responsible for the unsightly distribution of fat around your abdomen (aka the "fat tire") in order to provide your body with more energy reserves. Cortisol induces inflammation within your body and lowers blood calcium levels, affecting bone health.

Researchers have created studies surrounding the cortisol awakening response (CAR), the sharp rise in cortisol shortly after waking, to evaluate how the anticipation of daily events or stress predicts disease development. The CAR has received considerable interest in the research community and is the basis for many new studies currently underway. Researchers are finding that people who have higher cortisol awakening responses are more likely to experience multiple sclerosis flares, upper respiratory symptoms, severe depression, obesity, and metabolic syndrome in women. In addition, those with lower cortisol awakening responses are more likely to be diagnosed with type 2 diabetes, chronic fatigue syndrome (CFS), systemic hypertension, and gastrointestinal disease.

The theory is that those with abnormal levels of CAR are essentially adapting to the demands anticipated for upcoming events.[5] Returning to the bear scenario, consider this: Exhausted from running, you are finally safe from the bear and decide to sit down behind a tree to nap. As you close your eyes, you think you hear another noise and you startle. You don't see anything, but you anticipate another foe. As a result, your sleep has been interrupted and worry begins. What if the bear is hiding behind a tree? If he does pop out to chase you, where will you run? Just the anticipation of the bear sends your body into a reaction response that results in panic.

Most of us have felt this before. Think about when you are watching a movie and the suspenseful music plays. You can feel your body change in anticipation of what might be lurking behind the door, and you prepare to be startled. This is a prime example of your adrenal glands preparing your body for an anticipated response, which is as real to you as the actual event.

## Aldosterone

Aldosterone helps maintain your body's mineral balance via sodium and potassium, and it adjusts your blood pressure according to the situation in front of you. It also affects your parathyroid hormone, which is responsible for bone health. When elevated, aldosterone will excrete potassium into your urine and increase levels of sodium in your blood, resulting in higher blood pressure from sodium retention and muscle weakness from low potassium levels (also known as restless legs). Many doctors do not think about the effects caused by aldosterone when the body is under stress, and this means symptoms are often ignored or suppressed by medications that do not fix the underlying problem.

Because the release of aldosterone causes blood pressure changes, its relationship to the cardiovascular system is often acknowledged by conventional medicine. In fact, some of the commonly prescribed cardiovascular medications target aldosterone levels in order to lower blood pressure. If the research on how aldosterone affects the cardiovascular system were more linked back to aldosterone's source, the adrenal glands, doctors would be more apt to treat the source, ultimately reducing the use of medications and their side effects. If you read through all of the research on aldosterone, you would find a lot of food for thought when looking for the source of disease. Let's look at some of the current research and review how the adrenal glands might be linked to aldosterone.

Researchers have spent considerable time looking at the effects of aldosterone on cardiovascular disease. Basic physiology shows us that those with higher levels of aldosterone have higher incidence of hypertension, as it is aldosterone's "job" to raise your blood pressure when it's released. When scientists looked at high blood pressure in patients with elevated aldosterone and compared them with patients who also had elevated cortisol, epinephrine, and norepinephrine, the group with more than one elevated hormone had higher blood pressure and higher cardiovascular risk.[6] Now the study did not suggest a therapy for this, nor did they spend much time pointing out the inference. It was simply stated that cortisol, norepinephrine, and epinephrine will worsen the severity of symptoms.

So what does this mean? If other adrenal hormones will worsen the symptoms, then shouldn't we look to the adrenal glands as a possible *cause* of high blood pressure? Shouldn't your physician consider the stress response in your body before prescribing an agent that blocks aldosterone? Let's say that you have high blood pressure and took a pharmaceutical agent, such as Inspra, which is listed as a potassium-sparing diuretic and acts on aldosterone as its mechanism for lowering blood pressure. If the source of your high blood pressure was related to an increase in all of your adrenal hormones, would the drug work very well? No, not likely. Why not? Well, first let's look at what the drug's benefit would be. It would indeed lower aldosterone and your body would hang on to potassium, thereby lowering sodium, which in theory should lower blood pressure. But on the flip side, if your body is also releasing cortisol and epinephrine and norepinephrine, won't that promote the retention of sodium and result in a fight between your body and the drug? And won't that cause *more* stress, therefore raising cortisol further? Might this then promote further adaptations, such as swelling, inflammation, and blood pressure changes?

Often, this is when your physician would prescribe another blood pressure agent to lower your blood pressure even further by blocking your sympathetic nervous system. Wait! Did I just state that conventional physicians may add an agent that lowers the fight-or-flight response you get from seeing that bear in order to continue to lower your blood pressure? It is incredibly important to acknowledge that the

## CUSHING'S, ADDISON'S, AND ADRENAL FATIGUE: WHAT'S THE DIFFERENCE?

In the world of conventional medicine, adrenal gland issues are linked to two major conditions: Addison's disease and Cushing's disease. People are often born with Addison's disease, which is a disease that causes extremely low cortisol output by the adrenal glands. It's not something you can "catch," though it can be caused by damage to your adrenal glands due to tuberculosis, HIV, immune system attacks, tumors, use of drugs, or endocrine disease. Conversely, Cushing's disease is marked by an extremely high output of cortisol, often resulting from tumors or medication. Adrenal fatigue falls in between these two conditions. And while it's important that we don't confuse adrenal fatigue with these two life-threatening conditions, the seriousness of these diseases serves as a good reminder of how dangerous adrenal dysfunction can be when it goes on for too long.

standard medical treatment for managing blood pressure acts on adrenal hormone releases. So shouldn't we take some time to focus on the very likely source of high blood pressure and modify the treatment to support the adrenal glands, rather than just adding more drugs that will suppress adrenal function and bog down your liver? A study is simply a study, with controlled measures and funding. It is up to your physician to read the research and then extrapolate back to the basic biochemistry to draw a conclusion on treatment. I am asking you, as a patient, to challenge the norm and consider this point. The adrenal glands are involved in the process. Do not ignore them, as they will continue to try to get your attention.

As I mentioned, aldosterone is a big subject of research, but not only for hypertension. It is also being investigated due to its links to bone health and vitamin D. As your level of aldosterone increases, your bone health is affected by changes in the release of another hormone responsible for bone health—the parathyroid hormone. Many people at this point start to develop osteopenia (preosteoporosis) and vitamin D deficiency due to an excess of aldosterone. Studies have researched this phenomenon by looking at people with Cushing's syndrome, which is a disease in which the adrenal gland pumps out too much aldosterone. If these people, who have documented osteopenia, are affected by poor bone health due to aldosterone excess, why wouldn't someone with adrenal fatigue be affected?[7] When aldosterone is decreased, electrolytes are directly affected. Potassium levels will increase and sodium levels will decrease, resulting in overall low blood pressure. Parathyroid hormone is released, changing the levels of vitamin D and calcium, which results in bone health changes. These symptoms are all related and should be treated as symptoms of a common cause, not as independent disease developments.

## Sex Hormones—Progesterone, Testosterone, and Estrogen

In addition to production in the testes and ovaries, sex hormone production also occurs in the cortex of the adrenal glands. As we will discuss in more detail in subsequent chapters, progesterone and testosterone are highly regulated by your adrenal glands and are commonly affected by chronic stress, resulting in hormone imbalances. Reduced production of these two hormones results in a relative imbalance in estrogen, which can lead to estrogen-dominant conditions such as polycystic ovaries, endometriosis, uterine fibroids, and estrogen-based cancers.

## Epinephrine and Norepinephrine

The adrenal medulla releases epinephrine and norepinephrine, most commonly referred to as adrenaline and noradrenaline, respectively. Epinephrine and norepinephrine are released in response to acute stress but have different functions in your body. Epinephrine increases your heart rate and facilitates the movement of blood to your muscles and brain. It also causes your liver to release more glucose into your blood. Norepinephrine, however, narrows blood vessels with the goal of increasing your blood pressure in order to quickly get blood to the areas that need it most. Chronically elevated norepinephrine is a possible cause of numerous diseases, such as lupus, metabolic syndrome or type 2 diabetes, atrial fibrillation, and macular degeneration. Norepineph-rine is involved in many physiological processes, making it a key player in disease development.[8] In fact, the fear and excitement experienced during extreme sports, such as skydiving, directly result from the release of these two hormones.

The bottom line is this: Your adrenal glands are responsible for keeping you alive and prompting shifts in your biochemistry to ensure your survival. If you continue to put undue stress on your system, your adrenal glands will inevitably facilitate a permanent biochemical change, resulting in the development of chronic disease.

# THE THREE STAGES OF ADRENAL FATIGUE

There are three distinct stages of adrenal fatigue, as these glands relate to the development of disease. Determining your stage will help you decide which treatment is necessary. Each stage has some overlap in symptoms, but new symptoms always arise as a new stage is entered. So to begin, take this quiz to determine your stage of adrenal fatigue.

# DO YOU HAVE ADRENAL FATIGUE?

Rank each of these questions with the following scale:

| 0 | 1 | 2 | 3 |
|---|---|---|---|
| never | mild in severity and occurs occasionally (1–4 times each month) | moderate in severity and occurs moderately frequently (1–4 times each week) | intense in severity and occurs frequently (more than 4 times weekly) |

_____ When rising from a sitting or prone position, I get dizzy or see spots.

_____ I find myself getting up more than others in the middle of the night to urinate, or I urinate more frequently than most during the day.

_____ I feel faint, like I might black out.

__3__ I am fatigued.

_____ I experience heart palpitations.

__3__ I have to put in a lot of effort to get through my day.

__3__ I have a hard time getting up in the morning.

_____ I notice low energy right before my noon meal (around 11 a.m.).

__3__ I notice low energy in the late afternoon (3–5 p.m.).

__3__ I tend to feel better energy after 6 p.m.

✶__3__ My most energetic time of day is late at night due to an evening "second wind."

__3__ I have a hard time getting to sleep.

✗ __3__ I tend to wake in the middle of the night or early morning (2 a.m.–5 a.m.) and have a hard time going back to sleep.

_____ I have vague feelings of being unwell, with no apparent cause.

_____ I experience swelling in my extremities (legs, ankles, arms, or hands).

_____ I find that mental, physical, and emotional stress wear me out and make me feel like I need to rest.

_____ Exercise makes me tired or fatigued rather than energetic.

24

_____My muscles feel weak and heavy for no obvious reason.

_____I have chronic tenderness in my lower back.

_____I have a weak back and/or weak knees.

_____I have restless legs or arms.

_____I have a lot of allergies—foods, animals, pollens.

__3__My allergies are getting worse. (Rate 3 for "yes" and 0 for "no.")

_____I notice dark circles or bags under my eyes. They are typically worse in the a.m.

_____I have multiple chemical sensitivities, such as sensitivity to scented candles, perfumes, or even metal earrings.

_____I get regular lung infections (bronchitis, pneumonia, URIs) or have chronic asthma.

_____If I run my fingernail along my skin, a white line appears and persists for more than 1 minute. (Rate 3 for "yes" and 0 for "no.")

_____I notice an area of pale skin around my lips. (Rate 3 for "yes" and 0 for "no.")

_____My palms are red-orange in color. (Rate 3 for "yes" and 0 for "no.")

__3__I have dry skin.

_____I tend to have a sore neck and shoulders, often accompanied by headache.

__3__I am sensitive to bright light.

__3__I am commonly colder than those around me.

_____I do not like being cold, and I have a decreased tolerance to cold items.

_____I have been told that I have Raynaud's syndrome (characterized by extremely cold hands and feet). (Rate 3 for "yes" and 0 for "no.")

_____When I use a thermometer, my baseline temperature tends to be below 98°F. (Rate 3 for "yes" and 0 for "no.")

_____My temperature will fluctuate throughout the day.

__1__I have low blood pressure. (Rate 3 for low, 2 for low/normal, and 1 for normal/high.)

_____When I miss a meal, I notice that I become shaky, confused, irritable, or incredibly hungry.

__3__I crave sugary foods.

_____I use stimulants, such as coffee or tea, to get going in the morning.

_____I crave high-fat foods and feel better when I eat them.

_____I need caffeine (chocolate, tea, coffee, energy drinks, soda) in order to get through my day.

_____I commonly crave salt or foods high in salt.

_____I feel horrible when I eat sweets for breakfast without a protein source.

__3__I tend to skip meals.

_____I eat fast food on a regular basis.

_____My body is sensitive to pharmaceutical or nutritional supplements.

_____I have been prescribed and have taken high doses of steroid medications or low doses for a long period of time (prednisone, dexamethasone, etc.). (Rate 3 for "yes" and 0 for "no.")

_____I have some symptoms (like lack of energy or mental fogginess) that improve when I eat.

_____I have been diagnosed with depression or find myself feeling moments of despair and hopelessness.

__3__Due to my poor energy levels, I find that I have a lack of motivation to do anything.

_____I get easily irritated by others.

_____I get sick more than twice a year (cold, flu).

_____When I am ill, it seems to take me longer to recover than others.

__3__I have rashes, such as dermatitis, eczema, psoriasis, or other chronic skin conditions.

_____I have been diagnosed with an autoimmune disease (lupus, rheumatoid arthritis, Sjögrens syndrome, scleroderma, Hashimoto's thyroiditis). (Rate 0–3 for severity of condition, with higher numbers indicating greater severity.)

_____I have been diagnosed with fibromyalgia. (Rate 0–3 for severity of condition, with higher numbers indicating greater severity.)

_____I have had mononucleosis or have been diagnosed with the Epstein-Barr virus. (Rate 3 for "yes" and 0 for "no.")

__3__Amount of exercise: Enter 0 for 4+ days weekly, enter 1 for 2 to 4 days weekly, enter 2 for 1 or 2 days weekly, and enter 3 if you exercise less than once weekly.

_____Rate your long-term stress levels. (Rate 0–3 for severity of condition, with higher numbers indicating greater severity.)

_____I have perfectionistic tendencies.

_____My health is strongly impacted by stress.

_____I tend to avoid stressful situations for my health.

__8__I am less productive at work than I used to be.

__3__My mental focus has been impaired.

_____My ability to focus is hindered by a stressful situation.

_____I get anxious when faced with stress.

_____I startle easily.

_____I find it takes me days or weeks to recover from a stressful event.

_____I have IBS or digestive concerns related to stress. (Rate 0–3 for severity of condition, with higher numbers indicating greater severity.)

_____I have unexplained fears or phobias.

__3__My sex drive has diminished.

_____My personal relationships are strained.

_____My life does not allow me sufficient time for fun and enjoyable activities.

_____I feel "stuck" in my life, like I have little control.

_____I tend to get easily addicted to drugs, alcohol, or foods.

_____I suffer from post-traumatic stress disorder.

_____I have or have had an eating disorder. (Rate 0–3 for severity of condition, with higher numbers indicating greater severity.)

_____I have gum disease and/or tooth infections or abscesses.

_____For women only: I have symptoms of PMS.

_____For women only: My periods are irregular.

__60_TOTAL SCORE:

| Under 40 | 41–55 | 56–90 | Above 90 |
|----------|-------|-------|----------|
| very slight or no adrenal fatigue. Congratulations! | mild adrenal fatigue (Stage 1) | moderate adrenal fatigue (Stage 2) | severe adrenal fatigue (Stage 3) |

Note: If your score falls on the borderline of the next stage, review the descriptions below to see which stage best describes your current condition or health status to ensure that you've accurately assessed your level of adrenal fatigue.

(Adapted from M. Friedman and D. Wilson, Fundamentals of Naturopathic Endocrinology, Canadian College of Naturopathic Medicine Press, October 2005.)

# THE STAGE BREAKDOWN

Now that you know your stage, let's go through the stages and the physiological changes associated with each.

## Stage 1: The Initial Reaction

Stage 1 is that initial reaction to an event (such as the bear), where your senses heighten and you first become aware of the threat. Most people experiencing this stage of adrenal fatigue do not even realize they have a problem. At this point, your adrenal glands increase their production of cortisol. As a result, your cortisol remains elevated, causing you to feel "high" with energy from the adrenaline. You manage to cross off every item on your to-do list, without fail. Details are not missed. People in Stage 1 are often described as being "on top of their game."

Compare this to the bear scenario, and think about your senses in both situations. Your hearing is heightened, your sight is focused, and your muscles are primed and ready to go. Your biochemistry has shifted to manage anything that comes your way—you are "invincible." I find that many younger people live in this stage. They were raised with things beeping and blinking at them since birth. The technology age has made this a necessity. Seven-year-olds have cell phones, while teens now go to school, take early college classes, and have jobs, cars, iPads, and more. And they seamlessly pull it all off.

The downside—physiologically—to being in Stage 1 is that you are using all of the resources provided to you by your body. Nutritionally, your adrenal glands use vitamin C, $B_5$, $B_6$, and $B_{12}$, plus a variety of minerals to maintain balance and adapt to the situation at hand. Your body does this by altering your biochemical pathways to elicit an appropriate response to the threat ahead of you. During Stage 1, a person will usually have the nutrients available because they are typically young, and there is not a history, at that point, of prolonged stress. Some exceptions to this rule are those who have experienced eating disorders or a poor nutritional foundation during the previous years. Those people will have fewer nutrients available and therefore will progress to Stage 2 faster than someone with a sound nutritional base.

In either case, when experiencing the effects of Stage 1 adrenal fatigue, you are using up your stock of nutrients very quickly. If you are not replenishing what your body is using, you will eventually move along to Stage 2, where more troublesome symptoms occur.

## Stage 2: The Roller Coaster

Stage 2 is the most commonly diagnosed stage of adrenal fatigue, and it's often where disease development begins. I find that people in this stage spend a long time here, often 5 to 10 years, and that timeline alone makes it the most common stage that I treat. The difficulty with evaluation and treatment of this stage is that each person experiences different and variable symptoms.

This stage also has a progression associated with it that can change symptoms over time. For example, you may start with insomnia and anxiety as your only symptoms. Then, the following year, you may develop menstrual cycle irregularities and find that you are tired all the time. Soon after, you may develop high blood pressure, followed by elevated cholesterol. What may appear as "independent" symptoms developing over a period of time are actually quite commonly all part of the Stage 2 process. Why? Stage 2 involves fluctuations in cortisol, similar to the ups and downs of a roller coaster. You will go up a hill slowly, then come right back down quickly. You may turn a corner, experience a bump, and then come to a stop before the next hill. You are left constantly guessing what your next symptom will be, and as soon as you think you have one of the symptoms under control, you'll round another turn that causes another development. You may experience moments of extreme focus and good energy, but then, without warning, you will also have moments of insomnia, excessive fatigue, and depression. It is unpredictable. Most women at this point suspect perimenopause, as they feel like they are on an emotional roller coaster and immediately blame their reproductive hormones.

People in Stage 2 are also more prone to anxiety, as they will experience high levels of norepinephrine, epinephrine, and cortisol at various times, causing "attacks" or heart palpitations. Think about that roller coaster again: There is an anticipation of a fall, and when you do head down the hill, you feel a rush of adrenaline. Most physicians, when presented with this complaint by a patient, refer them to a cardiologist, who typically finds nothing wrong with the heart. They are then referred to a psychologist for antianxiety medication. The symptom is treated, but the underlying cause is not addressed. The medication they are prescribed then "dumbs down" their reaction to their adrenal output, so the adrenal glands become even more fatigued trying to elicit the appropriate response to what they see as a threat.

Keep in mind that your adrenal glands simply run off of input. The beep of a cell phone has the same effect on your brain and adrenal glands as a physical threat would. Anything that stimulates your brain to say, "look at me" in a quick manner will promote a response. Your adrenal glands do this to protect you from the effects of stress; unfortunately, you keep encountering bears to challenge your body. If you think of your adrenal glands as a friend, someone who warns you to slow down, you will fare much better during this stage. The more you ignore them, the more they will do to try to notify you of danger.

Imagine a toddler who is asking his mother for something. Mom keeps putting him off, telling him to wait. At some point, the toddler will throw a fit to get what he needs. Just like the toddler, when your adrenal glands are being ignored and suppressed with medications, they will overreact in order to be heard. They start to raise your baseline blood sugar, insulin, and blood pressure—or most commonly, they change your sleep cycles. Now you're not sleeping well, which means that your body does not regenerate during the night and has used up most of your nutritional resources. As a result, you begin to notice that you look tired. In addition, you may notice that your skin is sallow, you're losing hair, or you may even be gaining weight. And as a result of these changes, you have little motivation and begin to worry. People with Stage 2 adrenal fatigue often stew over what might be happening to their bodies. This causes further adrenal output and more physiological changes, resulting in high cholesterol (to make more cortisol) and potentially hypertension; thyroid changes; estrogen, progesterone, or testosterone changes; reflux; and changes in bowel movements (IBS).

At this point, many conventional medications are brought on board to treat the symptoms of these conditions that are related to your adrenal glands. Your doctor prescribes these and treats your issues as individual problems, not as symptoms of a whole. Unfortunately, these medications can then cause more nutritional deficiencies, furthering the adrenal cycle. This is the point at which you feel like you're running in a hamster wheel, without a clear explanation of why you feel like you do. Most of my patients have spent years in this cycle, desperately grasping for some answer. They try hormone therapy, thyroid therapy, and even change their lifestyles to abide by the conventional world's standard food pyramid (which does not address the massive loss of nutrients caused by adrenal fatigue). They try fad diets and stimulants, and reach for anything they can find to get better. Nothing works, and as a result, Stage 2 of adrenal fatigue produces a feeling of hopelessness.

Take a moment to imagine baking cakes in your kitchen. You have purchased plenty of flour, sugar, and eggs, and you've practiced the perfect technique for baking the cakes. You are so good at it that people start demanding your cakes. You decide to start a cake-making business and hire some employees to help out. Imagine that your thyroid, progesterone, estrogen, and testosterone are your employees. They are responsible for maintaining the supply of flour, taking orders, and performing customer service duties. Cortisol is your demand. The line of people is outside placing orders and expecting well-made cake. The hormones DHEA and pregnenolone are your supply (your flour, sugar, and eggs). As the demand for cakes increases, you require more supply to keep up with the demand. This system works great for a while, and you fulfill all your orders and produce incredible-tasting cakes (as in Stage 1).

Then the demand increases and you become a pioneer in cakes.

Everybody wants them. But you find yourself running out of flour on some days, so you put higher demand on your employees to fetch some. As a result of working so hard to meet your demands, they grow tired and fall asleep on the job. Sometimes they're so exhausted that they forget to even show up for work. Meanwhile, outside your shop there is a line of angry, impatient customers demanding more cakes. You start to feel overwhelmed with the responsibility of managing your employees and the constant customer demands. Ultimately, the quality of your cakes is affected. Some days, you run out of supplies and have to turn people away, causing you to feel lost and confused about why you started this business and what the purpose of it was. In addition, you worry about your future, experience depression, and sit up late at night wondering whether or not you can meet the next day's demands.

Before long, you're tired, frustrated, and just want to give up. Your employees eventually quit (this is basically what happens during menopause and andropause), and you are left with a low supply of flour and demand that waxes and wanes. People stop showing up to buy your cakes, and your business is failing. Think about how that feels: You have worked so hard to achieve success and have taken on everything yourself, resulting in failure. You want to stand in the kitchen and cry. You feel overwhelmed, exhausted, and frustrated. You lose interest in what you love to do because the stress associated with this failure is so overwhelming. You want to give up. This struggle to decide whether to give up or continue to fight may last a long time. It may last 2 to 3 years, during which you may experience a constant feeling of loss, lack of focus, and outright fatigue. At some point, if you don't change the way you do business, you will choose to quit. When you reach this point, you have progressed to Stage 3. You have given in to the demand and given up on the future.

This may sound grim, but this is today's society. With constant demands placed on your body, you struggle to keep up with your day-to-day responsibilities. There is no way your body can continue to run at such a fast pace indefinitely. The candle is being burned at both ends, and this results in burnout. Unfortunately, it's rare for a patient to express to me that they have good energy. Most are tired, napping in the afternoon, sleeping poorly, and so busy that they could barely take time to come in to my office. Many don't have the time or energy to commit to a supplement or exercise regimen due to their schedules. I can recognize my Stage 2 patients by how often they cancel or reschedule their appointments. I find that those running in a hamster wheel are constantly rescheduling due to being "too busy" to leave and come in for an appointment. How can I make someone better if they cannot find the time to commit to themselves?

Does any of this sound familiar? Ask yourself, when is the last time you simply sat down and relaxed? When was the last time you did nothing but be with yourself, away from electronics? How long does it take you to eat a meal? Is the meal about the food or the company? Throughout history, humans relaxed quite a bit. After catching our food and securing our shelter, we simply sat and enjoyed nature. We enjoyed our families and friends. We slept. We felt our feet on the ground. Have you done that recently? When asked this question, most of my patients say they relax all the time, but on further examination, they are usually watching television or surfing the Web or chatting on their phones. They are typically indoors on a couch. If this sounds like your life, I encourage you to go outside, sit in the grass barefoot, and simply watch the world. Let your mind go. Use your imagination. Make it a point each and every day to spend 30 minutes away from modern society. Sound crazy? Can't imagine taking the time to break away for some "me time"? If so, you are likely in the midst of Stage 2 and are quickly moving to Stage 3. And Stage 3 is not a fun place to be.

## Stage 3: The White Flag

The third stage of adrenal fatigue occurs when your glands have ceased to pump out hormones, causing low levels of those hormones—and low levels of cortisol, specifically. Your body has decided it is not worth the fight anymore. A person in Stage 3 of adrenal fatigue becomes depressed, begins to catch colds easily, and generally feels run-down. All of the conditions that develop during Stage 3 will be discussed in detail in subsequent chapters, but in summary, most people experiencing early Stage 3 adrenal fatigue will typically lie awake at night and sleep during the day. At the end of Stage 3, patients report feeling that they could sleep for 24 hours straight. They develop muscle aches and pains due to poor nutritional status that causes electrolyte imbalances and dehydration. In addition, they have a hard time focusing on their jobs and they lose interest in friends.

By Stage 3, all motivation to exercise and eat healthfully is gone. Most people at this stage have developed insulin resistance (type 2 diabetes), high cholesterol, low sex hormone production, low thyroid function, and hypertension. Many even develop cancer due to the demands constant cortisol output places on their immune systems. And just like during Stage 2, it is common for medications to be prescribed to help with the symptoms, without focusing on the cause.

Most people are toxic by this point, because the liver has been overworked for all those years. A recent study—the first of its kind—showed a connection between elevated liver enzymes and adrenal insufficiency. It was thought that liver enzymes only elevated with autoimmunity, fatty liver, or viruses. However, this study found that liver enzymes will elevate when someone has low adrenal function. This study found that if the patients' cortisol levels were increased, their liver enzymes regulated.[9] Those with bogged-down liver function due to adrenal fatigue will start reacting to items they never had trouble with before, such as particular foods, jewelry, cleaning agents, or scented candles. When you look at the entire picture, it makes sense that your body would give up. It used up all of its resources to keep up with the demand. It sacrificed its own nutrition, hormones, and immune function to give in to the constant stress. Going back to the cake analogy, your body, or the "boss," has been trying to communicate with you via its employees (thyroid hormones, sex hormones) for years, telling them that something is wrong by creating symptoms, but all of those symptoms were suppressed by medications.

Lifestyles were not changed to accommodate for this added stress. At this point, you're depleted, and you feel it. You may be plagued with diagnoses such as chronic fatigue syndrome or fibromyalgia, and conventional medicine cannot provide answers as to why. But studies have shown that two-thirds of chronic fatigue patients appear to have underactive adrenal glands.[10] And according to a study published in 2010, when compared with healthy women, those with fibromyalgia had significantly lower cortisol levels during the day and higher levels in the morning. In addition, the women with fibromyalgia reported experiencing more pain, stress, sleeping problems, anxiety, and depression, all of which mirror the symptoms of adrenal fatigue.[11]

Unfortunately, there aren't any medications available for fibromyalgia other than those prescribed for pain management, which further affect your liver and prevent your body from healing. By Stage 3, it is far more difficult to trace the origin and chronological development of disease because it is clouded by years of suppression. As a naturopathic doctor, I base a majority of my treatment around the idea of removing the obstacles that prevent healing. This involves finding the root cause of disease development and allowing your body to heal itself.

If you imagine your body as an onion, with a core and multiple layers, it is imperative that each layer be addressed individually and in the right order. Typically, a patient will present with a primary symptom, such as insomnia. By starting with that layer and recognizing the underlying stage of adrenal function, you can begin to support the adrenal glands while addressing the insomnia. Once the insomnia is resolved, another "layer" may flare up, and at that point it must be addressed. If adrenal function is treated throughout the entire peeling of the onion, you'll eventually reach the core, which will already have been treated. The result is that you cure the disease.

Our modern society places great demands on each of us, and these demands cause unlimited stress. If fear of a "bear" remains, your adrenal glands will spend more time allocating energy and deplete the nutrients you need for metabolic function. The process may take energy from you some days and provide it on others. Your body begins to reevaluate its situation and this starts the process of chronic disease development. As extreme as it may sound, one simple spike of reaction from your adrenal glands can set the tone for your future health.

# MY TURNAROUND
## JESSICA, AGE: 50*

For the last 24 years, Jessica has been working 12-hour days in a position she describes as exhausting. "I work 60-hour weeks on average. I was barely eating because I was so exhausted," she admits. "One of my colleagues was concerned because she knows how much I work. I knew I wasn't eating enough, but I was gaining weight instead of losing it."

After years of suffering, Jessica decided enough was enough. "I went to my conventional doctor, who had been my physician for 20 years, and the blood work came back that everything was normal. My intuition was screaming, 'No, it's not! I'm not okay. Something's not right and needs to be fixed.'"

Jessica knew she needed another approach, and that's when her coworker recommended Dr. Pingel. "I was always open to natural healing, and I knew I needed another approach and to find a doctor who would support me. When I saw Dr. Pingel, she said I had adrenal fatigue and that my body needed to calm down because it was in absolute survival mode. Dr. Pingel said it was because my hormones were out of balance," Jessica says. "I have also been overweight since I was a small child. If you name a diet, I've been on it. Before treatment, I weighed as much as 335 pounds. I had pain, exhaustion, and an utter sense of hopelessness."

Soon after treatment from Dr. Pingel, it was amazing. "I had an improved sense of well-being. I was calmer and more energized. My blood pressure, cholesterol, and blood sugar were all perfect. My weight was falling. My dress size was in the 24s, and now I'm in the 18s." Jessica's friends and family began noticing a difference, too. "At the gym, my trainer and the fitness director now call me a champ. A girl who was body building said I inspired her. My coworkers said, "'You look amazing.' That's huge—to have people come up and say that . . . it's amazing," she beams.

Today, Jessica has a positive outlook for the future. "I've lost 65 pounds, and now I'm thinking I can do anything I need to do. I can get the rest of the weight off—I can do it!" she says. "I had suffered for almost a year and a half before I found Dr. Pingel. I couldn't imagine living the rest of my life like that. Dr. Pingel's approach supports the whole person, not just a symptom. The change I've experienced is momentous—life-changing! I have my life back."

*The patient's name and age have been changed to protect the patient's identity.

# 2

# THE ADRENAL-DIABETES CONNECTION

Unfortunately, despite medical intervention, the number of people with diabetes grows with each passing year. And the disease itself is just the beginning, as this diagnosis comes with multiple complications that affect your entire body, including everything from cardiovascular to neurological issues. Standard treatment involves lowering the patient's blood sugar and improving insulin sensitivity, with the goal of preventing further damage. But what if we could not only prevent further development, but also reverse diabetes altogether? Despite what you may have heard about the disease, this is not an impossible goal. Your body is powerful, and you have the power to change your health and your future.

According to the Centers for Disease Control and Prevention, in 2010, 25.8 million people had type 2 diabetes and 79 million had the diagnosis of "pre-diabetes."[1] This is an epidemic that is not improving with modern medicine. Despite the efforts of conventional doctors to treat this epidemic, the incidence is rising. It is my experience that most patients, when diagnosed with type 2 diabetes, are told that the disease is irreversible. This simply is not true. How can I be so sure? Because I have seen this disease reverse. The key to reversing type 2 diabetes lies in the physician and patient both looking at all of the presenting symptoms when developing a treatment plan.

Diabetes rarely occurs alone; it is typically coupled with other symptoms. It is common for a patient to have a variety of doctors managing each symptom independently, but in the case of diabetes, the presenting symptoms are almost always related. I have seen many cases of diabetes that were the end result of adrenal fatigue. So often, the commonly co-diagnosed conditions of diabetes—fatigue, insomnia, myalgias, high blood pressure, high cholesterol, arthritis, gastroesophageal reflux, and irritable bowel syndrome—are part of the biochemical process that occurs as blood sugar levels are constantly challenged. In this chapter, you will discover the role that adrenal hormones play in the management of blood sugar regulation and how they make a drastic impact on the development of type 2 diabetes and its related conditions.

## STRESS AND YOUR BLOOD SUGAR

So why do we develop diabetes at such an alarming rate? Is it due to diet alone? No, it's physiology. Let's consider how diabetes begins in your body. Your blood sugar is ultimately controlled by the hormone insulin, which regulates glucose levels. Perhaps you didn't realize that blood sugar regulation is actually controlled by your hormones. Most people hear the word *hormone* and think of estrogen, testosterone, and possibly thyroid hormones. But it is important to realize that regulation of blood sugar is part of your hormonal system, also known as your endocrine system. This is why diabetes is typically treated by endocrinologists.

Diabetes is not simply the result of dietary sugar intake. Your body runs off basically three molecules to provide energy for you to live: glucose (sugar), protein, and fats. Glucose is the fastest responder, so when your body needs energy in a hurry, it is essential.

Think of that bear scenario again. You are faced with a threat, so you need two things. First, you need to get energy to your muscles so you can run. Second, you need to focus your mind on your target (in this case, a place far away from the bear). Glucose can be released quickly to accomplish this task. Fats and proteins are better utilized for long-term energy needs. For example, when you eat a piece of candy and it produces a "sugar high," you find yourself focused and energetic. Unfortunately, after about 30 minutes to 1 hour, you crash. That's because glucose is only a short-term energy provider. Conversely, it takes longer to get energy from fats and proteins, but they produce a longer response that avoids a crash.

The regulation of blood sugar is a physiological process of survival. Without it, we would not survive. However, if the sugars are too abundant or the threats are too constant (for example, if cortisol release is constant), it will cause an imbalance between glucose and insulin. Think of it like a scale: When one side is depressed with a weight, the other side has to carry more weight in order to achieve balance. Your body acts in the same manner. If you have too much sugar (glucose) and/or insulin, or too much cortisol, then all of the other endocrine hormones (such as thyroid, sex, and adrenal hormones) will adapt in an effort to become balanced. This imbalance in your endocrine system is the process of type 2 diabetes development resulting from adrenal gland malfunction, or adrenal fatigue.

## The Cortisol Trigger

When cortisol is released from your adrenal glands in response to stress, your body adapts its glucose (blood sugar) in order to react quickly to the stimulus. Your liver increases glucose production (it has the ability to generate its own sugar in absence of a dietary source), and any consumed glucose will rush into your cells so that you can respond quickly to the stressful situation. Have you ever noticed that when you starve yourself on a new diet, after a few days you don't seem to notice the hunger response as much as you did before and you seem to feel better? That's because your body has taken over the manufacturing of glucose.

But this won't happen for long, because your body means for this function to be used sparingly, like in times of stress, and cortisol controls this mechanism. Interestingly, researchers have found strong links between cortisol release, your brain, and the development of impaired glucose levels, yet treatment for the release of cortsiol is not currently considered an aspect of conventional treatment. A study published in 2013 showed that morning cortisol concentration was significantly associated with a higher prevalence of impaired glucose regulation and insulin resistance.[2]

Think of this biochemical process as a doorman standing outside of an apartment building in New York City. The doorman represents insulin, and he is responsible for letting people into the building. The street is your bloodstream, full of people (glucose). Every time you eat a meal, more people appear on the street. It is the doorman's job to keep the building secure and let in only those who are paying rent and contributing to the building's financial needs. In other words, he does not want loiterers or people who do not belong there to come inside.

In your body, the cell is like the building. On the outside of the cell is a receptor for glucose, a "door" that is controlled by insulin. It is insulin's job to regulate the amount of glucose that is let into the cell.

So imagine that all is working well. As people come to the door, the doorman opens it and lets them into their apartments. The streets remain clear and the rent gets paid. But now imagine that the street is loaded with people. The doorman goes to open the door to let people in, and it gets stuck. He can't open it. He pulls and pulls, but nothing happens. So he calls the other doormen to come help open the door. They get it somewhat open, and some people get in, but then it gets stuck again. They call on more doormen to help. Eventually, there are numerous doormen pulling on the door to allow renters into the building. The street starts to fill with people. They dump garbage outside the building. They hang out in the street. The integrity of the street has diminished. It looks horrible. The street is so full you can barely walk, which causes tension and irritability. It soon becomes so full that even if the doormen *could* open the doors, they would barely have enough room to do so.

This is a metaphor for insulin resistance, which is the foundation of the development of type 2 diabetes, or metabolic syndrome. You end up with numerous doormen (lots of insulin), yet you have minimal uptake of glucose. The insulin simply does not work. When your adrenal glands release cortisol, it sends the doormen (insulin) to the building's entrance to help let in the residents of the building. Unfortunately, many times, the streets are filling faster than the doormen can clear them. The residents get comingled with nonresidents of that building (in your body, these are fats, toxins, and excessive glucose), all of whom want to live in one of the apartments. But there is no space available. The littering of glucose, fats, toxins, etc., in the street represents the process of disease development as it relates to type 2 diabetes. And the excessive blood glucose increases, causing inflammation in your body, ultimately resulting in increased blood pressure, nutrient deficiencies, elevated cholesterol, and further disease development.

Think of inflammation in your body as an overcrowding of the street. Everyone is pushing against each other, angry and irritated. Some will charge ahead and cause trouble (such as cancers). Some will sit back and hang out along the outer wall of the building (like plaque in arteries), making it more difficult for others to pass. The harder it is for people to pass through, the more pressure increases and the flow thickens. This represents the significant cardiovascular decline that occurs in those with type 2 diabetes. Once your blood thickens, your blood pressure elevates and your arteries fill with fatty deposits. Eventually, the excessive sugar will be deposited onto your nerves, causing neuropathy (nerve pain or loss of feeling) in your feet. All of these symptoms are known side effects of diabetes and are what drug therapies attempt to treat.

# TREATING DIABETES WITH MEDICATION

Now, you can go about treating diabetes in numerous ways. A conventional physician may prescribe a drug, usually metformin, that attempts to make your body work more effectively with insulin so glucose moves into your cells and out of your bloodstream. Along with prescribed dietary changes, which decrease the amount of glucose in your blood, the medication may work to prevent further decline; however, it will not reverse the process because the signal (cortisol) is still being released, causing the insulin to keep trying to help.

Metformin is designed to reduce the amount of insulin that comes to help. The most common side effects of metformin are diarrhea, nausea, headache, vomiting, abdominal discomfort, and rashes.[3] This is incredibly tiring to your body and although fatigue is not listed as common side effect, I speak from experience when I tell you that patients who take this medication are incredibly tired. They are simply worn out.

The two more serious side effects of taking metformin are $B_{12}$ anemia and lactic acidosis, which is a serious condition affecting your muscles and their ability to contract. In fact, I give any patient who wishes to continue taking metformin regular $B_{12}$ injections to help them avoid developing anemia, and therefore fatigue and neuropathy development. I also recommend exercise; if you keep your muscles moving, it helps avoid the muscular side effects. But simply treating the high amounts of insulin does not address the root cause of the issue. The insulin is coming to help because cortisol is asking it to. Removing the insulin because there is too much is not the answer. You must first find out why your cortisol continues to call insulin to the scene and consider the impact of your liver's attempt to provide your cells with energy.

Metformin is reported to lower your liver's production of glucose and improve the sensitivity of insulin receptors.[4] But if this is true, why is your liver increasing the endogenous production of glucose in the first place? Is it due to poor diet? No, not in the case of adrenal fatigue. If it were due to dietary factors alone, your body would not feel the need to produce more glucose from your liver, as it would have enough from your intake. Your liver makes glucose and releases it via a process called gluconeogenesis when your brain signals that it does not have enough sugar to complete a requested job.

Now here's the confusing part: If your bloodstream is littered with glucose molecules already, why would your liver then be signaled to release more glucose into it? There are a few possibilities. Perhaps this is because your insulin is not getting the glucose into your cells, so your brain calls more potential glucose to enter your bloodstream. After all, it does not want an empty apartment building, and your brain does not understand why it is empty. Your brain sees that insulin is there and assumes that insulin is allowing glucose inside. So when it senses an empty apartment, it presumes that there are not enough potential renters (or glucose) available, and it calls on the liver to bring more.

The brain cannot "see" who is lingering in the street, only who was let into the building. The way your body works in general, and particularly your endocrine system, is that your brain responds to signals *inside* the cells (buildings). If the substance (in this case, glucose) never gets *inside*, your brain will assume it is not there and find another way to get it. Your brain cannot see outside the cells. Diabetes is an endocrine abnormality that is a result of poor signaling between your brain, sugar, and insulin. This is why dietary changes can help prevent further diabetes complications—changing what you eat simply reduces the amount of extra glucose coming in from sugary dietary sources. But this alone does not (and cannot) reverse the process because your liver is still being signaled to generate more sugar. And in order to reverse diabetes, you must be able to stop this signaling.

## Medication versus Adrenal Support

This is what makes the difference between a reversal of diabetes and maintenance of the disease. Your adrenal glands play an integral role in your liver's production of sugar. The reason why your liver continues to slowly raise your blood sugar, regardless of dietary changes and the use of metformin, could be that your brain is calling on insulin to signal more glucose so that you can run from a frightening bear. You cannot run without sugar, and your brain can hear the call from cortisol loud and clear. One simple "Help!" and it can respond by creating sugar via your liver and releasing it into your blood.

Another reason your liver might be responding with glucose production is a personal history of continuous yo-yo dieting. If you do not eat regularly or you've tried a bunch of yo-yo diets that resulted in bouts of low blood sugar (hypoglycemia) over the years, your body will signal for more sugar production in order to remain alive. If you gave your body a choice between having high blood sugar or low blood sugar, it would choose high. Why? Because low blood sugar can kill you. You could go into a coma and possibly never recover, which is why low blood sugar is considered to be a medical emergency.

If the stimulation from cortisol becomes a chronic situation, your liver begins to release glucose more regularly out of fear of repeated hypoglycemia episodes. This results in a slow increase in blood sugar. So maybe this year it normally runs around 75, then next year it's 80, then 85, then 90, then 95, and then bingo! You hit "prediabetes." With high blood sugar, you fill your bloodstream with sugar, and yes, it can cause a variety of complications, but it is not an immediate death threat. Any variety of things can happen during this process of developing diabetes, but they all start with your adrenal glands signaling your brain to request more sugar. This explains cravings for sugar during times of stress. Many people suppress these cravings, but your body will get the sugar somehow—if not from food, then by getting your liver to release it. And this makes your adrenal glands, not medication, the proper focal point if you want to reverse diabetes.

## The Vicious Cycle of Suppressive Therapy

So let's say that you have been placed on metformin to treat your type 2 diabetes. Your blood sugar is dropping slightly from the metformin, as expected by your physician, and is holding steady at around 100 each morning. You continue to go about your life, playing with your children or grandchildren, having nice dinners with your spouse, playing golf, watching TV, etc. Your routine does not change much, and you are hardly affected by the symptoms that generally accompany diabetes. Sounds great, right?

Then one day, during your annual checkup, your doctor informs you that your cholesterol and blood pressure have risen. Your blood work reveals that your inflammatory markers are increasing, but you can't understand why and think that it must have happened overnight. But why? You are on medication and your blood sugar levels are decreasing. Your hemoglobin A1c (or HbA1c, a test used to diagnose diabetes and record your average blood sugar over a 3-month period) is improving. Your doctor had said that as long as your blood sugar numbers decreased, you would be considered stable. Metformin was supposed to help! What is going on?

These new findings are ultimately deemed a cardiology issue by your endocrinologist, so you are sent to the cardiologist and he or she performs an EKG and an angiogram. They find plaque development on your arteries and you are placed on a statin drug and a blood pressure medication. No one connects your diabetes with your development of cardiovascular symptoms because the endocrinologist is only reviewing and treating your sugar levels and the cardiologist is only reviewing and treating your heart and blood vessels. And that's a shame, because what is happening is a direct result of not investigating the original cause of your insulin resistance.

If you continue to treat these medical conditions independently rather than addressing the stress on your adrenal glands, your body will continue to release cortisol in response to stress. But every time it does, with the full intent of raising insulin and blood sugar, it will be blocked by the metformin. Your liver will try to produce more sugar in response to the cortisol output, but the drug will not let it. So a tug-of-war ensues between the cortisol (trying to produce glucose) and metformin (trying to block glucose). And as a result, your liver becomes inflamed due to overactivity. If you run an engine for too long, it will eventually overheat. Well, you liver works the same way. In fact, most commonly prescribed drugs, in particular statins and diabetic drugs, require regular screening of liver enzymes to avoid "overheating" and ultimately destroying the liver itself.

So what does this mean? Think about what happens any time something gets "stuck" or blocked in your body: The area swells. Think about how it would look if a sliver of something became lodged in your arm. If you left it there, the tissue around it would swell. The same thing happens with your liver. It becomes bogged down and tries to overcome the effects of the drug therapy, and then it becomes inflamed, and possibly enlarged, and can even form fatty deposits. All of this raises the amount of inflammation in your body, worsening the plaque buildup in your arteries. It's the vicious cycle of suppressive therapy.

## The Risk of Elevated Blood Pressure

Unfortunately, when you consume sugar, even if it's within the American Diabetes Association's recommended guidelines, it causes inflammation and can result in elevated blood pressure. Now, blood pressure is actually a survival mechanism for your body. If blood is needed in your muscles or brain quickly, say in response to a powerful stimulus, your adrenal glands can raise your blood pressure to accomplish this. They can also lower your blood pressure to avoid excessive bleeding during an injury. Your adrenal glands can change your blood pressure at a moment's notice, and this has likely saved you numerous times.

Imagine seeing a dog in the middle of a busy street. A car is coming, so you quickly dash out into the street, almost without thought, and scoop him up, saving his life. How did you get the ability to quickly move your muscles, considering how quickly you had to get to the dog and successfully get to the other side of the road without causing further accidents or being hit yourself? Your adrenal glands released norepinephrine, epinephrine, cortisol, and aldosterone to raise your blood pressure, send blood to your brain and muscles, and increase your blood sugar (via your liver) to accomplish the task. Once accomplished, these hormone levels return to normal and your blood pressure and blood sugar regulate, assuming there is no further threat.

Your blood pressure can also become elevated because your adrenal glands are overproducing aldosterone in an attempt to get your liver to produce sugar. Research has revealed links to metabolic syndrome development and aldosterone release. In a study published in the *Diabetes Care Journal*, 278 out of 1,215 participants (or 22.9 percent) who were negative for metabolic syndrome (diabetes type 2) at the beginning of the study developed metabolic syndrome by the end of the study. The cause? Aldosterone was positively associated with the change in metabolic syndrome status. In fact, the researchers concluded that elevated aldosterone levels can predict the incidence of metabolic syndrome.[5] Remember that aldosterone is often released when cortisol is released, particularly when cortisol is being called upon by the body on a regular basis due to stress. As mentioned previously, there are clear links to adrenal function, elevated blood pressure, and blood sugar increase, yet many still are not connecting the dots when it comes to therapy.

## Blood Pressure Medication and Your Liver

It's important to know that your liver plays many roles in physiology. It is responsible for the breakdown and synthesis of blood sugar, therefore making it a key player in carbohydrate metabolism. It also breaks down dietary fats and turns them into energy. Your liver can synthesize cholesterol to be used as the backbone for building hormones, vitamin D, and phospholipids, which are the primary fats that make up your cell walls. Your liver builds proteins, breaks down proteins into amino acids, and removes toxic waste via your urine.

Your liver aids in the secretion of bile, which helps with the digestion of fats and removal of toxins via feces. Your liver also plays a huge role in the development of lymph, which aids in the removal of toxins from all areas of your body. It is critical in your day-to-day function, and without a well-functioning liver, numerous diseases can develop. Once anticholesterol and antihypertensive drugs are in your body, your liver has an even bigger job to do, as it now has to work on clearing medications, in addition to its usual jobs. Your liver attempts to perform its intended role, typically resulting in hypertrophy (overgrowth) of the liver and further fatty deposits. Your liver normally breaks down fats, but if your body continues to add more toxins (in the form of medications), your liver will address the toxins first, leaving the fats to go unprocessed. This results in fat deposition in your body and on your liver. The excess work causes liver enzymes to increase, causing further inflammation. It is now a downward spiral of side effects that leads to diabetes.

## The Rising Cost of Diabetes

While medication is costly, it is only one of the expenses diabetics face. In 2012, the total cost of treating diagnosed diabetes in the United States was $245 billion. Of that, $176 billion was for direct medical costs, such as hospital or emergency care, office visits, and medication, and $69 billion was due to indirect medical costs, such as absenteeism, reduced productivity, and unemployment due to diabetes-related disability. Medical expenditures are 2.3 times higher for those with diabetes than for those without. Now those statistics were for diabetes alone, not including the costs associated with diabetes-related diagnoses, such as hypertension, high cholesterol, neuropathies causing amputation, blindness, kidney disease, liver disease, and the need for emotional support.

In 2004, heart disease was noted on 68 percent of diabetes-related death certificates among those 65 and older. Stroke was listed on 16 percent. Adults with diabetes have heart disease death rates that are two to four times higher than for those without diabetes. In addition, between 2005 and 2008, 67 percent of diabetic adults ages 20 and older reported high blood pressure. Diabetes is the leading cause of kidney failure, accounting for 44 percent of the new cases in 2008. And if that's not enough, 60 percent of all nontraumatic limb amputations are due to diabetes.[6] Another important fact to consider is that diabetes is not the direct cause of death in people. As the statistics show, the majority of diabetics die of cardiovascular complications.

According to the Cleveland Clinic, you can calculate your risk of experiencing a cardiovascular event based on your cholesterol, blood sugar, and medication use. One such calculator is available on their Web site.[7] These calculators are provided to patients to help them predict their risk of mortality from disease. Reducing mortality is an emerging area of science, yet the proposed treatment results in further complications, which result in more health-care spending. By combining the research of endocrinologists with that of cardiologists, we would get a better grasp on what therapies would actually reverse mortality without the complications and side effects of medications.

# THE CONVENTIONAL APPROACH TO DIAGNOSING DIABETES

Type 2 diabetes is a condition where blood glucose (sugar) levels rise above a recommended level. Normal blood sugar levels after fasting for 8 hours are between 70 and 100 mg/dL, impaired or "prediabetic" levels fall between 101 and 126 mg/dL, and diabetes is diagnosed at above 126 mg/dL. It is recommended that those with levels falling within the prediabetic range begin a diet and exercise program to reverse the developing diabetic state. Physicians recommend a low-sugar, low-fat diet combined with exercise and often drug therapy.

The first recommendations by most physicians to reverse the signs of pre-diabetes are changes to diet and lifestyle, yet once someone has been officially diagnosed with type 2 diabetes, they state that the condition is permanent. What changed? Why do diet and lifestyle changes reverse the condition of prediabetes but not diabetes? Is your body responsive to diet and exercise at lower blood sugar levels and not at higher levels? I ask this question because most people don't. What happens between 115 and 126 mg/dL? Does your body change?

Type 2 diabetes is the result of poor lifestyle, malnourishment, and stress. Therefore, it can be reversed if you reverse the cause. In my opinion, it is critical to also run blood work that measures HbA1c and insulin prior to officially diagnosing diabetes, and here's why: Typical

HbA1c ranges fall between 4.5 and 5.6 percent. Once someone reaches 5.7 percent, they are considered prediabetic; at 6.4 percent, they have diabetes. This lab value is typically used for monitoring drug therapy. Some physicians diagnose based on this number alone. But let's think about the adrenal roller coaster scenario in Stage 2 of adrenal fatigue for a moment.

Many people in Stage 2 skip meals, binge eat, yo-yo diet, crave sugar, and reduce their water intake. If your body is fluctuating between low and high blood sugar, based on the above situations, your blood sugar will race up and down, depending on your current level of stress and diet. This will result in a higher average HbA1c. So is this diabetes? The answer is no, because I find that those with adrenal fatigue will commonly have an increased HbA1c, but it will be coupled with normal insulin and glucose. In fact, in this situation, insulin and glucose levels are often low. During a diagnosis of diabetes, insulin and glucose numbers will be impacted. Why? Because we ask you to fast for the test. Your body has 8 to 10 hours to regulate your blood sugar before the test. Those who already have diabetes would be affected by this, as the liver is affected during that time, so their tests will still show high glucose. In the early stages of development, however, your liver can still produce sugar via gluconeogenesis, so it has plenty of time to produce a normal fasting glucose level. The HbA1c lets us see an average over time. It tells us if someone has fluctuating blood sugar levels, giving more insight into whether the development of diabetes is adrenal related or dietary related.

Another test commonly run for the evaluation of diabetes is a 2-hour postprandial glucose test. For this test, you have your blood drawn an hour or two after eating. Those with diabetes will show an abnormally high level of glucose, whereas those with adrenal fatigue will commonly show low blood sugar levels. This helps determine whether adrenal fatigue is the source of blood sugar irregularities. But if these irregularities are left unchecked for long periods of time, it will start to develop into diabetes.

Very rarely is insulin tested by endocrinologists for evaluation of type 2 diabetes. Doesn't this test, called a fasting insulin test, seem like a valuable tool? If type 2 diabetes is a process of insulin resistance, then it makes sense to always know someone's baseline insulin. If it increases every year, and the HbA1c is affected, you can start to reverse the development of diabetes immediately.

## The Problems with Recommended Dietary Guidelines

The recommended diet for people with type 2 diabetes is adapted from a base of carbohydrates, fiber, fish, and good fats. Now, I am not opposed to carbohydrates for diabetics, but when reading the descriptions of what qualifies as an acceptable carbohydrate, I find the recommended carbohydrate suggestions to be poor in nutritional value. For example, one sample menu had the person eating beef stroganoff and a side salad for dinner.[8] They do not mention portion size and they state that the salad is the "side dish." Now, if you are trying to reduce inflammation and lower overall sugar levels, why would the main dish be made up of carbohydrates and inflammatory meat? Shouldn't the salad be the main dish? How about 4 to 5 cups of vegetables and ½ cup of stroganoff? How many Americans do you know who eat like that?

The recommended diet also mentions that those with diabetes should get carbohydrates and fiber from whole grains. Unfortunately, they do not mention quinoa, buckwheat, amaranth, and other alternative grains; they only suggest whole wheat. Have you ever read the labels on the whole wheat breads at your local grocery store? Take a look. They're typically full of additives and sugar. And the meal I mentioned above was stroganoff, which is pasta. Pasta is made of semolina flour—processed white flour. Without having a doctor to explain this diet, it is very easy to follow it incorrectly and end up in worse health than when you started.

Furthermore, meat is not limited on this diet, and the recommended vegetables are typically tomatoes, carrots, green peppers, and spinach.

And while you may love those veggies, doesn't it seem like something's missing? What about veggies with more nutritional value, such as kale, collards, radishes, squash, and asparagus? As an alternative approach to conventional dietary recommendations, perhaps we should take note of each food's impact on the adrenal glands and look more at the nutrient content, rather than just the glycemic index (GI) or calories. And even if we did base this recommended salad meal on the glycemic index, we would find that it contains the vegetables with some of the highest values. Tomatoes fall at 35, carrots at 16 to 92 (depending on the cooking method), and peppers at 50. Compare this to kale, cucumbers, Brussels sprouts, spinach, asparagus, and squash, all of which have a GI between 0 and 15. (Not to mention that they're far more filling.)

The Mayo Clinic guidelines mention that you should eat good fats, but to be cautious of the calories in avocados and nuts and avoid going overboard. Now, if your diet in general is primarily vegetables, you don't need to worry about the calorie content. But if you are having a 6- to 10-ounce steak for dinner every night, you do have to worry about it. They also mention fish consumption, which is incredibly healthy and not very inflammatory, but the size of the serving is a concern. How much fish is the right amount? (See Chapter 11 for complete dietary guidelines and sample meal plans.)

With proper nutritional education, one could follow the guidelines given by the Mayo Clinic with great success—unfortunately, no one is discussing the different sources of carbohydrates, fiber, fats, and protein. All foods are lumped into one category. When looking at the glycemic index, potato chips have virtually the same rating as a banana and a Snickers bar.[9] Which is more beneficial to your body? Which do most choose? And why is a candy bar even listed as an option? And why does the glycemic index list ice cream as comparable to oatmeal? Every time you bring a piece of food up to your mouth, ask yourself, where did this food come from? If the answer is a plant, eat it. If the answer is a factory or a box, don't eat it. And if you are someone who is incorporating meat into your diet, ask yourself where that meat came from. Was it wild caught, or was it raised on a factory farm where it was treated with hormones and confined to a small pen? Did your fish come from the ocean, or was it farmed? The bottom line is that it is possible to reverse diabetes, as long as you have a strong dietary commitment and a physician's watchful eye on your adrenal health, nutritional status, and blood sugar control.

## The Inevitable Cycle of Diabetes and Resulting Malnutrition

Nutritionally, your body absorbs the foods you eat and uses the minerals and vitamins from those foods to complete everyday functions. In order to absorb the nutrients, your cells require some key factors. The outer layer of each cell is composed of fat. That's right, I said fat. This layer of fat is necessary for proper mineral absorption. Sodium, potassium, calcium, and magnesium, for example, are needed for normal cell function. When your body is starved of nutrients, and fats in particular, you will start to become dehydrated due to mineral imbalances. The first sign of dehydration is thirst. You drink more water, and then you'll urinate 10 minutes later.

This malnutrition and dehydration starts to affect your energy, resulting in fatigue. If you have a high-stress lifestyle, running from bears at every turn, your body will start to dump potassium and retain sodium. This further worsens the mineral imbalance and typically causes a rise in blood pressure. Your body then starts to retain water, and at this point, weight gain commonly begins.

Now, a typical person in this situation will begin a diet regimen recommended by his or her physician. And this diet typically encourages low-fat, low-sugar, high-protein, and complex carbohydrate foods. The result? Your poor cells begin to shrink, worsening your metabolic status. Your body becomes malnourished, tired, and frustrated. And this state only worsens your adrenal fatigue, causing your body to use its resources to maintain energy production. You begin to store fat around your abdomen for backup energy. Cortisol increases your pancreas's output of insulin, which initially lowers your blood sugar, making you feel lightheaded, fatigued, and foggy.

Most type 2 diabetes cases begin with episodes of hypoglycemia (low blood sugar), eventually leading to increases above normal levels. This makes sense from the adrenal perspective, as it is dropping blood sugar, commonly from the release of cortisol and insulin, that signals

## THE VICIOUS CYCLE OF CARBOHYDRATE CRAVINGS

Think of health as a spectrum. On one end, you have optimal health. On the other end, you have disease (and diabetes is considered a disease). Let's say that you have a fasting glucose of 90, which is considered to be normal. Then, the following year, it lands at 92. Then 95, and then 98. Still normal, but when compared to previous years, it has increased. This process is very common. Most physicians simply look at the range and not the trends of blood work. Then, finally, your blood sugar lands at 102 and your physician says, "You are now prediabetic. You need to change your diet or start taking metformin."

At this point, it is much harder for you to change your ways, as you have developed an addiction to carbohydrates. Why? Because during the slow process of developing diabetes, you have become dehydrated, tired, and malnourished. As a result, you crave carbohydrates to give you a feeling of energy, and when you don't eat them, you feel exhausted, hungry, and simply miserable. By this time, a layer of fat around your abdomen has usually developed, and losing weight is a daunting task to say the least. You cannot understand why you do not lose weight by following standard healthy eating guidelines, and you give up. The weight loss simply does not come as quickly as it did before.

Dieting has become a chore, so when given the option to start metformin, you feel that you must choose to take it, as your physician tells you it is the only other solution. It's ironic that, during a time when the media and health care are focusing on preventative medicine, it's not actually being practiced. Diabetes is preventable if the appropriate labs are run before the condition is diagnosed. HbA1c, insulin, and glucose should be drawn every year and compared to previous years. Dietary changes need to be implemented before diseases are present.

your liver to produce more sugar to compensate. Let me reiterate from the previous chapter that your body wants to keep you alive. If it has a choice between an insulin (hypoglycemic) coma or a slow decline in bodily function (hyperglycemia), it's going to pick the latter. After all, it is better for your body to lose function progressively than all at once. Your body makes a choice to become diabetic. Diabetes is not a virus; you can't catch it. It does not develop out of nowhere. It is a slow-developing, easily prevented disease—if your physician is watching.

# THE STEPS TO BECOMING DIABETES-FREE

So all of this is fine and good, but the bottom line is, America is sick with diabetes and obesity. What do we do with all of these cases? It has become clear to me that unless you restore normal cell function, you will not cure a disease. Diabetes is not simply about avoiding bad food. How many people have you come across who follow their doctors' recommended diets and exercise programs and yet continue to be plagued by diabetes? It is not simply about sugar consumption—it is about malnourishment. It is about dehydrated cells and poor mineral status due to adrenal fatigue. And until you restore the way your body takes in and processes nutrients, a diet will not make much of a difference unless it focuses on replenishing those lost nutrients.

Good fats are essential, and increasing your intake of foods with high concentrations of omega-3 fatty acids is the first step in a multi-step process. Many people's cells are so dehydrated by the time they come see me that I will start with a series of nutritional IVs to restore hydration, minerals, B vitamins, and vitamin C levels. Patients will begin to feel better, have more energy, and feel more motivation to get well. Many of my patients have felt poorly for so long that they do not remember what it feels like to have proper nutrition. Without that knowledge, the patient feels lost and hopeless, and gives up.

I see this often in my patients with type 2 diabetes. Many of them say they are not willing to give up the food they like in exchange for reversing—or curing—their disease. And many tell me that they feel fine. Yet upon further examination, they admit that they don't play golf as much as they'd like to, due to joint pain, or they find themselves taking naps in the afternoon. They cannot play with their children or grandchildren or walk long distances with them at the zoo. If you have developed these symptoms over time, it is likely that you don't fully remember what it felt like to be your normal self. These aches and pains have been attributed to "normal aging" for so long that it's hard to associate lifestyle as a cause. It always amazes me how much proper nutrition can change a person.

Once I've restored a feeling of wellness through nutrition, the next step is to address adrenal function. If cortisol levels continue to fluctuate, so will insulin and glucose. Not only will adrenal support provide even more energy and motivation, it will actually assist in lowering insulin levels and therefore reducing the demand on glucose to maintain balance. If the demand on insulin is reduced by regulating cortisol, the insulin resistance will halt. And if a proper diet is maintained, the glucose in your bloodstream will be controlled. Aldosterone will no longer surge, causing increased blood pressure. Cholesterol, which makes cortisol, will also be decreased, inflammation will lessen, deposition in the arteries will improve, and the massive domino effect started by the adrenal glands will be slowly halted and reversed.

So what is more dangerous—prolonged stress levels or a poor diet? There's no clear answer. It's likely that a combination of the two is the most dangerous of all, but the stress component has to be addressed in addition to diet modifications, or the progress of stress-induced diabetes will continue.

# MY TURNAROUND
## LIZ SNELL, AGE: 24

At age 21, Liz Snell knew something was wrong. "I had chronic fatigue and was exhausted all of the time. Even so, I couldn't stay awake at work in the middle of the day. When my blood sugar would fluctuate, I would experience dizziness, mental fogginess, irritability, low sex drive, etc. I was on the verge of depression," she says. "My family doctor told me I just needed to 'exercise more and watch what I eat.' Soon after, I was diagnosed with type 2 diabetes and high cholesterol by an endocrinologist."

After a year of taking medications for her diabetes and high cholesterol, Liz didn't feel any better. "The medications just masked my symptoms. It didn't make them go away," she explains. "I didn't want to be taking prescription medications for diseases I knew I wasn't supposed to have. I was stressed every single day. I knew I had to do something."

On a mission to discover what was really causing her symptoms, Liz scheduled an appointment with Dr. Pingel and was immediately diagnosed with late Stage 2 adrenal fatigue. "I never suspected the real cause could have been adrenal fatigue, and the doctors I was seeing weren't interested in digging deeper to figure it out," Liz says.

Liz soon began following Dr. Pingel's plan, and within 2 months, she saw results. "It was scary at first. I thought that I needed those prescriptions to function like a human, and I was so wrong. After getting on Dr. Pingel's all-natural plan, I had more energy. I was weaned off of my prescription meds for diabetes and cholesterol. The lab work showed I didn't need them anymore."

Liz's sleeping and eating habits also improved. "Now, I sleep 8 to 10 hours each night and can get through the day with only one cup of coffee! I also eat less meat and dairy and more greens and carbs," she states.

Liz's only regret is not finding Dr. Pingel sooner. "I wish I wouldn't have let myself become so engulfed and saddened by what the other doctors told me. Dr. Pingel was incredibly thorough, and the plan was easier than I expected. I can't imagine myself ever taking another prescription," she says.

Today, Liz is happier, healthier, and more energized. "It's really changed my life—saved my life. If not for figuring it out, I would still be on prescriptions for the next 50 years."

# 3

# ADRENAL FATIGUE AND YOUR HORMONES

In recent years, you've likely heard more and more talk about hormone imbalances: Ads on TV are selling testosterone to men; books on the uses of hormone therapy are being published; medical studies are evaluating the risks and benefits of different hormone therapies; celebrities like Suzanne Somers have begun speaking out about using bioidentical hormone replacement therapy (BHRT) and its incredible effect on energy, even after bouts of breast cancer. As you probably know, hormone-based cancers are continuing to increase in America, and there is a lot of fear in the medical community surrounding the use of hormones and cancer risk.

With all of this new awareness (and fear and concern), many are left wondering why these hormone-based cancers are happening and how to treat hormone imbalances. But has anyone asked, what did our ancestors do? Did they have such a high incidence of cancer? Were their periods painful? Did they suffer from erectile dysfunction? What is changing in our society that is allowing these developments and diseases?

Your hormones are designed to work together in harmony. When we look at other mammals, such as dogs, cats, and cows, which were built with similar endocrine systems, do we commonly see infertility? Do we see them in pain while menstruating? Do we see them experience a lack of erectile function? I pose these questions to you because there is one dramatic difference that affects our physical health: The lifestyles to which we subject our bodies. As humans, we place a higher demand on our systems.

# THE ENVIRONMENT OF HEALTH

Comparing our lives to those of animals may seem pointless to you, but it is a useful exercise that is often overlooked. Having a history in veterinary medicine has opened my eyes to the differences in conventional medical models. For example, let's imagine two plots of land, each with an assortment of cows. On one plot of land, the cows are producing calves with significant birth defects, and on the other plot of land, the cows are producing healthy calves. If you were asked to solve this problem, what would you do? Most medical doctors would start running genetic tests on the cows to find the source of the adaptation. Conversely, most veterinarians and agriculturists would suggest running tests on the soil. It comes down to this: Is it a problem with the cow, or is it a problem with the environment?

Well, it may surprise you to learn that the veterinarians and agriculturists are right. The soil in the plot of land that contains the cows with birth defects is deficient in minerals, while the soil where the healthy cows live is highly nutritive. As it turns out, numerous agricultural studies show links between mineral levels in the soil and poor milk production, development of birth defects, poor reproductive health, and disease development in cattle. These defects result from a change due to a lack of minerals, not due to a problem with the cows themselves.

So how does this relate to our topic of sex hormones and stress? Conventional physicians seem to look at the individual hormone, or the cancer gene, or they pump your body full of hormones in order to induce pregnancy. They prescribe birth control pills to hide the symptoms of endometriosis and irregular menstruation and they give testosterone to fix erectile dysfunction. But have we considered that perhaps this is not the best approach to treating these issues? Maybe we need to take a look at our soil—our environment—to find the reasons why our bodies are giving us these symptoms.

# THE ADRENAL-HORMONE CONNECTION

The adrenal glands make hormones—plain and simple. So this is logically a good place to start the discussion of your environment. If your adrenal glands are affected by your environment, then so are your hormones. And if your sex hormones change, your other hormones will change, too. There is an inevitable domino effect that occurs in your endocrine system, and it needs to be considered when evaluating hormonal symptoms.

Let's start by talking about how sex hormones work together to keep everything in balance. In men, the primary sex hormone produced is testosterone; however, they also produce estrogens and progesterone. The endocrine system is considered a feedback system, meaning that your brain signals the release of testosterone, and when levels hit an elevated amount, your brain turns off the signal. Imagine a fountain with a balloon shut-off valve: When the water level gets high, it shuts off. When the level gets low, it turns back on to add more water. This is the same way a hormone feedback loop works.

## Men: The Endocrine Secrets

In a healthy male, baseline testosterone levels increase by 10 to 20 times during puberty and typically start to decrease once he hits his forties. By the time a man is 50 years old, the amount of testosterone in his body is often about 50 percent less than it was during puberty. Testosterone is made in both the testes and the adrenal glands, and the decline that occurs with age can happen due to destruction of the cells that produce testosterone. This reduces the amount of bioavailable testosterone (the amount specifically made for your body to use) to be absorbed by the tissues. In situations of adrenal fatigue, your body will decrease the production of bioavailable testosterone and will do one of three things with the testosterone it has left: It will store it, remove it from the system, or convert it into estrogen. This last scenario poses a problem in males because excess estrogen will not only cause enlargement of the prostate, but will also commonly cause men to show signs of weakening muscles, breast development, softening of the testicles, fatigue, insomnia, and truncal obesity. In addition, it increases the risk of developing estrogen-based cancers.

So let's say that a male named Bob goes to his doctor, complaining of erectile dysfunction (ED), lack of sleep, and low libido. He states that his buddy gets testosterone shots and he would like to chat about that possibility. The doctor runs a blood test called "total testosterone," which shows that Bob has borderline low testosterone, and the doctor agrees to place him on weekly testosterone injections. At first, Bob feels great! His ED is gone, he is raring to go (sexually), and he is sleeping like a baby. He starts hitting the gym every morning, getting great efficacy from his workouts. He couldn't be happier.

Fast-forward to about a month later, and Bob doesn't feel the same. He is starting to feel tired and he is noticing that his libido is variable on a day-to-day basis. He notices that he's starting to wake up at 2 a.m. again. His starts to gain some fat around his waist despite all the exercise he has been doing. He returns to his doctor, who runs another blood test for total testosterone and sees that it is lower than it was originally. So the doctor increases his dose. But Bob doesn't notice a difference from this increased dose. In fact, a few months later, he is even more tired, cannot seem to get rid of the fat around his belly, and is now becoming depressed.

What happened? If you are replacing testosterone, then why are your levels still dropping? Why doesn't Bob feel great anymore? The first problem here is that we do not know what Bob's body is doing with the testosterone it makes and is receiving from the injections. All hormones have a total number, which is the total amount of hormone produced or replaced in the body, as well as a free value, which is the usable or bioavailable amount. The remainder will either be stored or converted into another hormone—in this case, estrogen.

When Bob first visited the doctor, he was told that his total testosterone level was borderline low. But no one checked his free (bioavailable) levels. Why does this matter? Well, if you were given ten jellybeans and only ate two of them, you only have two that were providing you with sugar and eight left in the bag. So if your total testosterone levels happened to be normal (600 to 1,000 ng/dl) but your free levels were low, then you would know that your body was producing testosterone, but not using all of it. On the flip side, if your total levels were borderline low (say 400), but your free levels were in the average-to-high range, you would know that even though your body is producing less overall testosterone, most of it is being used.

The mistake here is that no one looked at Bob's free levels. So two things could be happening: Either the extra testosterone raised the free levels too high and therefore down-regulated the signal from his brain, lowering the amount of testosterone produced, or the testosterone being added is being converted into something else. Think about the fountain we discussed and its shut-off valve: If it is too full, the valve will shut off. Why should your body make more testosterone if it already has too much? And what will happen to the excess testosterone being "poured" into your body? When a man asks me about testosterone replacement, I have to take into consideration a variety of numbers before responding. I need to know his total and free testosterone, of course, but I also need to know his estrogen and DHEA levels. Why? Because DHEA makes testosterone, and testosterone can turn into estrogen. By looking at the entire picture, you can see whether the testosterone is not being utilized or not being produced, and then you can come up with an appropriate dose or treatment to improve the symptoms.

If Bob has adrenal fatigue, these conversions of DHEA, testosterone, and estrogen will be affected. Depending on the stage, he will experience a number of different things. If he is in Stage 1 or early Stage 2, the testosterone made in his body can turn into estrogen or be stored, which lowers his free levels but maintains his total levels. If he is at the end of Stage 2 or has progressed to Stage 3, his DHEA will be lower, meaning that his body is less likely to stimulate production of testosterone, resulting in lower levels of both total and free testosterone.

When a man is given testosterone at this point, he often feels better for a short time but then feels worse because the hormone becomes an additional stressor on his body. Plus, if he chooses to use a high-dose shot rather than a lower-dose daily cream or sublingual therapy, it will induce even more stress and encourage storage due to the excessive amount given at one time. Why? Because that large shot of testosterone is more than his body can handle at that moment. Consequently, the excess gets converted into estrogen and innate production is shut off. This is why steroid abusers tend to develop female characteristics and become dependent on testosterone supplementation after extended use.

Physiological stress on your body has a gigantic impact on how you use testosterone because sex hormones and cortisol are both made from the hormones DHEA and pregnenolone, as well as cholesterol. If cortisol is being overproduced, sex hormone production will decrease—and vice versa. Every aspect of hormone use and production is affected by adrenal fatigue, and that results in physical symptoms.

## Hormonal Rhythms in Women

Women experience a similar situation when it comes to testosterone. It's common for women to have perfect levels of total testosterone and low levels of free hormones. Think about it: If you are busy running from or anticipating the appearance of a bear, you don't make time to have sex in order to reproduce. Instead, you just run.

Women also tend to convert a lot of their testosterone to estrogen and experience complications from that, such as irritability, excessive menstruation, premenstrual syndrome (PMS), painful periods, fibroid and ovarian cyst development, weight gain, and more. But unlike men, they have a great mechanism for observing hormonal balance: the menstrual period. You can tell a lot about the rhythm of your hormones based on menstrual symptoms alone.

Hormonal imbalances are accompanied by symptoms. For example, hot flashes can occur if estrogen is too high or too low in comparison to progesterone. Again, the greater the imbalance, the more severe the symptoms. Many perimenopausal women are given supplementary estrogen when they complain of hot flashes; this often happens without their doctors even looking at their hormone levels. And their symptoms worsen! How could that be? Because their baseline estrogen was already too high in comparison to their progesterone, and then their estrogen levels increased, so their symptoms worsened.

Hormone therapy is not only a science, but also an art. Your hormones have to be perfectly balanced in order for you to feel well. This "art" is why it is so difficult to perform studies on bioidentical hormone replacement therapy. Every person is different, with a different starting point. In order to conduct a randomized, controlled trial, you need control groups of people who are all exactly the same. How many women do you know who are exactly the same? Treatment is tailored to individuals, and that makes the studies very difficult to complete.

## Symptoms of an Unbalanced System

Some common symptoms of having too much estrogen in relation to progesterone are excessive or heavy periods, painful periods, hot flashes, weight gain around the abdomen, ovarian cysts, uterine fibroids, estrogen-based cancers, menstrual migraines, insomnia, irritability, PMS, and miscarriages. An imbalance resulting from too much progesterone in relation to estrogen presents as excessive breast tenderness, weepiness, bloating, fatigue, and fogginess.

Testosterone plays a role here, too. Remember that every hormone can convert into another hormone, so let's say that there is too much estrogen in relation to the amount of progesterone in your body. That excess estrogen can convert into testosterone and vice versa. Many women think that testosterone is the primary player in libido, but that's not always the case. Women with hormone imbalances typically need to prepare themselves for sexual activity by perhaps taking a bath, relaxing, or having a glass of wine. Only then, when they have reduced the impact of stress, are they able to unwind enough to access that hormone and enjoy sexual activity.

Why is that? Well, if your body is under adrenal stress, your free levels of testosterone can be compromised, making it unusable. If you're in Stage 3 adrenal fatigue (when DHEA is scarce), your adrenal glands may not make testosterone at all. Estrogen also drives sexual desire. In fact, many women report being more interested in sex when they're ovulating. Why? Because estrogen levels are highest at that point, which prompts higher libido, or a desire to reproduce. But if your body is under stress, it may not recognize those signals because it is too concerned about the bear it thinks you're running from.

Recall that if you want to make hormones, you need DHEA. And when you're in Stage 3 adrenal fatigue, you don't have enough DHEA to make cortisol (or other hormones). A 2012 study on monkeys being given estradiol (estrogen) supplementation evaluated the sexual desires of those in stressful versus nonstressful environments. Researchers found that those who were under less stress had higher sexual desire, regardless of the dosage of estradiol. Alternatively, the ones under greater stress had lower levels of sexual desire, even when supplemented with more estradiol.[1] This goes against the belief that supplementation with hormone therapy in postmenopausal women will increase their sexual desire and supports the idea that the stress response and adrenal function have more impact on sexual desire than the hormone itself.

When it's in balance, progesterone calms us down, makes us feel warm and fuzzy, and helps us sleep. If you have ever been pregnant, you may have felt this effect. You may have found yourself lounging on the couch instead of cleaning the dirty kitchen. And you didn't care; you were just rosy and happy. Without progesterone, your body may not calm down enough for you to want to engage in sex. Moreover, irritability caused by excessive estrogen production may also turn you, and your partner, off! Many women also complain that in the week before their cycle they feel more emotional, fearful, or snappy.

A recent study published in the *Journal of Psychoneuroendocrinology* investigated the relationship between progesterone and cortisol and their association with fearful memories. When progesterone is high, cortisol levels are increased and correlate with emotional memory. Remember that cortisol and progesterone are derived from the same hormones, DHEA and pregnenolone, and that your body can convert all of these hormones into one another. This study suggests that progesterone mediates cortisol response to stress, confirming the link between these two hormones and confirming that this could result in higher anxiety and fear levels during the peak of progesterone levels (7 to 10 days prior) of a woman's menstrual period. This shows how emotions are directly linked to hormonal status.[2] The bottom line is that you cannot link a symptom to just one hormone. They all play a role.

## The Dominance of Estrogen

Let's discuss the role of estrogen dominance a little more because it is strongly associated with many of the symptoms typically experienced by women with hormonal imbalances. Estrogen starts off the menstrual cycle by slowly increasing until ovulation around day 14 (in a 28-day cycle). During those first 14 days, this increase in estrogen prompts the building of a uterine lining. Progesterone, which has the job of balancing out estrogen, is primarily made in your adrenal glands from pregnenolone and DHEA, which were made from cholesterol. During the second half of your cycle (days 15 through 28), called the luteal phase, progesterone increases to its highest levels. Its primary job is to prepare your uterus for implantation of a fetus. Once your body realizes that it does not have a fetus to implant, your progesterone levels drop and that causes you to shed the uterine lining, or menstruate.

So imagine that your estrogen level is higher than your progesterone level. Even with that spike in progesterone during the luteal phase, it still cannot reach as high as the estrogen. When progesterone drops, a woman experiences heavier bleeding because the lining was built up so much by the higher levels of estrogen. In some women, this bleeding will last a long time, because the progesterone never gets high enough to stop it. What does this mean? Well, if you have heavy periods, you have excessive estrogen relative to progesterone.

Now, this could be due to one of two things: Either you have high amounts of estrogen or you have low amounts of progesterone. The common therapy at this time is the birth control pill because it keeps your levels from fluctuating. It holds them steady so that your body cannot build up as much lining and the shedding is diminished, resulting in lighter periods. But is this healthy? Shouldn't we consider why the levels are so imbalanced? What will happen when the risk of oral contraceptives becomes too great to continue? Will your heavy periods return? Of course! Your body will return to its original state, unless you have addressed your adrenal fatigue.

## Stressed Hormones

As I mentioned, stress plays a huge role in sex hormone balance. Your adrenal glands are responsible for managing your endocrine system, and they will move hormones around depending on your stage of adrenal fatigue. During Stage 1, hormones are overproduced and the demand for DHEA is increased to handle the synthesis of sex hormones and cortisol. By Stage 2, DHEA is normal or elevated, but the production of sex hormones is reduced in lieu of making cortisol. And by Stage 3, DHEA is low, leaving your body without the tools it needs to synthesize any hormone. These stages will affect the day-to-day function of your menstrual cycle, resulting in symptoms such as PMS, excessive or lack of menstruation, mood swings, and disease development. And in men, low DHEA results in low libido, energy, sleep, and even mental fogginess.

PMS is a condition where a woman experiences a group of symptoms in the time leading up to her cycle. These symptoms may include food cravings, mood swings, depression, bloating, or fatigue, and they typically occur the week prior to the start of her cycle. Once the cycle begins, the symptoms go away. Progesterone is meant to rise to meet estrogen during the 7 to 10 days before menstruation begins, but if the woman has an imbalance (more estrogen than progesterone) and it can't, the woman will experience PMS symptoms. Then, once the cycle starts, all of the hormones drop, so the symptoms go away.

The question to address is, why is the progesterone unable to meet up with the estrogen? Is there not enough progesterone being produced due to adrenal fatigue? Is it an irregularity in the thyroid? Is estrogen being overproduced or stored? Find the answer, find the cure. The process is not overly complicated; you just have to get to the bottom of it. Take the time to find the answer and your symptoms can be resolved.

When I ask women if they have menstrual cramps, they often reply, "Not more than normal." But what's normal? Did our ancestors stop working the in the fields because they had such severe cramps that they could not go on? What about our grandparents or great-grandparents? Did you ever ask them? I rarely find a woman over 65 who had horrible periods. But the baby boomer generation is bombarded by these pains. The change seemed to start with them and has worsened over time. What changed around that time? Well, we started to use more technology, eat more processed foods, use inventions to make things faster and easier, and more women joined the workforce. We turned to factories and businesses to provide goods and services, theoretically giving

## STRESS AND PROGESTERONE PRODUCTION

Adequate progesterone levels are often a casualty of adrenal fatigue. In times of stress, your adrenal glands cannot make this hormone as effectively, possibly because your body figures that in times of chronic stress a fetus would not be safe. Or it could be that your body senses that under your current levels of stress, you may not have enough nutrition for a fetus should you become pregnant. Regardless of the reason, progesterone production suffers. Your progesterone levels decrease and your relative estrogen levels increase. This will promote cyst development, uterine fibroids, endometriosis, and potential cancer development.[3]

everyone more leisure time. And while some of these changes are positive, they all resulted in additional adrenal stress. More stimulation forced us to get more done in a shorter amount of time.

## Adrenal Fatigue and Polycystic Ovarian Syndrome

Another common disorder linked to adrenal fatigue is polycystic ovarian syndrome (PCOS). The condition is commonly believed to have an "unknown cause." Doctors agree that it's due to a hormonal imbalance, but no one knows for sure why this imbalance causes PCOS. They also state that it is linked to development of type 2 diabetes and is commonly treated and reversed using the diabetic drug metformin. Now, if a diabetic drug will actually reverse the symptoms of PCOS, then it seems to me that we should look at the association between blood sugar regulation and hormone development to find a cause. Some studies have begun to do this. A study published in the *Journal of Women's Health* showed a connection between PCOS, type 2 diabetes, and how the body uses insulin. Both conditions stem from insulin resistance, but in PCOS this insulin secretion results in the formation of estrogen and testosterone, whereas in type 2 diabetes it results in the destruction of pancreatic cells. The researchers in this study state that further investigation is needed in order to determine why the body chooses to do different things in the same situation.[4]

So let's consider the role of the adrenal glands in this situation. Type 2 diabetes can be caused by numerous factors. First, we have the dietary link, where poor diet leads to excessive sugar levels. Then there is the idea that someone with adrenal output issues will release insulin in response to the "bear," resulting in baseline sugar increases. Both situations result in hyperglycemia, and therefore diabetes, but it was arrived at by different mechanisms. Different pathways were affected, so different outcomes will occur. If cortisol is affected by adrenal fatigue, it would not only raise insulin, but would also affect the production of sex hormones. In fact, a 2004 study showed that cortisol abnormality

*(continued on page 66)*

# WHAT'S YOUR TYPE?

Depending on the extent of your adrenal fatigue and the relative compensation by your body, a number of hormonal changes can occur. There are a few common scenarios in women.

**THE TESTOSTERONE-DOMINANT WOMAN.** This woman has relatively high amounts of both estrogens (particularly estrone) and testosterone, with low amounts of progesterone. She enjoys working out and is successful at it. As a result, she has a muscular build. She finds herself with good energy, but she can easily become irritable. She notices fibrocystic breasts (which contain dense tissue that can inhibit proper screening and give breasts a "bumpy" appearance) or diminishing breast size. It's also likely she has a history of ovarian cysts. In addition, the testosterone-dominant woman commonly shows signs of oily skin, may sweat more than usual, and often complains of black hairs on her chin. She reports a healthy libido. However, she may come to her doctor concerned with heavy, painful periods, and her doctor will typically recommend using the birth control pill to control cyst development.

**THE EXHAUSTED ESTROGEN-DOMINANT WOMAN.** This woman has increased amounts of estrone and estradiol, low free testosterone, and low progesterone. She reports having had horrible, painful periods since she was a teenager. She tends to spot between periods or bleed for excessively long periods. She has used the birth control pill to control her periods. She typically has early breast development, is exhausted, and complains of excessive weight around her abdomen. She may have had a live birth and a couple of miscarriages. This woman felt great while she was pregnant, but now her libido is low and she feels flabby. Her gynecologist recommends the pill, but she does not feel well when she takes it, so she may seek alternative options but is afraid of how her periods might respond.

**THE PERIMENOPAUSAL STRESSED WOMAN.** This woman has normal estrogens, low progesterone, and low testosterone, and she comes to the doctor's office for hormone therapy because she knows something is wrong. She still bleeds occasionally, but it is erratic. Sometimes the bleeding is heavy (sometimes excessively so), sometimes light, and sometimes it doesn't happen at all. She is snappy, reports no libido, and feels foggy. Her periods were never a problem before and she has always been able to get things done, as she is normally well-organized and clear thinking. She is typically fit but is noticing changes in her figure, despite a normally healthy weight. She simply does not feel like herself and tells her doctor that she feels like she is going through menopause.

**THE NATURAL MENOPAUSAL WOMAN.** In this woman, all hormonal levels are equally low. She is typically over 50 and is in good spirits. She reports that she always had a normal menstrual cycle and that one day it basically just stopped. It has been more than a year since she last had a period, and despite some mild hot flashes and gray hair, she feels fairly good. She would love to look younger but does not have any overwhelming complaints besides lack of overall wellness.

**THE PREMATURE SURGICAL MENOPAUSAL WOMAN.** This woman's estrogen may be normal or high, while her progesterone and testosterone are low. She recently had a hysterectomy and likely had an endometrial ablation in the past due to heavy periods. Her cervix and uterus were developing fibroids and her periods were a hassle, so surgery was recommended to solve the problem. She reports being an emotional mess, crying at virtually everything and snapping at her loved ones. She isn't sleeping and lacks motivation. Her hair is falling out. She feels ugly, run-down, and foggy. Her doctor placed her on estrogen therapy after surgery, but her symptoms just seemed to get worse.

**THE PSEUDOMENOPAUSAL WOMAN.** This woman's estrogen level is normal or slightly low, possibly due to high levels of stored estrogen, low progesterone, and low testosterone. She has not had a period for about 9 months, and the last period she had was light or barely there. She is certain she is in menopause. Her hot flashes are severe, occurring both during the day and at night. She reports changes in mood, lack of sleep, and a change in libido. Her prior periods were variable, and they changed after she had children. Her periods slowly tapered off over the years, appearing less and less often, with diminishing flow. She feels like a different woman and does not like how snappy she has become. She is uncomfortable during her hot flashes.

Each of these women needs to be treated differently. Keep in mind that all of these women are presenting for "hormone issues." It would be wrong to simply assume that each woman's symptoms are due to low estrogen. It is imperative to run blood tests to confirm all of their hormone levels and to assess adrenal function to determine the causes of these imbalances and restore balance.

was directly linked to elevated estrogen levels and immune destabilization in animals. Additionally, the author of the study identified the adrenal cortex as the source of the hormonal imbalances and strongly recommended further human research on the impact of cortisol defects.[5]

We should also consider that if someone eats an excessive amount of sugar and develops type 2 diabetes, they will usually suffer from obesity, which results in excessive fat deposits. This puts more stress on the body and induces storage of hormones, resulting in the development or worsening of PCOS. A study investigated the effects of higher fat levels in relation to production of androgens and insulin resistance in those with PCOS. It found that those with a higher percentage of body fat have higher sex hormone production and worsening insulin resistance. The researchers evaluated adrenal cells and discovered that when fats were added and adrenocorticotropic hormone (ACTH) was stimulated (which is the signal to release cortisol), DHEA levels increased by 38 percent. DHEA is the backbone of androgen production, and therefore androgen production was increased.[6] The adrenal glands are the ruler of this phenomenon. Whether insulin resistance is developed through diet or chronic stress, the adrenal glands decide whether to induce further disease development via hormone production mechanisms.

## CALMING YOUR STRESSED HORMONES

Can stress really have such a great impact on your body? While studies support that both PCOS and diabetes are mediated by the adrenal glands, conventional treatment does not include stress management and adrenal gland support. A study published in *Psychoneuroendocrinology* noted that those with PCOS have significantly higher cortisol levels, increased heart rates, and increased inflammatory responses when exposed to stress compared to those who do not have PCOS.[7] In addition, the *American Journal of Obstetrics and Gynecology* found that those with PCOS experienced higher psychological stress than a control group of women without PCOS. They deduced that the elevated levels of stress must contribute to the hormone irregularities associated with the development of PCOS.[8] This study intrigues me as a physician because it clearly states that the severity of a hormone imbalance as it relates to PCOS is determined by stress. What does stress do to your body? Why isn't stress management a part of standardized PCOS treatment? We are simply looking at the insulin, not the environment. Let's look at the soil and rid these women of the symptoms of PCOS.

We cannot lose sight of this medical fact: The adrenal glands make hormones. By assuming that menopause is simply about estrogen, we are doing ourselves an injustice. We are also putting people at risk with hormone therapy that may not be needed. When I look at a perimenopausal case, I take a look at the patient's stress response first. I do this because if I prescribe a hormone, bioidentical or not, the body will interpret it as a stress if the adrenal glands are not primed to handle it.

Many physicians would suggest adding DHEA to a hormone formulation, as it is considered to be the "fountain of youth" by many anti-aging specialists. But if we do this, we are then adding a hormone that will react to excessive stress. If we add DHEA to a body that is using cortisol, the DHEA will support the cortisol, not the testosterone. Or it will make the testosterone, but then store it or convert it because the body is not calm enough to use it. This can pose a problem in the future because the information then feeds back to your brain that DHEA is not needed. At that point, your body stops making it and becomes dependent on hormone replacement for survival.

It would be wiser to try to restore the function of your adrenal glands through herbal or glandular therapy prior to supplementing with DHEA. That would allow your body to decide what it needs to produce and use, which restores normal balance. Once this is accomplished, if certain hormones are still imbalanced or deficient, then BHRT could be considered and would be well received by your body. Bottom line: Your doctor needs to consider the whole picture before running to prescribe hormones. If this is not done, hormone therapy can actually cause more symptoms and worsen your adrenal fatigue.

# MY TURNAROUND
## JOHN MARCUS, AGE: 53

John Marcus had been healthy and active all his life, but a few years ago, stress and a lack of energy began to take over. "I was having sleep issues and working 16-hour days. I'm a very busy and very regimented person who has a certain way of doing things. And in the course of being busy, those things—plus added stress—exacerbated the issue. The lack of energy was just killing me. It was like I woke up one day and I was a different person in a different body," he explains.

John decided to go to a men's clinic and have some tests done. "When I had my labs taken, the men's clinic only checked my testosterone, estrogen, and PSA (prostate-specific antigen test) levels. I kept telling them something's not right. The doctor ran the typical tests based on my complaints, and while my sugar had never been high before, it came back at 101, and the dropoff was 100. That concerned me," he says.

A friend's previous experience with natural medicine inspired John to see a naturopathic physician. "When I was in college, a friend of mine was diagnosed with a brain tumor. After he received herbal treatment, his tumor shrunk about 30 percent in 3 months. A doctor was eventually able to remove the tumor, and he's fine now," he shares. "It made me think that I should stop counting on the traditional medical community for the answers." Soon after, he scheduled an appointment with Dr. Pingel.

As part of Dr. Pingel's plan, John began taking a testosterone supplement and saw results within a few days. "My testosterone levels had gone up 100 points, and I was able to go back to the gym," he says. "While I've never been a heavy guy, I've since lost 40 pounds and feel so much better. My business partner even remarked that it was amazing how much both my energy and strength have changed. In fact, he's interested in seeing Dr. Pingel as well!"

Today, John has his stress under control and feels much better. "I'm a type A personality and a very driven guy, and the way I pushed myself was linked to my adrenal fatigue," he admits. "But I wanted to feel better and be better. I wanted to reverse anything that had gotten out of sequence before my body couldn't handle it anymore. You owe it to yourself to ask questions, do you own research, and not settle until you feel better and have answers."

# 4

# FIGHTING THE BATTLE WITHIN

My mother, Robbi, has been an incredible inspiration to me not only because of her devotion to my success, but also due to her ability to keep an open mind and heart while fighting cancer. She was diagnosed with non-Hodgkin's lymphoma (NHL) almost 10 years ago and just 6 months ago was told that she is entering remission. Despite our entire family's input, she opted to stick with natural therapies and avoid chemotherapy. Her quality of life was more important to her than any "assurances" chemotherapy could have given her. She has lived a very wonderful life, playing with her grandchildren, enjoying her hobbies, exercising, and traveling—all in the face of the dreaded "cancer."

Now, being her daughter, I also provided input on how to address this disease, and we have been going about this in a rather unconventional way for the last several years. My mother had a long history of continual external stress. She snapped at everything, hardly slept, and consumed poor food and alcohol regularly as a result of these stressful situations. There was no obvious sign of this cancer in previous routine checkups, although her oncologist suggests it was likely there long before her diagnosis.

Her cancer was diagnosed shortly after she retired, and I believe it developed because her body was so used to being in a high-stress (or sympathetic) state that even when she removed the external stress, her body continued to run in a high-stress state, essentially anticipating upcoming stress. This created inflammation, which progressed to lymphoma, which is considered an overactive immune response. I am sure you can imagine our devastation when the surgeon informed us that her biopsy was positive for cancer and was incurable. But instead of putting all of her affairs in order and giving in to this grim diagnosis that conventional medicine still claims has no cure, we started addressing her adrenal function, hormone deregulation, and elevated sympathetic output. We also began detoxifying her liver. She started sleeping better, had more energy, improved her mood, and started exercising more. She also snapped less, smiled more, and genuinely enjoyed every moment.

Every 6 months she would go for a PET scan, and the doctors would be shocked. Her lymph nodes were either shrinking or were not changing at all. They had told her that most NHL cases result in significant life impairment within about 10 years, but hers was not progressing. Six months ago, her white blood cell counts returned to normal and her lymph nodes are still shrinking. I will be honest with you: I don't know how this will progress. By the time this book reaches your hands, her life may have changed. But I cannot ignore the amazing improvement that occurred after simply addressing the nutritional and hormonal fallout that resulted from the adrenal impact of chronic stress. When I ask my mom now what she thinks "cured" her current state, she always tells me that she has never considered herself a cancer patient. She spent each day living it to the fullest and managing stress—and continues to do so. Her mind-body outlook is inspiring.

I share this story with you because I want you to consider the role your immune system plays in your overall health. Most people consider cancer to be an invading organism, something we "catch," but we all actually have cancer cells in our bodies all of the time. The truth is, if your immune system is functioning properly, your body will kill the disease before it progresses. But if your immune system isn't doing its job, the disease will progress and you'll receive that devastating diagnosis.

# THE ROLE OF YOUR IMMUNE SYSTEM

Your immune system is responsible for keeping you safe from invading organisms, just as our front lines protect us from enemies in a war. They may fire warning shots or send out a bunch of troops to warn the enemy, or they may hide and secretly attack when the impact is greatest. And like our armed forces, your body has intelligence (your adrenal glands) behind the front lines that determines which threats are the most dangerous and attacks the greatest threats first.

Some common warning signs of attacks on your immune system are eczema, hives, psoriasis, diarrhea, mild colds and flus, swelling of your lymph nodes, and seasonal allergy flare-ups. Threats may sneak up slowly and catch you off guard, such as many cancers, HIV/AIDS, and other diseases. In any case, whether it's a stealth attack or a full-on assault, there is always an enemy. Something triggers your body to plan an attack. And if you pay attention, you can usually find the cause.

Unfortunately, conventional medicine simply attacks back, and that is not always curative. If your body has been attacked by a cancer and you retaliate with chemotherapy, you may slaughter the enemy, but you will also kill a lot of helpful cells. When that happens, you may damage other areas of your body, prompting further attacks at a later date. If you use a steroid to eliminate a rash, all you've really done is temporarily restrain the enemy. But at some point he will probably get away and retaliate. It is more important to look to the intelligence of your body, such as your adrenal glands, to find where these attacks are coming from, predict where they will happen next, and stop future attacks.

## The Team of Defense: Your Personal Army

Think of your lymphatic system as your own personal army. Some key players in lymphatic function are your thymus, bone marrow, spleen, lymph nodes, and lymphocytes. Each fills a specific role in the chain of command.

- **YOUR THYMUS** is where your body grooms and begins to train its team for future battle. It is active when you're young, and T-cells you create there make up your future immune system. It is essentially a "recruiter" gathering its future team for attack.
- **YOUR BONE MARROW** is the yellow substance in your bones. It is almost like a boot camp because it's where your body makes white blood cells and prepares them to be released for battle.
- **YOUR SPLEEN** is the commander and decides which cells need to be released for battle. It calls upon your bone marrow to deliver cells for specific duties.
- **YOUR LYMPH NODES** trap viruses, bacteria, cancer cells, and more, holding them so that your white blood cells can get to each node and kill off the enemy. When a lymph node has trapped something, the node typically feels enlarged and is often tender. (Most people have had an infection, flu, strep throat, or other mild illness that has caused an enlargement in the nodes of the neck and below the chin. That swelling means you have trapped an invader.)
- **YOUR LYMPHOCYTES**, which are a type of white blood cell, at that point, are released in order to begin to kill this invader, or pathogen. Your body has different types of lymphocytes for different jobs, similar to soldiers in an army. There's the macrophages, which capture the enemy and determine the threat and the location. This then prompts the T cells to send a signal to the spleen asking it to recruit the appropriate type and number of cells to defeat this particular enemy. The response is faster if this enemy has been encountered before, as your body has a team already assembled. (By the way, this

is the theory behind vaccinations or immunity developed by exposure to a particular virus. Once the army has killed a particular enemy, it assembles a preventative team in case that enemy returns; this process is called adaptive immunity.) Finally, the B cells are our troops and are released to begin killing the enemy. Once the attack of the enemy is complete, a signal (called the suppressor T cell) is sent back to stop the attack. This avoids any unnecessary casualties among our own troops, and the attack is then over. It's called a suppressor cell because it does just that: It stops, or suppresses, your body's own attacking force. The lymph nodes are emptied and drained, and your body reverts to normal immune function because the threat has been eliminated.

## Adrenal Fatigue and Your Immune System

Now let's talk about how your adrenal glands are connected to your immune system. Your adrenal gland works in your body's intelligence department (along with your brain). It receives a threat and determines its value. For example, let's say you think you hear a bear in the woods. Your immune system quickly starts to mount a response via cortisol release, as it senses the bear might become a valid threat. But no enemy appears, so your immune system relaxes. Then another sound may prompt an alert, so your immune system gets called again. But if no invader appears, your immune system relaxes, waiting for another potential attack. You can think of this as the story of the boy who cried wolf. In the beginning (Stage 1), your immune system will respond to every signal, whether it is a valid threat or not. After so many false alarms, your immune system will change its response (Stage 2) and you will start to notice immune system effects. Let's take a look of how this process of immune function evolves in relationship to the adrenal fatigue stages.

In Stage 1, when the threat of a bear is there consistently but your body is still in a functional state, your immune system stays on alert and you rarely get sick. Every single threat is immediately demolished. You may have heard yourself say, "I haven't had a cold in years!" As great as this may sound, it is not always a good thing—at some point, your "soldiers" will get tired. It is important to have some trial missions. It is important for the soldiers to face some small threats in order to train for larger ones—especially threats that might hide in your lymph nodes for a long time before being discovered.

As you hit Stage 2 of adrenal fatigue, you may get sick or be hit by a horrible case of the flu once a year or so. Typically, it will happen when you are on vacation. Why? The threat is lower on vacation, which means your adrenal glands calm down. As a result, your soldiers sit back and start to relax and *wham!* Seemingly out of nowhere, the flu takes you down. It takes a while for the soldiers to attack for two reasons: First, they have not had practice, and second, they have been resting.

Recent studies have connected the dots between stress and a compromised immune system. Researchers surveyed 176 men and women about difficult situations they had experienced in the preceding year before administering nasal drops containing the common cold virus. After checking the subjects to see who actually caught a cold, the researchers noted that those who had experienced stress were twice as likely to develop the cold. But here's the really interesting part: Additional tests showed that the immune systems of subjects who had developed the cold virus had grown less sensitive to cortisol. This decreased sensitivity to cortisol allowed inflammation to thrive, resulting in increased likelihood of developing the cold.[1]

In Stage 3, your immune system is simply not as effective. The soldiers react to things they shouldn't and begin to attack their own people. Signals get confused. As a result, those in Stage 3 adrenal fatigue often develop hives, even if they've never had them before. Maybe this has happened to you and you couldn't figure out why. You cannot connect the hives to a specific lotion you used or a certain food you ate, but the hives are there and seem to come out of nowhere. And although they do occur during the day, they often happen at night, while you're at rest.

The majority of my Stage 3 adrenal fatigue patients report developing rashes, hives, or allergic responses at night, during rest. Then those symptoms disappear in the morning. So why does this happen? Well, those "soldiers" can no longer decipher what is a real threat and what isn't. Their bodies have been tricked so many times that they attack things that do not need to be attacked.

For example, someone in Stage 3 may suddenly develop a rash whenever she eats blueberries because her immune system is attacking the blueberry, thinking it is harmful. When you lie down to rest, the soldiers are not used to the quiet after going through the previous adrenal fatigue stages. They are used to the stimulation in Stages 1 and 2 and expect to hear those cries for help. But in Stage 3, adrenal function is low and the signals from cortisol are hindered, or perhaps delayed, causing an attack on the wrong item.

Your soldiers start to anticipate that they may be missing signals and do not want to let anything through by mistake, so they send a signal to attack randomly once you relax. They start attacking things they should not. Imagine how much damage someone could do if he ran into the middle of the forest and opened fire on the wildlife in absence of an actual threat. When this happens in your body, it causes inflammation, which can result in a skin lesion or pain. At this point, a conventional physician would prescribe a steroid or an antihistamine to put out this inflammatory response in your body. However, if your body is trying to attack an unknown enemy and keeps getting shut down by a steroid, what is the long-term effect? If your adrenal fatigue is not addressed, your immune system will eventually be defeated, and further diseases of the immune system will develop.

# MAJOR THREATS: THE DEADLY DISEASES OF THE IMMUNE SYSTEM

Have you ever known someone who is constantly mildly sick? Does she always carry tissues in her pockets? At this point, her immune system has stopped reacting and has given up. Only some of your defensive cells are sent into battle, so the invaders are kept at bay, but not killed. If these cells aren't paying close attention, this chronic mild illness sometimes allows a major enemy to get through the trap and grow unchecked. Take a look at some of your body's major enemies.

**CANCER.** Let's say your "soldiers" have allowed cancer to get past the traps. Imagine that the cancer gets ahold of a lieutenant colonel and takes him hostage. The cancer starts directing your immune system, telling the soldiers to abort the orders to kill. Cancer takes control of your body and starts calling the shots. As I mentioned earlier, cancer is not something you can catch; you have cancer in your body right now. But your immune system has it under control, and hopefully it has the intelligence to predict—and avoid—a hostile takeover.

This sneak attack by cancer when your immune system is not paying attention is why stress is commonly linked to cancer development. If your body is constantly busy addressing stress, it will likely miss the real threat of cancer. In fact, there is a link between higher-stress jobs and women with breast cancer: A 2013 study showed that those with prolonged deregulation of cortisol due to high-stress jobs had at least a 57 percent higher risk of developing breast cancer.[2] Cancer creates a problem with your body's signaling ability and a physical change in an antigen (immune response system). It changes the signal and immune response so that your immune system misses the signal.

So if we all have cancer cells in our bodies all of the time, what do our immune systems do to those cells? Are they destroyed before they can replicate? Or does the cancer sneak past our barricades and replicate, ultimately changing the internal structure of our immune systems?

Think of cancer as a terrorist attack. The terrorist always exists, but if it's caught, it won't cause destruction. When missed, it causes political, structural, and emotional changes to our system. When the World Trade Center was attacked, America felt defeated. We were angry. Our economy was affected. Our sense of trust was altered. Our border patrol was changed. Even our standards for flying were changed. We took action to prevent a future attack. And despite the deaths of the attackers on those planes, we still felt the lingering effects.

This is how it is with cancer cells in your body; they are hidden and you are on alert. Now imagine that you kill those attackers yourself, with chemotherapy. How many good cells will you kill in order to eliminate the threat? You cannot prevent cancer, you can only be better in tune with your body so you can recognize it, attack it at first sight, and avoid sideline casualties (such as killing your noncancerous cells). Bottom line? You need to minimize false threats promoted by stress so that you are better able to attack the real threats to your system.

**HIV/AIDS.** Another silent attacker is HIV. According to the Centers for Disease Control and Prevention, there are about 50,000 newly diagnosed cases each year, and around 1.1 million people are currently living with the disease in America. HIV development occurs because your T cells, which are responsible for signaling the B cells to attack, are affected. This allows HIV to replicate and take over. In fact, HIV can even destroy the helper T cell that is involved in this immune attack. And similar to cancer, HIV also changes the actual structure of your immune system, which allows the virus to hijack your system and develop into AIDS. Both cancer and AIDS slowly attack your body by taking nutrients, oxygen, and blood cells from your army—holding you hostage. Without more boot camps, more "soldiers," and stronger defensive lines, you cannot hope to defeat either disease.

This is actually the basis for naturopathic therapy for these diseases. In the naturopathic world, we use high-dose vitamin therapy to create a stronger immune system. We use lymphatic drainage, a method for moving killed invaders out of the body, to drain the traps and attack the unsuspecting invaders with the rebounding immune function. We build, rather than destroy. We plan the attack by putting in the nutrients needed to form white blood cells, red blood cells, T cells, and B cells. Then the body drives the enemy into plain sight, where it can be attacked. This is against the conventional model that destroys every cell, good or bad. Without replenishment of the good cells, your body is left depleted, which often results in Stage 3 adrenal fatigue. It is a vicious cycle. And depression, loss of hope, pain, and further toxicity are all common results. Many studies boast of vitamin C's antioxidant activity and its ability to help destroy cancer cells. This ability presents us with alternative avenues of therapy that are much less stressful than chemotherapy. Not only will vitamin C kill the cancer cell, but its antioxidant effects will also strengthen the army backing up your body.[3] These recent studies have prompted more focus on using nutrition as an adjuvant treatment for cancer over traditional chemotherapy methods.

## MY STRESS-RELATED ILLNESS

There was one especially stressful year, early in my practice, that I'll never forget. I had been working really long, hard days, and I had some tough cases that took up a lot of my thoughts. I had a 1-year-old and a 4-year-old at the time, so they demanded all of my attention when I was home. Needless to say, I had adrenal fatigue. I was exhausted, but I had no time to worry about it. Ultimately, I decided that I should take a week off around Christmas, as I missed my kids and needed some rest.

I was home for only 1 day before I was hit with the flu, and it lasted a full 7 days. Unbelievably, it went away the day I was to return to work. I kept wondering where I had contracted it from. Well, being a doctor, I am exposed all of the time. I had seen numerous flu cases in the weeks prior, but my immune system never gave me the hint that it was coming. The minute I shut off my brain, it hit me—and it hit me hard. I could barely walk and my fever was up above 103°F. My "soldiers" were so overworked from keeping minor threats away that when a big threat snuck past the trap, they completely missed it.

I had tricked my body so many times with silly worries of a "bear attack" that when I needed my immune system the most, it failed to catch the flu before the flu caught me. If I had not been in a state of adrenal fatigue, I would have likely developed a small cold, maybe a runny nose, or perhaps a light fever for a few hours instead of the flu. One quick day of rest, and I would have been downstairs enjoying my family at Christmas. I encourage you to remember that your immune system is there to help you, and it needs to be rested and on alert to keep you well. If you find that when you get sick you are severely sick, it's time to address your stress response and think about your adrenal glands.

**AUTOIMMUNE DISEASE.** According to John Hopkins University, at least 10 million Americans suffer from more than 80 different autoimmune illnesses. And approximately 75 percent of these sufferers are women. Autoimmunity is recognized as the immune system attacking itself. It's important to note that there are both genetic influences and environmental triggers related to the development of these conditions. And although we cannot change our genes, we can do something about those environmental factors.

The treatment for most autoimmune diseases is corticosteroid therapy. Conventional medicine does not see cortisol release as a causative factor in autoimmune disease, yet the treatment involves a corticosteroid that is similar to what your adrenal glands make in times of stress. If cortisol is not acknowledged to have an impact on immunity, then why is treatment centered around cortisones? Because they suppress your immune system. The theory is, if you suppress your immune system, the autoimmune illness will not progress. But by suppressing what your body is trying to say, you aggravate your body, allowing other diseases to develop. Anyone with a toddler knows that when toddlers demand something and you ignore them, they throw a tantrum. They hit you, or throw something at you, or throw themselves on the floor in anger. Over time, they give up. The same is true for your body: It gives you small warnings of disease development by exhibiting mild symptoms. When you suppress those symptoms, it gets angry and causes havoc. And after long periods of time, it gives up— and so do you.

I've noticed a couple of distinct trends in my autoimmunity patients, regardless of what particular disease they may have. First, I usually find a hormonal imbalance that favors estrogen and a depletion of adrenal DHEA. Patients usually fall somewhere between Stage 2 and Stage 3 adrenal fatigue and also have a history of symptoms pertaining to estrogen dominance (such as heavy and painful cycles, fibroids, cysts, infertility, or easy miscarriage). I also usually find some sort of toxin in their systems, most commonly in the gastrointestinal (GI) system. We will speak more specifically about the GI system in Chapter 7, but when there is an overgrowth of bad bacteria and a depletion of good bacteria, it can affect your endocrine system and result in problems such as unbalanced hormones. It can also present as toxicity to your liver, which is extremely stressful to your body, further impairing your endocrine system. This toxicity sends a signal to your lymphocytes to destroy the toxin. However, over time, in the presence of stress, your immune system changes and promotes an attack on itself. It cannot distinguish the good from the bad anymore.

I do not treat the particular diseases of my autoimmune patients directly. Instead, I treat the underlying hormone imbalance and gastrointestinal system, since it is always affected. And oddly enough, symptoms disappear. There is not a lot of research on the effects of the adrenal glands on autoimmunity, but there is research on the effects of corticosteroids on halting disease. So if we increase cortisone, we lower inflammation and improve immune function? Great. If a patient with an autoimmune disease is exhibiting symptoms of Stage 3 adrenal fatigue, supporting adrenal function and increasing cortisol release will support her recovery.

However, if the person appears to be in Stage 2, it is a bit trickier, as her cortisol levels are changing daily and we risk overstimulation. By calming the system and then supporting regular adrenal function, she can find relief from symptoms without using pharmaceuticals. Some of the research that does exist on this topic explores the connection between adrenal function and the development of rheumatoid arthritis (RA). Studies have shown that patients with early RA have lower levels of cortisol and DHEA, and the idea of using those markers to predict the development of RA is now attracting interest.[4] They have also found altered cortisol release and circadian rhythms (sleep–wake cycles) in those with RA.[5] If cortisol levels are flipped, becoming higher at night and lower in the morning, and it has been shown that low levels of cortisol will worsen RA, this may explain why those with RA complain of worse pain in the morning. By altering the sleep-wake cycles, it is theoretically possible to reduce the symptoms of rheumatoid arthritis.

## INVEST IN YOUR DEFENSE

Your immune system is your defense; it is your protection against invaders. If your "soldiers" are distracted by false threats, they will not be as successful at protecting you from invasion. Your adrenal glands largely aid in your defense due to their role in anticipating and securing a threat. Each cortisol output is a response to the anticipation of a possible invader. You need your adrenal glands to be sharp, focused, and able to correctly identify those threats that will be detrimental to your system.

# MY TURNAROUND
## TANYA MATT, AGE: 51

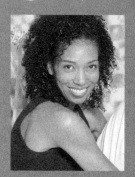

After spending 30 years working in the fashion industry, Tanya Mall was running on empty. "I was juggling modeling and producing shows, which was a lot of pressure. My name was on the job, and it was really important that I was flawless," she explains. "I was so busy that I would only eat one big meal a day."

In addition to her hectic work schedule, Tanya had a lot of additional stress on her plate. "I had a miscarriage in 2005, and it was really devastating for me," she says. "A few years later, I jumped into an online master's program, and it was the longest 2½ years of my life. The only way I survived the sleepless nights was with a big bag of almond M&Ms next to me."

She knew she needed to do something, and that's when she turned to Dr. Pingel. "She told me that I had lupus and that my organs were shutting down on me because I wasn't eating and I was doing too much," Tanya reveals. "My body was essentially feeding off itself, and my adrenal glands weren't working." But after several months on Dr. Pingel's plan, Tanya began to notice some changes. "The supplements and Mediterranean diet have made a huge difference. According to my blood work, I'm improving and regaining my energy."

Thanks to Dr. Pingel and the support of her family and friends, Tanya has taken back control of her life. "It's important for me to take care of my body so I don't wake up with something else. Now, I feel like I'm being sheltered from stress and that I'm being helped and protected. I don't know where I would be at this point if I hadn't found Tricia," she confesses. "It's really all about learning to destress. And my husband and parents helped me do that. Even though teaching is more stressful than I thought it would be, I love the children and I love the energy they bring me."

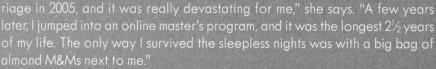

# 5

# TAKE ADRENAL FATIGUE TO HEART

Your adrenal glands have a direct, undisputed link to your cardiovascular system. As we've discussed in earlier chapters, when you are confronted with a stressful situation, your adrenal glands release cortisol, epinephrine, norepinephrine, and aldosterone in order to increase your blood pressure and deliver more blood to your muscles so you can run from or react to the stressful event. Your cardiovascular system is responsible for moving blood to your tissues, and your adrenal glands can control that mechanism at a moment's notice. In this chapter, we will explore the responsibilities of your cardiovascular system, the common clinical conditions associated with cardiovascular complications, and how addressing the health of your adrenal glands may be the missing link to finding proper treatment and reversing the development of heart disease.

## UNDERSTANDING YOUR CHOLESTEROL

Your cardiovascular system is responsible for moving blood and oxygen around your body, which is crucial for survival. Your body is filled with receptors that can respond to danger in an instant. So if you have an injury, your body moves more of your blood supply to that area so your blood cells can help the wound heal. When confronted by a "bear," your blood pressure changes in order to get oxygen to your muscles so that you can run. It is a finely tuned system that is highly susceptible to symptom development, as 68 million Americans suffer from hypertension and 71 percent have high cholesterol.[1] This results in a lot of medications being prescribed, yet cardiovascular disease is still one of the top killers. Despite our medical efforts, the medication is not working, and the death rates from cardiovascular disease continue to rise.

With almost three-quarters of the American population suffering from high cholesterol, we have to ask ourselves why this is the case. Do these same people also have heavy plaque deposition in their arteries and an incredibly high risk of heart attack? Not necessarily. Before you can figure out their risk, you have to find out why a person's cholesterol is elevated in the first place.

Cholesterol was never intended to be a bad guy. In fact, cholesterol is essential to your body's ability to manufacture hormones, maintain cellular integrity, and form bile from your liver; it's even involved in vitamin D production. I see numerous patients who were put on statin drugs because their cholesterol went up following menopause or andropause. Well, of course it did! If your hormones drop rapidly, your body attempts to make more of those hormones and increases the production of cholesterol to facilitate this. This usually results in a small increase, typically around 10 points, but that seems to be enough to warrant statin therapy by most practitioners.

## Is Your High Cholesterol Really That High?

Let's put this diagnosis of high cholesterol into perspective. Many people are unaware that the desired ranges of low-density lipoprotein (LDL) have changed over the last 10 years. Currently, it is recommended that LDL should fall below 100, and some doctors suggest an even lower number if someone has had a previous cardiovascular event, such as a heart attack or stroke. Recently, the ideal number was anything under 130. And a couple of years before that, they wanted it below 150.

So who sets these standards that treat everyone as having equal risk, without regard for diet and lifestyle factors? The American Medical Association (AMA) sets these guidelines based on research studies. Many of these studies are performed on patients who have had cardio-vascular events in the past, have high levels of inflammation, and are considered "high risk." So let's say you have an LDL of 130. Many physicians will prescribe a medication to lower your cholesterol based on that number alone. But the use of a medication with such high-profile side effects, such as a statin, should be regulated a bit more closely.

As you can see, these "reference ranges" have changed a lot over the course of a few years. The desired range was designed based on the risk of heart attack or stroke. If a person's risk is low, meaning that they have low levels of inflammation, eat a good diet, have a reasonable body weight, and have no other complications (such as diabetes or a previous cardiovascular event), the AMA actually suggests that LDL be lower than 160. That's 60 points higher than the "range" on your lab test.

Now, let's say you have a couple of risk factors. If that's the case, the AMA recommends keeping your LDL below 130. If you're high risk, essentially meaning you have had numerous cardiac events, the AMA suggests keeping LDL below 70.[2] You should know that your lab report will simply state a range for those at high risk, so it may say that your LDL needs to be below 100. But if you are low risk, you should techni-cally fall below 160 without medication therapy being indicated. It is up to your doctor to weigh your risk factors and decide on an appropri-ate treatment range, so don't worry about what the paperwork says. Just because your LDL displays as "high" at 130, that doesn't mean that it's high for you. When I evaluate cholesterol, I look at a few factors. First, what is the risk of the patient? And second, what is the trend in the patient's cholesterol level over a period of years? For example, if you are at 130, and have always been at 130, that's not a concern. If you had been at 160 the previous year, you should be pleased. However, if you were at

85 the previous year, there could be a strong risk factor at play. Lab tests are meant to evaluate trends, not state absolutes. Therefore, your whole history (not just your current number) should be reviewed before a physician decides whether or not medication is indicated.

## Cholesterol and Inflammation: What It Means for Your Health

Here are my primary concerns with cholesterol therapy: If your LDL falls below 70, what will happen to your hormones? What will happen to your vitamin D supply? What will happen to the cholesterol-based cell membrane that is responsible for maintaining electrolytes, water, and nutritional balance within your cells? It's no wonder that medications that block LDL formation cause numerous side effects.

One of the things I focus on is how much inflammation a patient is experiencing. This evaluation is becoming more widely used by cardiologists, but it is not considered strongly enough as a risk factor. High sensitivity C-reactive protein (HSCRP) is a blood marker that identifies inflammation in your body and is a key diagnostic marker for risk of cardiovascular disease. Most cardiologists state that your HSCRP should be below 3.0 mg/L, but I believe it should fall below 1.0 mg/L. That's because the lower the number, the lower the inflammation, and lower inflammation equals a lower risk. But more importantly, it should not be widely variable.

For example, if you have a value of 2.0 mg/L, but it remains stable year after year, then you have a lower risk of developing cardiovascular disease than someone who has an HSCRP of 0.5 mg/L one year and a value of 2.0 mg/L 2 years later. Once again, the trends shown by test results need to be taken into consideration. If your inflammatory marker goes up by 200 percent in 2 years, that is more dangerous than one that starts a little higher but has 0 percent change.

Quite simply, inflammation causes disease. Think about it: If you had a cut on your arm, it would swell and become inflamed. This then creates more opportunity for infection, lack of healing, scarring, and discomfort. The only difference between this cut and cardiovascular inflammation is that we can see the cut and we cannot see the insides of our bodies. If you have an inflammatory process going on inside your arteries, that causes them to swell and become more prone to infection, poor healing, and scarring, which ultimately will "catch" more cholesterol deposits as they pass through your bloodstream. This causes a buildup of plaque, which puts you at risk for developing a clot.

Cholesterol deposition in your arteries is due to inflammation. The diseases that plague our society are inflammation related. In fact, two of the most common and prevalent health issues today, cancer and diabetes, are both inflammatory diseases.[3] So who is at greater risk of a cardiovascular event, someone with low cholesterol and high inflammation or someone with high cholesterol and low inflammation?

The issue is not how much cholesterol you have, but what your body does with it. If your arteries are inflamed, they become "sticky," and cholesterol will be more likely to build up on them (a condition known as atherosclerosis). And if your blood is not flowing quickly through your arteries, such as when you're dehydrated, it has more time to "stick." This dehydration will also result in mineral imbalances, which can cause heart rhythm changes (known as arrhythmia). It can also cause an increase in blood pressure (hypertension) over time, as that buildup and dehydration together mean that your blood has increasingly smaller passageways to pump through.

So I just named three cardiovascular conditions—atherosclerosis, arrhythmia, and hypertension—that are all regulated by something as simple as water. Should you take medications to lower your blood pressure, reduce your cholesterol, and block signaling from your heart to cure these afflictions? Or should you increase your consumption of water and minerals? These examples show how finding the cause of your cardiovascular complication is imperative if you want to avoid medications. Most patients I see want to stop taking statins and hypertension drugs, but they are fearful of doing so. They're concerned about having a heart attack or stroke. By determining the cause of your condition, it is easier to find support for going off of these drugs and reversing cardiovascular complications through more natural methods.

# INDEPENDENT SYMPTOMS OR PART OF A WHOLE?

Why is it that when someone has one cardiovascular disease, they tend to develop more cardiovascular complications? How many people do you know who are on both cholesterol and high blood pressure medications? Which condition developed first? I ask because the history of development is very important. In the majority of the cases I see, the process began with high blood pressure. I also tend to find that these people are in some stage of adrenal fatigue. After years of running from bears, their bodies have evolved to raise their baseline blood pressure so that they always have blood supply when they need it to run. In the process, they've also changed their mineral balance. That's because when your body responds to a bear, it raises your levels of the hormone aldosterone, which retains sodium and dumps potassium in an effort to raise your blood pressure. This tends to raise your baseline blood pressure over time, until finally a medication is prescribed. Unfortunately, the medication then suppresses your body's attempts to raise your blood pressure and it fights against the desired effect from your adrenal glands, causing inflammation in your body due to the resulting imbalance. The process goes on, and eventually you develop other diseases.

## The Effects of Aspirin

If your body is under stress, from life or even from the addition of blood pressure medication, your cholesterol will rise in an attempt to make more cortisol. This has a further inflammatory effect, eventually resulting in a heart attack. In fact, the Normative Aging Study showed that negative emotions associated with high stress levels are significant risk factors for heart disease. When compared with men reporting no symptoms of anxiety, those reporting two or more anxiety symptoms had more than three times greater risk of developing fatal coronary heart disease. In addition, they were almost six times more likely to experience a heart attack.[4]

But does taking medication actually prevent a heart attack? Take a survey of those you know who have had heart attacks. Were they on medication at the time? Odds are they were. How many were taking aspirin? (Aspirin is often prescribed as a blood thinner.) The theory is that if your blood is thinner, it is less likely to clot. But aspirin can't work miracles. And the biggest mistake I often see is that conventional physicians prescribe aspirin as this "magic pill" to prevent a heart attack, but they neither explain why it works nor give the patient the opportunity to change his or her lifestyle to achieve the same desired effect.

Some of commonly reported side effects of aspirin include diarrhea, heartburn, dizziness, rash, vomiting, abdominal pain, constipation, and gout. An anti-inflammatory diet full of good fats and oils will help you avoid all of these complications and keep your blood moving (see "Natural Alternatives to Aspirin Use," on page 90). In fact, a 2013 study published by the Agency for Healthcare Research and Quality stated that aspirin had no effect on peripheral artery disease in asymptomatic patients. This means that in those who are not showing obvious complications from narrowing arteries, aspirin will have no effect. Yet it is still prescribed as a preventive therapy! The study also showed that exercise had a better impact on prevention than drug therapy.[5] And if you are still not convinced that aspirin isn't your best option, another study published in the *International Journal of Food Sciences and Nutrition* concluded that dietary antioxidants should be investigated as preventative therapy for atherosclerosis.[6]

So if dietary measures and exercise can drastically reduce your chances of experiencing a major cardiovascular event, why are we not stressing diet and exercise as the primary treatments for cardiovascular disease? Some may argue that this is being addressed: If you have seen a cardiologist, he or she likely mentioned lifestyle improvement. But were you actually shown *how* to implement these changes? Did your doctor

## NATURAL ALTERNATIVES TO ASPIRIN USE

Despite what you may have heard, you're not stuck taking aspirin to minimize your risk of having a stroke or heart attack. Here are some other ways you can keep your blood thin and less likely to clot.

- **EAT AN ANTI-INFLAMMATORY DIET.** A diet low in inflammatory foods will also keep your blood thin because it promotes free-flowing blood. When you have inflammation, your blood is sticky and turbid as it slowly moves through your veins. Vessels with lower inflammation have faster, less-dense blood.
- **INCORPORATE MORE MOVEMENT AND EXERCISE.** Just moving more plays a huge role in getting your blood going. When you exercise, your heart rate increases, pumping more blood to your tissues.
- **CONSUME MORE FISH OIL OR PLANT OILS.** These can work just as well as, if not better than, aspirin because oils thin out your blood and help it flow through your vessels more easily. (This makes sense, because oils are slippery.) The blood will slide right over any nicks in your vessels that could otherwise promote plaque formation. Additionally, these oils have been shown to have other health benefits, including increased skin health, better brain health (such as sharper focus and reduced depression), improved blood sugar, lowered cholesterol, and even reduced inflammation.

have in-depth discussions with you concerning what dietary and exercise measures needed to be addressed? The commitment required from both the practitioner and the patient is substantial. Both have to be willing to commit to each other to reverse disease, because it is possible.

# ADRENAL FATIGUE AND LOW BLOOD PRESSURE

Most people aren't aware of the sheer number of patients with low blood pressure, which is a major concern. Those with severe adrenal fatigue (ranging from late Stage 2 to Stage 3) usually have abnormally low blood pressure due to the retention of potassium and dumping of sodium; this is because their adrenal glands cannot release aldosterone as well as they used to. Subsequently, the relatively high level of potassium can cause heart palpitations and arrhythmias. A patient in this situation usually states that he or she has always had low blood pressure and commonly feels dizzy after standing up too quickly. Though patients are usually dismissed as normal or are advised to "avoid standing up quickly," this condition should be recognized as a sign of adrenal fatigue.

Let's look at the example of a woman with low blood pressure who goes into menopause. Her blood pressure moves into the normal range, meaning it's now 120/80. The doctor thinks this is fine, but the patient knows it is high for her. Should it be ignored? Most likely, her hormones are shifting as her adrenal fatigue is progressing, and her body is adjusting to her low blood pressure to keep her alive. This change should not to be ignored, nor should the initial typical low blood pressure reading.

## YOU ARE WHAT YOU EAT: HOW DIET IMPACTS CARDIOVASCULAR HEALTH

The diet most commonly recommended for cardiovascular health by the American Medical Association is the DASH (Dietary Approaches to Stop Hypertension) diet. The DASH diet focuses on low sodium consumption and encourages you to make the largest portion of your diet consist of carbohydrates and animal proteins. It also allows sweets, alcohol, and caffeine on a daily basis. Knowing what you now know about sodium and potassium, do you think a diet focused around low sodium intake will fix the problem? Not to mention that this diet allows two alcoholic drinks a day for men and one for women, coupled with sweets as a recommended option. It even states that artificial sweeteners are acceptable and that you can substitute a diet cola with artificial sweetener for a regular cola.[7]

The diet states that trans fats and animal fats contribute to heart disease and therefore should be limited, yet they still advise you to eat them. If animal fats are linked to cardiovascular disease, why are they recommended at all? Does this seem logical? What nutrition does your body get from a cola? What about a diet cola? If you are trying to change blood pressure and cholesterol and lower your cardiovascular risk, should you be consuming empty calories that your body does not know what to do with? Should you be loading your body with carbohydrates and animal fats? Think about it this way: If you had a splinter in your arm, your body would swell around it because it is foreign. What is cola to our body other than foreign?

So if the DASH diet isn't you best option, what is? Vegan diets have been the most successful in eliminating cardiovascular disease.[8] But what is it about a vegan diet that virtually eliminates not only cardio-vascular disease, but also diabetes, cancer, and autoimmune disease? Simply put, it is anti-inflammatory. The research supports both vegan and vegetarian diets as the most successful at not only controlling, but also completely eliminating, cardiovascular disease. For a country so dedicated to research, we sure are not focusing much on this data.[9]

There are some studies combating this theory, saying that vegans and vegetarians have higher levels of homocysteine, an inflammatory marker linked to high blood pressure.[10] These studies are meant to combat the idea that vegans and vegetarians have better cardiovascular health. Homocysteine is regulated by vitamins $B_6$, $B_{12}$, and folate, which are commonly deficient in vegetarians who eat poor diets. For example, a vegetarian could eat French fries and processed soy burgers all day, with minimal legumes, plant-based proteins, or nuts. That particular vegetarian will have more nutritional deficiencies than one who does research and eats a well-balanced diet.

Also, consider this: The adrenal glands use vitamins $B_5$, $B_6$, and $B_{12}$ in order to operate. So anyone, vegan or not, who has adrenal fatigue and burns the candle at both ends will likely end up with a vitamin B deficiency (see Chapter 9). Vitamin B deficiency results in elevated homocysteine, low serotonin production, nerve pains and neuropathies, extreme fatigue, anemia, and mental fogginess. So what does all of this mean? Adrenal fatigue is the cause of all disease. The reason that poor-eating vegetarian is eating that way is likely due to stress and time restraints. He doesn't have time to make a meal; French fries are easier and faster. Couple his poor diet with the impact on his cardiovascular system via his adrenal glands (in relation to sodium and potassium), and we have a pretty poorly nourished person. And you can see how this poorly nourished person could become a very sick person—one dealing with diabetes, gastrointestinal disease, immune status, and hormone irregularities.

## REVERSING CARDIOVASCULAR DISEASE THROUGH ADRENAL SUPPORT

So if diet and lifestyle changes can truly reverse cardiovascular disease, then we can reverse cardiovascular disease in America simply by changing our focus. Cardiovascular disease develops from inflammation, and inflammation is a primary adaptation to stress. A 2013 study published in the *Proceedings of the National Academy of Sciences* found that chronic exposure to stress increases pro-inflammatory markers, which are the causative factors in disease development.[11] Another study published in 2012 in the same journal also investigated this link. Researchers found that chronic stress results in a decrease in the immune response and that those with chronic stress were more likely to develop illnesses (such as the common cold) than those who weren't stressed. This supports the belief that inflammatory responses associated with the immune system were affected by chronic stress, making the body susceptible to disease development.[12] Stress promotes poor eating habits by occupying your time. And this, in turn, increases your level of inflammation via cortisol, altering your nutritional status and causing further inflammation. It is a cycle that is easily broken if you are willing to commit. And it all begins in your adrenal glands.

# MY TURNAROUND
## SHEREE HARTWELL, AGE: 35

"I own and run a model and talent agency and represent 350 people. I manage a lot of personalities, lives, and finances, and I have a 3-year-old, so each day is very demanding," Sheree Hartwell says. "I was making time for everyone but myself. And I had trouble sleeping. I used to wake up at night and couldn't go back to sleep."

But after fainting one morning, things changed. "I felt light-headed and dizzy. When my husband asked me what was going on, I brushed it off because I thought it was a fluke. He was very adamant about me finding out what the true situation was, so I had my blood pressure checked, and it was extremely low: 80/60. If he hadn't pressed me, I probably wouldn't have gotten the help I needed."

Shortly after, Sheree made an appointment with Dr. Pingel and was diagnosed with adrenal fatigue. "I had very high cortisol levels. I went to Dr. Pingel for cardiovascular symptoms due to a high-stress job. Today my blood pressure is fine, my cortisol levels are balanced, and my diet is much better," she says. "Now, thanks to treating my adrenals, my sleep is 110 percent better. I would have times when I would wake up at night and it would be very difficult to go back to bed. Now I wake up rested and not fatigued. I was feeling a little spacey and forgetful in the weeks leading up to the fainting spell, but now I definitely feel better and not so frazzled and run down."

Managing her adrenal fatigue has made a huge impact on Sheree's life. "My husband sees me every day, and he has definitely noticed a change. He said, 'It seems like you're feeling better as a whole,'" she shares. "I grew up dancing, but I hadn't done it in 10 years. Now, I'm dancing again and it's great!"

Sheree's advice for anyone in her situation? Listen to your body. "I knew I was running myself ragged, but I pushed myself. I lost my mom about 4 years ago to cancer, and she burned the candle at both ends quite a bit. I'm trying to take better care of myself now so I know how to prevent this from happening in the future. Your health is the most important thing you have."

# 6

# ADRENAL FATIGUE AND YOUR THYROID

In any business, there is a chain of command. There is a boss, an assistant, a receptionist, a production line, and so on. Your body is no different. Every part has its function and a way to communicate effectively in order to get the required business done. Imagine each respective body part as a member of a business team. Each has a desk, phone, filing cabinet, and inbox.

Suddenly, an urgent phone call comes in to the front desk. There is a strong demand for the product and it needs to be handled immediately. Andrea (adrenal glands) the receptionist, shoots off an e-mail, a text message, and a phone call to the members of the team to get right on this order. Tyrone (thyroid), Ted (testosterone), Esther (estrogen), Al (aldosterone), Pam (progesterone), Ina (insulin), and Greg (glucose) jump right on it, completing the order in no time by pulling workers off the standard production line (GI tract, liver, and parasympathetic activity) and accommodating this urgent request. The thrill of working so well together excites them, and they thrive on it. They continue to handle orders in this fashion and bring in large amounts of product. The boss (brain) is pleased, as he has not been called on to do any additional work. His team is handling it all.

Let's fast-forward to 1 year later. Esther is working on a new project (creating follicles to achieve pregnancy), and Pam and Ted are assisting her with this. They have a lot going on, and occasionally Andrea attempts to call them about other urgent matters. Andrea sends out excessive e-mails and texts, and even demands their help over the loud-speaker. Although Esther, Pam, and Ted hear these calls, they are simply too busy to assist. They contribute small amounts at a time, moving between existing projects (getting pregnant) and urgent orders, trying to multitask. As a result, their inboxes are filling up and their quality of work is diminishing.

Ina (insulin) and Greg (glucose) work differently. With all this added stress, they have been given pay cuts and no longer have all of the nutrients they need to work efficiently. The consistent cortisol output lowers their nutritional resources, which has a significant impact on their jobs. As a result of this, they start altering their work schedules to accommodate for the lack of resources. Ina responds to the immediate demand and Greg picks up the slack of daily maintenance tasks (such as regulating blood sugar) and attempts to keep the production line stable while Ina addresses urgent matters. What was once a team for management of blood sugar is now two individual workers who are unable to easily work together. In the midst of this chaos, Andrea is having a hard time getting the responses she needs to complete her job. She knows that customers drive the business, and they are calling her with complaints. People are yelling at her, and she is becoming emotional. She finds herself feeling overwhelmed and is blowing up at people on the phone. She cries when they yell back at her.

Ultimately, she decides to call the boss (brain) for help, and this makes the boss unhappy. He has enough to do without having to deal with everyday tasks. So he calls his right-hand man, Tyrone (thyroid), to help out. Tyrone is reliable and is always there to help. He has the unique ability to sort through what is and is not important for everyday function. He listens to Andrea's calls and swoops in to protect her job and get things done. He also attempts to call the hormone three, but usually finds that they disappoint him, as Ted and Pam often avoid his calls and Esther is too fiery and overwhelming. (He usually finds himself cleaning up her messes.)

Despite Tyrone's efficiency, he is constantly fielding follow-up calls from the boss via a signal called thyroid stimulating hormone (TSH). Tyrone starts to put some tasks aside and forces the production line to slow down during the day to accommodate only the urgent requests, and then he has the workers come in at night to complete the daily operations. This slows day-to-day operations (metabolism) and increases the speed at which the workers handle urgent calls. Because the workers start taking on night shifts to finish what they used to accomplish during the day, they're not sleeping, and they're eating on the go. They are tired. Sensing a lack of efficiency, the boss releases more TSH to force Tyrone to come up with another solution. He starts seeking outside workers to assist. This is the development of subclinical hypothyroidism (or the inability to properly use the thyroid hormone due to stress).

The new workers demand more resources from the boss, who gives them some medicine (levothyroxine, a synthetic form of the thyroid hormone T4) to assist Tyrone. Tyrone is offended by the assistance, as he makes plenty of his own product—he just spends so much of his time accommodating everyone else that he can't properly use it. He knows he does not need that extra T4 so he starts storing the levothyroxine to use later, and the entire company experiences worsening "symptoms." The company is in decline, and poor Tyrone gets blamed. Esther, Pam, and Ted soon reduce their hours due to the stress. Ida and Greg increase their hours to assist, but they are not a productive pair. They seem to cause more headaches than anything else. How long can this go on before the company dies? How much can Andrea and Tyrone continue to bear before the boss gives up and starts finding other ways to get the projects done?

# THE PREVALENCE OF THYROID MALFUNCTION

As you can tell from the story above, your thyroid is a compensation organ. When other hormones are not working to their full extent, your thyroid steps in to help. It can change the status of your body quickly by stimulating or inhibiting production of the thyroid hormones (T4 and T3) and by altering the way your body uses calcium to function. It also aids with maintenance of your skin, nails, metabolism, bones, and more.

It is reported that 30 million Americans have Hashimoto's thyroiditis, an autoimmune disease caused when your body attacks its own thyroid gland, resulting in poor thyroid function. But this is only one cause of thyroid malfunction; other causes range from damage due to exposure to radioactivity to autoimmune diseases to a simple nutritional deficiency. More commonly, in my practice, I find that the thyroid itself is producing T4 just fine, but the *use* of this hormone by the body is affected by situations related to adrenal stress.[1] This condition is called subclinical hypothyroidism (or low-functioning thyroid) and is commonly missed by standard screening tests (see "Could You Have a Low-Functioning Thyroid?" on the opposite page). And since 1 in 500 people have low thyroid function, this is a pretty common issue.

In fact, levothyroxine, the primary conventional treatment for low thyroid function, is one of the top prescribed drugs in America.[2] But despite therapy, people are not feeling better. Patients are still concerned with fatigue, hair loss, weight gain, slow metabolic rate, low body temperatures, joint pain, and other symptoms of low thyroid function. The question remains: Why are people not feeling better when they are being treated by the standard conventional model? This has been the topic of numerous books and articles and lots of research, as patients are coming forward and admitting to this lack of improvement in symptoms while receiving thyroid therapy.

A study published in the *Journal of Endocrinology* in 2013

recognizes that the standard range for thyroid screening may not be appropriate for evaluating symptoms. After monitoring patients' symptoms and relative TSH levels, researchers determined that even the slightest variation is TSH levels can be associated with negative symptoms, even when those levels fall within an acceptable range. They suggested that physicians more closely monitor patients with varying TSH levels to avoid worsening symptoms.[3] This is a new area of research being pursued due to the constant complaints of patients with thyroid symptoms after a screening reveals a normal TSH.

# THE BASICS OF THE THYROID GLAND

Your thyroid gland is located in your neck and is shaped like a butterfly. In some people, this gland will be enlarged if it is either deficient in iodide or overstimulated for production. This enlargement can cause a hoarse voice or difficulty swallowing.

Your pituitary gland, which is located in your brain, releases TSH in

## COULD YOU HAVE A LOW-FUNCTIONING THYROID?

The symptoms of low thyroid function (hypothyroidism) are as follows:

- Weight gain or inability to lose weight
- Hair loss
- Dryness of the skin
- Muscle or tendon aches and pains
- Depression
- Irregular sleep cycles
- Constipation
- Fatigue
- Poor growth in children
- Mental fogginess or lack of intellectual ability
- Deep, hoarse voice
- Trouble swallowing
- Puffiness around the eyes
- Low body temperature
- Cold sensitivity (always cold)
- Irregular menstrual periods (either lack of or excessive)

response to the levels of thyroid hormone floating around in your bloodstream. TSH simply tells your thyroid whether or not your body is in need of thyroid hormones; it is not responsible for energy production itself. Instead, it is simply a signal or a phone call from your brain stating the recognized need for supply. Doctors typically run a TSH screening test each year to access thyroid function. The level of TSH is also normally within the acceptable range in most subclinical hypothyroidism cases. After stimulation from TSH, thyroxine (T4) is produced in your thyroid gland with the assistance of the mineral iodine. T4 is not overtly responsible for the symptoms we relate to thyroid function. It is an intermediary hormone, as it is then further converted, based on your body's needs, into one of two other thyroid hormones: T3 or reverse T3. T3 is our active hormone and reverse T3 is a storage hormone.

## The Thyroid Hormones: T4, T3, and Reverse T3

After it's created from iodine, T4 is released into your bloodstream and your peripheral tissues decide whether to use the hormone as T3 or store the hormone as reverse T3 (see Figure 1). The conversion of T4 to T3 requires vitamin A and minerals, including selenium, zinc, and iodine. If you are in adrenal fatigue, your body will convert T4 into a storable or inactive form like reverse T3. High levels of reverse T3 will

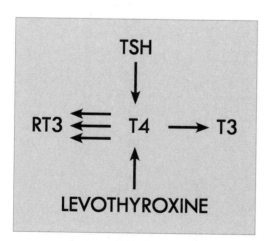

Figure 1: TSH stimulates the release of T4, which can be converted into either T3 (active) or Reverse T3 (inactive). Keep in mind that levothyroxine, the most commonly prescribed thyroid medication, is simply a synthetic form of T4 and also is subject to conversions.

produce the same symptoms as low levels of T4, yet T4 and TSH levels will appear normal in standard lab screenings. So, in this case, TSH and T4 are normal, but the use of the hormone is reduced.

This storage of T3 as reverse T3 results in the *exact* same symptoms as hypothyroidism, but when screened, the thyroid is deemed "normal." I see numerous patients who have been to doctors about symptoms of low thyroid function only to be dismissed with "all is in the normal range" reports. Are these patients imagining their symptoms? Of course not. Most likely, the T4 they are making is simply being stored due to excessive cortisol release. Think back to our story and how your thyroid steps in to help when needed by your adrenal glands. The thyroid stores the excess T4 in order to help with other projects and reserve energy for future urgent requests. This process is part of our survival mechanism and what makes our species so incredible. We adapt to survive, and that's why your thyroid is so adaptable.

Here's another example: If every time you were given 10 jellybeans as a snack you only ate 2 and stored 8, you would eventually end up with a stash of jellybeans and very little in your system to provide you with quick energy. Even more important to recognize is that the standard treatment for low thyroid function is levothyroxine, or Synthroid, which is a synthetic form of T4 (thyroxine). So if your body is under stress, it will convert most of the T4 into reverse T3 (instead of T3) and store it, which results in worsening symptoms while on thyroid therapy.

Many people complain that they feel great on levothyroxine for only a few weeks before their symptoms worsen again. Why? Because their bodies are storing it due to adrenal fatigue. When a conventional doctor only looks at TSH levels, they may even *reduce* the levothyroxine, further worsening the patient's symptoms. It is incredibly important to review the usage and storage of the thyroid hormone before addressing any sort of therapy. In many cases, the prescription will worsen symptoms rather than improve them.

In many of my patients, I find that their original doctors increased the dosage in an attempt to remedy the symptoms of hypothyroidism. If the patient also has adrenal fatigue, they will find that as a result of this increased dosage, the symptoms of low thyroid function, such as fatigue and inability to lose weight, will worsen from the increased conversion to RT3. To make matters worse, they will notice the development of hyperthyroid symptoms (see "Could You Have a High-Functioning Thyroid?") from the high levels of T4 being put into their bodies. They will have increased anxiety, insomnia, and hair loss. As a result of treating based only on symptoms and TSH levels, instead of the entire picture, they now have additional symptoms. This will usually result in extreme frustration for the patient. No one likes to feel bad, and many doctors do not understand their patients' frustration with the standard treatment.

In other cases, T4 levels are normal and T3 is low or low to normal, with a normal or low reverse T3. In these cases, your thyroid is not storing the T4. Instead, this is typically a result of low mineral levels. As you may recall, low mineral levels can also result from adrenal fatigue, typically in an earlier stage, such as Stage 1. These cases still present with symptoms of a poorly functioning thyroid, but the treatment is different because the biochemistry is different. It is simply a lack of supply, not your body's tendency to store excess hormone. In this case, your body is properly producing T4 (with iodine) but is unable to convert it into T3, typically due to low levels of selenium or zinc or both. If your doctor does not screen your levels of all of these nutrients, then he or she cannot tell you that your thyroid is working "fine"—all they can tell you is that the signal or production of T4 is appropriate.

Another important thing to note when it comes to any hormone test is that the ranges are highly variable. The "normal" range of TSH is from approximately 0.5 to 4.5 uIU/L, but I have found that once the TSH moves above 2.5, the thyroid is usually not working optimally. Typically, I find that there is some sort of subclinical hypothyroidism going on, meaning that T4 is not being converted appropriately into T3. And researchers agree. A study published in 2012 assessed the relationship between TSH levels and cortisol in 54 healthy young men and women without clinical evidence of hypothyroidism. The scientists

## COULD YOU HAVE A HIGH-FUNCTIONING THYROID?

The symptoms of hyperthyroidism are as follows:

- Insomnia
- Tremors
- Nervousness
- Excessively high body temperature
- Rapid heart rate
- Frequent bowel movements
- Excessive sweating
- Joint pain
- Enlarged eyes
- Chest pain
- Osteoporosis

discovered a significant positive relationship between TSH and cortisol in the study's subjects. As a result, they suggested that any TSH greater than 2 uIU/L should be considered to be a possible sign of abnormal thyroid function.[4]

# DEVELOPING HASHIMOTO'S THYROIDITIS

The most common situation I find in a patient who is complaining of fatigue, weight gain, menstrual irregularities, hair loss, and dry skin is that she has a TSH around 2, a low-normal T4 (0.9), a low level of T3 (2.0 to 2.3), and a high reverse T3 (greater than 20). I will also typically find a slight elevation of TPO antibodies, which are indicators of Hashimoto's thyroiditis.

Hashimoto's is an autoimmune condition of the thyroid. Antibodies (TPO and thyroglobulin) form, causing low thyroid function. Hashimoto's is the most common cause of hypothyroidism in iodine-sufficient areas, such as the United States.[5] Conventional medicine believes that Hashimoto's is genetic, although it is recognized that environmental factors can cause it to develop. It is commonly accepted that the trigger of this autoimmunity is "unknown." In any autoimmune disease, your immune system overreacts and attacks a local material, thinking it is foreign. In the case of Hashimoto's, the immune system attacks your thyroid gland, causing inflammation, reducing thyroid function, and potentially enlarging the gland.

As you may recall from our earlier story, the thyroid was so bogged down that the brain called upon some outside workers (in this case, the immune system) to assist with the high demand. They worked all day and all night. Autoimmune conditions do just that: They overwork the area under attack and cause destruction. In this case, they destroy the thyroid gland itself.

## Hashimoto's and Adrenal Fatigue

It is also reported that the complications of Hashimoto's disease are increased cholesterol, irregular heartbeat leading to failure, significant depression, decreased sexual desire, and slowed metabolism. Now, let's think about this for a moment. When someone develops thyroid antibodies, they have cardiovascular effects, mental and emotional effects, menstrual irregularities, immune dysfunction, and weight gain. Doesn't this sound a lot like what happens when we run from a bear all of the time? Isn't that an environmental cause? Yes it is, because it is situational.

If your adrenal glands are stressed, the number of antibodies produced increases and symptoms worsen. Naturopathic physicians typically disagree with the conventional wisdom that Hashimoto's is primarily genetic. I find it to be primarily environmental in origin. Consider this: Your thyroid gland does not produce estrogen or progesterone or testosterone, so why is it recognized that it will affect menstruation? Your thyroid does stimulate fat mobilization, and levels of triglycerides are commonly inversely related to thyroid function. Does this promote the increase of LDL cholesterol? Or could it be the stress on your body as it attempts to raise cholesterol in order to make more cortisol, progesterone, or testosterone?

To treat these systems independent of one another is a mistake. Your thyroid is involved in the control of every system in your body and must be properly evaluated whenever you develop a chronic symptom or disease. In my experience, there are two types of Hashimoto's patients. One has the genetic form of Hashimoto's, where their antibodies fall well above normal levels. You must have 35 IU/ml TPO antibodies in order to be officially diagnosed with Hashimoto's thyroiditis. These genetic patients will typically have well over 1,000.

This diagnosis is independent of your T4 levels. Many Hashimoto's patients have normal levels of T4 and a slightly elevated TSH. I find that only a small percentage has ridiculously high quantities of antibodies. The majority of patients I see have low levels—less than 300, with the majority below 100. And when adrenal fatigue is treated, the number of antibodies decreases, T3 levels increase, and symptoms resolve many times without the use of thyroid medication. If the disease were genetic, this would not happen. By treating the adrenal glands, we are treating the environment and reversing disease. When the entire thyroid is evaluated, one can usually see a pattern of a normal to high TSH, a normal T4, a low T3, and a high reverse T3 with high antibodies. When this happens and your body favors storage for long periods of time, it becomes inflamed and promotes the development of an autoimmune response.

This is true for any autoimmune disease, not simply Hashimoto's. A high reverse T3 tells us that your adrenal glands are under stress and are calling on your thyroid to help out with energy storage. In Figure 2 on page 106, if you were to draw a line from the top to bottom just to the left of TSH and T4 (see dotted line), anything on the right would amount to an issue in your thyroid and anything on the left would be related to poor adrenal function. This is how treatment is constructed. If the issue is conversion to reverse T3 or antibody development, you need to focus on your adrenal glands. The exact treatment will depend on other adrenal markers, such as DHEA and cortisol. It's also advantageous to evaluate the sex hormones to rule out the possibility that

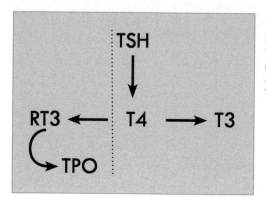

**Figure 2:** When the conversion of T4 consistently goes to RT3, it will usually induce the formation of TPO antibodies, resulting in Hashimotos Thyroiditis

they're having an impact on your thyroid. If the right side of the figure is affected, you may contemplate thyroid support directly, either via nutritional support or thyroid gland supplementation.

Keep in mind that if your body is converting most of the available T4 into reverse T3, then taking levothyroxine (synthetic T4) will worsen the conversion. Your body will just take most of the medication and turn it into reverse T3, unless your adrenal glands are being supported. I prefer to use either a combination of T4 and T3 or simply a sustained release T3 medication to help ease the symptoms while the adrenal glands are healing. I can often lower or eliminate thyroid support once the adrenal glands are healed enough for the patient's body to convert more T4 to T3 than to reverse T3. Although there are always exceptions, I disagree with the conventional medical assumption that once you require thyroid medication you will require it for a lifetime.

## THE RULER OF THE THYROID GLAND

So why do the adrenal glands rule the thyroid gland? Look back at the opening scenario. The adrenal glands made the decision that something was urgent and the thyroid stepped in to help. The adrenal glands made the choice to live or die. When that bear is upon us, the adrenals choose to either run or lie down. When they run, they call on one of the most important glands in your body to mobilize fat for energy: your thyroid. If the demand continues, your thyroid gland will be overworked, causing inflammation, which leads to further hormonal changes, health conditions, and diseases.[6] When someone runs a business, if they overwork their employees, at some point the quality of work will decrease. Overtired workers will take days off, be distracted during work hours, and become agitated. Your body is the same way, and this state of health is, unfortunately, incredibly common in the United States.

Some investigation of the links between thyroid and adrenal function has been conducted. A study published in *Rheumatology International* discovered that a patient with an aldosterone-producing adrenal tumor and Hashimoto's disease had a reversal of Hashimoto's after the removal of the tumor. Before this, it had not been thought that hyperfunctioning adrenal glands would cause an autoimmune disease like Hashimoto's, but this study confirms that there is a connection.[7]

This also relates to our discussion of people who are progressing from Stage 1 to Stage 2 and whether or not they will have a higher output of adrenal hormones, including aldosterone. It's accepted that these increases cause inflammation and elevated blood pressure,[8] but conventional medicine had not recognized aldosterone's connection to the thyroid. This supports the argument that prolonged stress increases conversion to reverse T3 and the development of Hashimoto's antibodies. Wouldn't it have been interesting to see a subsequent evaluation of this patient's reverse T3 and T3 levels during this study? A decrease in reverse T3 and a stabilization of T3 supports the idea of treating the adrenal gland for Hashimoto's in addition to thyroid levels, if appropriate.

## Emotional Side of Your Thyroid

There is also a connection between thyroid function and mental or emotional symptoms. People with subclinical hypothyroidism (which is defined by conventional medicine as elevated TSH with normal T4 levels) will have heightened responses to stress and more depressed moods.[9] So if we take a look at my proposal that subclinical hypothyroidism can be caused by prolonged stress to the adrenal glands, it would explain why that person is more on edge and experiences more negative emotions. There is a bear chasing them and it has been chasing them for quite some time. They anticipate running and fear being eaten! It would have been interesting to see this study with the addition of laboratory evaluations of T3 and reverse T3, because while subclinical hypothyroidism patients have elevated TSH and normal T4, they also tend to have low T3 and high reverse T3. By supporting your adrenal glands, you'll also lower reverse T3, subsequently raising T3.

Your thyroid also has an impact on calcium metabolism. Calcitonin, a hormone released from the thyroid, affects how we utilize calcium. When stimulated, it lowers our serum calcium by changing how it is absorbed by our bones and by promoting calcium excretion via urine. Therefore, when someone has an issue with low thyroid function, they typically also have low vitamin D levels and osteopenia (preosteoporosis) or osteoporosis.[10]

Researchers have found a link between low thyroid function and the expression and conversion of vitamin D in the kidney, resulting in lower serum vitamin D levels in those with diagnosed hypothyroidism.[11] A study released in 2013 found an inverse relationship between free T3 levels and vitamin D levels. The researchers drew an association between subclinical hypothyroidism and low vitamin D levels, suggesting that thyroid function should be assessed when vitamin D levels are shown to be low.[12] Vitamin D is also affected by digestion, as D is a fat-soluble vitamin. So if digestion is slowed due to adrenal stress, that will also have an effect. Also, remember that vitamin D is made from cholesterol, which is typically affected by poor thyroid and by adrenal malfunction. These systems are all related; they are not independent. To treat them as such is malpractice. As I have stated previously, whenever a person exhibits symptoms or is presented with a diagnosis, the question is not how to suppress the symptom, but why the symptom developed in the first place. Find that answer, support that system, and you can reverse the cause and eliminate the symptom.

# GRAVES' DISEASE

Less commonly, a patient may present with elevated thyroid function. This situation promotes agitation, anxiety, and weight loss. There are a few reasons for this scenario. Some are born with Graves' disease, which is an autoimmune condition that attacks your thyroid. This is the most widely known reason for hyperthyroidism. But I want to introduce you to something I see more commonly but that is missed by many practitioners. It is common for your thyroid to surge before it fails. Just as adrenal gland function rises and falls after prolonged stress, so does thyroid function. If you experience heart palpitations, hair loss, weight loss, skin changes, and lack of menstruation, you may have your thyroid checked and be told that you have hyperthyroidism. The doctor may recommend a medication that blocks thyroid function. These medications can permanently damage your thyroid, so this is not a decision to make lightly. It is incredibly common for a *low-functioning* gland to have a final surge of thyroid hormone before its function slows.

Going back to the original story, just before the thyroid considers giving up, it puts in numerous hours trying to improve the situation. It works nights and pushes itself to correct the problems. The thyroid overfunctions until it quits from exhaustion. In Chapter 1, we discussed how your adrenal gland experiences surges in output during Stage 2, causing heart palpitations, anxiety, and insomnia prior to crashing and burning in Stage 3. Beware of this phenomenon. If you are not 100 percent certain that what you have is true hyperthyroidism, either through a diagnosis of Graves' disease or by confirmation of high antibody counts, wait it out before treating your condition with medications.

Most of these surges last only a couple of weeks before you experience low thyroid function. If the adrenals are properly treated, many people will regain normal thyroid function again after a few weeks, and those patients could avoid any type of therapy. But, if you use the suppressive medication too soon, it is almost guaranteed that you'll require medication for a low-functioning thyroid gland in the future. Viruses and toxins can also cause temporary hyperthyroid symptoms. In these cases, inflammatory markers will increase, the patient will have had a viral illness within the last few months, or the white blood counts will be affected. It is *imperative* in all thyroid cases that the patient's overall health be evaluated. If the doctor does not screen for viruses, white blood counts, and inflammatory markers, how would he or she know if the situation is temporary or permanent? How could a physician put you on a thyroid-blocking medication without confirming that you need it? To do so would put you at risk of further thyroid problems.

## STRESS AND YOUR THYROID FUNCTION

Your thyroid is your body's right-hand man when it comes to your metabolism, immune function, skin, hair, nails, and energy. It helps your heart beat regularly, shifts your endocrine system to accommodate stress, and is essential for day-to-day functioning. But the impact of your adrenal glands on your thyroid gland cannot go without notice. If you do not find a way to handle your stress, you will ultimately end up with thyroid disease, and the Cleveland Clinic reports that the incidence of hypothyroidism increases with age. Why is that? If you were not born with the disease, why does it develop over time?

Your thyroid is a compensation gland, meaning that it adapts to the situation surrounding it. As you age, you introduce more stress and toxins into your system, and your thyroid has to manage those changes. Thyroid function is related to your stress response from your adrenal glands, and it needs to be treated with these associations in mind. If treated correctly, your symptoms will disappear and your diagnosis of hypothyroidism will be in the past.

# MY TURNAROUND
## ERIN MULKINS, AGE: 40

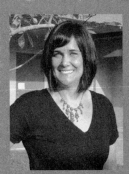

For most of her life, Erin Mulkins suffered from exhaustion and never knew the reason why. "I had taken thyroid medicine since I was 16, and I had been on antidepressants for 14 years. I'd been on these medications hoping to feel better, but I was always tired and irritable," she says. "I would go to bed at 8 p.m. and sleep until 12 or 1 p.m. the next day—and I'd still wake up tired!"

About 10 years ago, Erin was diagnosed with Hashimoto's thyroiditis, and the exhaustion persisted. "I couldn't find the energy to do anything other than work. I would join and quit the gym, and my weight would fluctuate up and down. And my hands were always swollen from the Hashimoto's," she shares. "I was under an endocrinologist's care for years, and no one ever said anything was wrong, because my levels were 'fine.' I knew something wasn't right, because I kept saying that I didn't feel right, but no one would listen to me."

After her friends recommended Dr. Pingel, Erin decided to take action. Dr. Pingel diagnosed her with adrenal fatigue and immediately began to wean her off her medications. "I was really focused on my thyroid, so I had no idea that it had anything to do with my adrenal glands. Everyone thinks exhaustion means thyroid problems, and it's not always the case. If your adrenal glands aren't producing the hormones you need, you're not going to get the adrenaline boost—and that's what was making me exhausted," Erin explains. "I went off one medication right away, and I'm now off Prozac, too. I love not having to pop that pill every day. Before, all my doctors just tried to fix my problems with a pill, but I'm a prime example of how that isn't always the answer."

Today, Erin's adrenal fatigue is under control, and she says her life is better as a result. "Now I wake up in the morning and I'm not tired at all. My teaching assistant said she can't believe the change in me. I feel like a different person," she exclaims. "Now I'm looking forward to going to the gym 5 days a week, and my trainer said you would never know what I was like before. The plan was so easy—and quick! I was skeptical at first, but this has changed my life in a mere month or two. Dr. Pingel saved my life!"

# 7

# STRESS AND YOUR DIGESTIVE SYSTEM

As you may recall, in Chapter 1 we said that the rate of misdiagnosis for those with adrenal insufficiency, or Stage 3 adrenal fatigue, was 68 percent. Well, would it surprise you to hear that the most common false diagnoses were of psychiatric and gastrointestinal (GI) origin?[1]

In the world of conventional medicine, your gastrointestinal system is considered to be separate from your endocrine system. When you complain of GI distress to your primary care physician, you are typically sent to a specialist, known as a gastroenterologist, who *only* looks at your GI system.

During your exam, the focus is on that system alone, and other systems are rarely investigated. The signs of adrenal fatigue are usually present, but they're rarely investigated by a GI specialist. If your gastroenterologist does ask you further questions that don't relate to your GI tract, you may reveal additional symptoms such as insomnia, fatigue, hormonal irregularities (heavy periods, for example), or mental fogginess. You may also mention signs of nutritional deficiencies, such as ridges in your fingernails, brittle nails, hair loss, dry hair, dry skin, and even small bumps on the backs of your arms or legs.[2]

According to many patients, the most common experience at the gastroenterologist's office consists of a 5-minute exam, the recommendation of an endoscopy, and a prescription for medication. But over time, these medications cause side effects and patients often seek a second opinion. Many ask to come off of the medication and find the cause of the imbalance in the first place.

# STRESS AND YOUR GI ISSUES

Gastroesophageal reflux disease (GERD) medication is one of the most commonly prescribed medications in the United States. And as a result, it is making a huge impact on the health of our society. You may complain of a cough, or chest pain, or heartburn after eating. Immediately, you are given an endoscopy exam and told that you have reflux. You are then given medication to block stomach acid and are told to lose weight.

It is fairly common knowledge that irritable bowel syndrome (IBS) is caused by stress; however, physicians rarely treat your body's stress response in order to relieve IBS. Most IBS patients are given steroids and a prescription for an antidepressant, and they are referred to a psychologist. Here's the problem: Steroid therapy can actually worsen adrenal fatigue, causing further flare-ups and the need to take even more medication. But if stress is a trigger for the main symptoms of IBS, such as chronic diarrhea, why aren't physicians investigating the adrenal gland component—especially when science is beginning to make this important connection?

In a recent study, 53 college students were divided into two groups (those with and those without IBS), and each group was given stressful tasks to complete. The researchers measured their stress and adrenal hormone levels before, during, and after the tasks and found that adrenal hormone levels were significantly lower in the IBS group than in the control group. In addition, throughout the experiment, the IBS group experienced a higher cortisol-to-DHEA ratio than the control group, displaying cortisol dominance during stressful situations. The researchers concluded that this adrenal hormone imbalance may exacerbate abdominal symptoms in those with IBS.[3]

The real question that we should be asking is *why* does digestive function change? Your body's acid production was not excessive when you were a child, so why is it excessive now? What happened? To give you a better example, imagine the bear scenario again. The bear appears and your sympathetic nervous system begins to take over. Your eyes focus, your energy is diverted to muscles so that you can run, and your blood pressure rises. As a result, your parasympathetic system and its functions are put on the back burner. (Digestion is a parasympathetic response.)

Think about it: When you run from the bear, you do not stop to use the bathroom. And depending on how long you've been running from that bear, it may be days before you are able to have a bowel movement. When you finally have time to relieve yourself, your body is unsure as to when the bear might come back, resulting in either a quick release of loose stools or further retention (or minimal excretion) of stool, resulting in chronic constipation. This then predisposes your body to a higher toxic load, and therefore more symptoms such as gas and bloating, abdominal pain, hemorrhoids, changes in acid production, malabsorption, muscle aches and pains, headaches, mental fogginess, weight gain, sensitivity to substances (such as chemicals, perfumes, medications, smoke, and so on), allergic hive development, memory loss, hair loss, skin changes, dehydration, nutritional deficiencies, and more. The list just goes on and on.

# THE INS AND OUTS OF YOUR GI SYSTEM

Taking all of this into consideration, let's discuss how a normally functioning digestive system works. The purpose of your digestive system is to take ingested food, break it down, and provide nutrients for your body. It consists of a long tube, or GI tract, that starts at your mouth and ends at your anus. Along the way, various sources aid in digestion. These include saliva from your mouth, your teeth and tongue, your gallbladder, stomach acid, your pancreas, and your liver.

When food enters your mouth, your salivary glands release saliva to begin to break down carbohydrates, and you begin to absorb the nutrients from your food. Your teeth assist in chewing and your tongue helps move the food to the back of your mouth. The food then travels down your esophagus, through a "trapdoor" called the esophageal sphincter, and into your stomach. Hydrochloric acid and enzymes are then released from your stomach to break down your food. The food is moved into your small intestine, which is about 10 feet long and performs the bulk of the digestion process. Your pancreas, liver, and gallbladder then release enzymes and bile into your small intestine to break down all remaining food into its chemical building blocks. The further breakdown of food happens in your stomach, but the majority of nutrient absorption occurs in your small intestine. What's left moves into your large intestine, which then absorbs vitamin B and vitamin K before eliminating feces from your body.

## The Impact of Probiotics

Another very important part of your gastrointestinal system is your intestinal flora, or "probiotics," which assist in the digestion of food and prevention of disease development. Numerous studies have cited the impact these flora have on diseases and ailments such as irritable bowel disease, autism, allergy development, cancer development, autoimmune disease, cardiovascular disease, and more. Probiotics have been an emerging area of research, which has lead to numerous probiotic products being released into the general market and heavy marketing dollars driving people to these products. The links between intestinal flora and potential disease are statistically strong and warrant strong consideration in all patients.

# IS YOUR GI ISSUE A SYMPTOM OF ADRENAL FATIGUE?

The list below contains GI conditions commonly linked back to your adrenal glands.

- Heartburn, gastroesophageal reflux disease (GERD)
- Gas, bloating, distended abdomen
- Abdominal pain or discomfort
- Constipation and diarrhea, or alternating bouts of each
- Food allergies
- Leaky gut
- Irritable bowel syndrome (IBS)
- Colitis
- Celiac disease (present in genes, but worsened by adrenal fatigue)
- Crohn's disease (present in genes, but worsened by adrenal fatigue)
- Ulcerative colitis (present in genes, but worsened by adrenal fatigue)
- Intestinal overgrowths of yeast, bacteria, parasites, or viruses
- Hemorrhoids

Here are surprising symptoms related to both poor GI function and adrenal fatigue.

- Insomnia
- Depression or anxiety
- Seasonal allergies
- Poor recovery from common colds or flu, or constant reinfection
- Joint pain
- Estrogen dominance
- Hot flashes
- Headaches
- Mental fogginess
- Sensitivity to substances
- Autism and ADHD
- Obesity
- Chronic rashes

## Probiotics throughout Your Life Span

Studies on microflora have shown links to the development of allergies in infants. A study published in the *Journal of Allergy and Clinical Immunology* found that infants who had higher colonization by particular probiotics were less likely to develop allergies than those who had lower colonization levels. They also found greater growth of bacteria, such as staph, in those who were not highly colonized with probiotics.[4] This article is particularly pertinent to our discussion because it supports the idea that our health path begins at birth. What happens to you as an infant influences your health as a child and an adult. Most allergies in babies and children are treated with suppressive medications, such as antihistamines or steroids. If your GI system is evaluated at the first sign of an allergy, it is highly possible, according to this study, that allergies can be avoided. I commonly recommend that all babies be placed on a probiotic at birth to improve immune support and to avoid further allergy development.

The benefits of probiotics have been linked to the prevention of aging and disease development, and to longevity. When bacterial flora was evaluated in the elderly population in a 2007 study, links were found between disease development and quality of life in those with certain bacteria populations—specifically, decreases in lactobacilli and bifidobacteria (beneficial) and an increase in facultative anaerobes (harmful). As a result, the study suggests that by providing the elderly with strains of pre- and probiotics to address bacterial flora, we can improve their quality of life by lowering their chances of disease development.[5]

## The Neurotransmitter and IBS Connection to Flora

Even the mainstream medical community recognizes the strong links between intestinal health and autism. It has been observed and documented that children with autism have a higher incidence of gastrointestinal symptoms. And the more severe cases of autism were associated with more severe GI distress.[6] With these observations, autism specialists have begun to focus more on gut flora, diet, and GI maintenance as a treatment for autism. And these medical advancements have made a huge impact on this disease. The idea that by simply changing the gut flora in your GI system you can change the neurotransmitters in your brain is incredibly exciting.

In alternative medicine, some specialized labs perform testing that assesses your levels of good and bad bacteria, yeast, parasites, and markers for digestion and inflammation in your intestines—all of which have become crucial to the treatment of autism.[7] When your gut flora is out of balance, the overgrowth of certain strains will affect the development of neural, immune, and endocrine functions. The florae send out neurotoxins, which can be a source of numerous neurological disturbances ranging from depression and anxiety to autism and schizophrenia.[8]

In addition, links to IBS and neurological function have been well documented.[9] It is known that the cause of IBS has something to do with neurological function, and that is the basis behind its treatment with antidepressants. When you look at the production of serotonin (a neurotransmitter responsible for mood), the majority of it occurs in your intestine, so it makes sense for the treatment to address neurotransmitters. But let's take it a step further: If the imbalance of flora is the cause of the neurotransmitter changes, then why not start by treating the flora and see if neurological function improves?

## Take Probiotics to Heart

Probiotics have even been linked to your cardiovascular system. A recent study in the *New England Journal of Medicine* linked microbial flora to an increased risk of a cardiovascular event. They compared those with suppressed levels of beneficial bacteria to those with normal levels, and in both groups they monitored a metabolite that is responsible for plaque deposition. They found that those with suppressed levels of beneficial bacteria had higher levels of this metabolite and therefore higher risk of a cardiovascular event.[10] One interesting aspect of this study was that the researchers gave the participants antibiotics in order to suppress the beneficial bacteria. Knowing this, it seems that those who chronically use antibiotics would also be at higher risk of a cardiovascular event. Makes you think twice before jumping to use antibiotics for every sniffle, doesn't it?

# PROBIOTICS AND WEIGHT LOSS

With the current epidemic of obesity, most Americans are focused on losing weight but finding that they cannot, despite the dietary advice being given by their physicians. A recent article in the *New York Times* summarized a link between obesity, an inability to lose weight, and intestinal flora. They found that certain strains of flora actually prevent weight loss.[11] Another study supported this by stating that small intestinal bacterial overgrowth leads to inflammation and disease development. The researchers stated that obese people have a greater degree of bacterial overgrowth because the bacteria is harvesting energy via the person's fat cells. They related the imbalance to endotoxemia, systemic inflammation, further obesity, and nonalcoholic fatty liver disease.[12]

Many articles have been published discussing the intestinal bacterial differences between lean and obese people and the imbalance in flora that results from consuming processed foods.[13] This supports that idea that your entire body must be functioning properly before you can lose weight. It also forces us to take a closer look at the fast foods that we're consuming due to our lack of time. These processed foods have more preservatives, which affect our bacterial flora. If your body is under stress due to GI disturbances, it will hold on to weight more than it would if it were not stressed. Your adrenal glands react when your GI tract is disturbed, and your GI tract reacts when your adrenal glands are disturbed. These systems are interrelated.

Intestinal bacteria are also essential to such processes as removing waste from your body; supplying vitamin K; deconjugating and converting bile acid; fighting infections related to the bowel; counteracting malabsorption and other bacterial overgrowth syndromes; and preventing hepatic coma.[14] Without a good balance of these organisms, your system cannot function efficiently.

## The GI Apartment Complex

Let's imagine that your GI system is an apartment complex. In apartment A you have the Streptococcus family, apartment B has the Candida family, apartment C houses the Ecoli family, apartment D houses the Pseudomonas, and so on. This apartment complex is huge, consisting of many (bacterial) families who live and coexist with one another. The office of the complex has a large staff of landlords (probiotics) who keep order in the complex. They collect the rent, evict those who misbehave, and maintain the property. Things go along well until something disruptive happens.

So imagine that a little hoodlum, we will call him Amoxicillin, comes along and burns down the property office. Half of the landlords are lost, leaving the other half to run the property. Now the remaining landlords are doing twice as much work and things get overlooked. The grass starts to grow too tall. The light bulbs don't get changed. The Streptococcus family in apartment A are street-smart and see that the landlords are bogged down. Taking advantage of this, they start to plan an attack to take over another apartment. When the landlords aren't looking, they barge into apartment B and take over the Candida family's apartment. The Candidas are not happy about this and decide to barge into apartment C. The pattern continues until you have an unruly complex with holes in the walls and families in the wrong apartments. They finally all come together and take over the office. The remainder of the landlords are destroyed and the complex is now ruled by a variety of families that have overgrown their respective apartments.

So antibiotic use is one way to find yourself with an overgrowth of bacteria, but this situation can also occur when you are in a constant state of sympathetic response. Enzymes from your mouth are not released because you scarfed down your meal in between bear attacks. The food lands in your stomach, but your stomach enzymes are withheld due to a lack of parasympathetic activity. So the food just sits there, causing inflammation. Over time, your intestinal lining breaks down, causing "leaks" in your intestinal wall; this is commonly referred to as "leaky gut syndrome." Particles from food leak into your bloodstream, and your immune system attacks them, causing food intolerances. Food intolerance then leads to other symptoms, such as gas and bloating, headaches, joint aches and pains, changes in bowel function, and endocrine and hormonal imbalances. In fact, these symptoms were discovered in soldiers who were under constant stress and developing worsening intestinal symptoms. A 2013 review showed that the stress the soldiers were under had an impact on their neuroendocrine systems, immune activation, and intestinal permeability.[15]

In terms of the apartment complex scenario, this permeability relates to tenants not cleaning up after themselves. They bring in all their groceries, garbage, and dirty clothes, and they just leave them in the apartments. Over time, the stuff exceeds the space and starts to push on the walls to the adjoining apartments. This means that in your intestines, bacteria and yeast start destroying the walls to make more room. As they destroy a wall, they release the bacteria on the other side, eventually creating co-mingling among all of the tenants. At some point, the bad bacteria will kill off all of the good bugs. And until you kick them out, repair your intestinal walls, and reestablish some good bacteria, your GI tract is going to be a mess.

Destruction of property, regardless of how it occurs, often brings in some outsiders from another community, and your body is no exception. Invaders such as parasites will take this opportunity to attack your system. By this time, you probably have numerous symptoms and a gastrointestinal doctor will finally agree to analyze a stool sample to search for parasites.

All of these scenarios result in the same thing: symptoms. Many patients have spent countless hours on the Internet looking up candida, bacterial overgrowth, and poor flora, and many have tried numerous diets to kill off these organisms. You may have gone on a strict candida diet, only to find that you did great until you had one tiny spot of sugar—and then all of your symptoms flared. You may be desperate, tired, and hopeless. At this point, you may decide to get food intolerance testing to find all of the reactive foods you should avoid in an attempt to decrease your symptoms. Avoiding those foods will temporarily relieve your symptoms, until you develop another intolerance to another food and the cycle continues.

## Which Came First: The Stress or the GI Imbalance?

As I mentioned before, the only way to treat these imbalances is to kill the excessive bacteria, repair your intestinal walls and the damage to your GI tract, and restore the beneficial bacteria. In the early stages of treatment, you may choose to minimize your symptoms by avoiding certain foods that cause reactions, but you must "clean up the property" to get long-term relief. But you also have to consider the adrenal fatigue or stress on your body that started this process in the first place. You have to ask *why* this destruction happened the first place. Was your body in constant sympathetic response? Did it experience excessive antibiotic use? Consider the long-term effects of antibiotics. If the good flora are constantly being killed off, how stressful is that to your system? It makes absolute sense to assume that using antibiotics can worsen adrenal fatigue and therefore weaken your immune system.

There is an immune complex called IgA that is present in your mucosal membranes and assists with your immune function. It is also highly present in your GI tract and is your first line of defense for your immune system, meaning your intestinal flora is the first thing to attack an invader that's been ingested. In those with leaky guy syndrome, IgA levels will be very low, while those with autoimmune diseases, such as lupus, rheumatoid arthritis, Sjögren's syndrome, and so on, will have very high levels. I like to think of IgA as an outside management company that may assist the landlords when needed once a building has been affected. If you have adrenal fatigue, the management company employees are either incredibly hard working (overproductive) or lazy (underproductive).

Either way, their job is to back up your immune defense in conjunction with the probiotics. If they aren't doing their jobs, items may "leak" into your bloodstream and create an immune reaction. For example, let's say you eat a blueberry and develop a headache shortly thereafter. Why? Think of it as a piece of blueberry leaking through your intestinal lining, landing in your bloodstream, and being attacked by an immune complex to be removed by your immune system. This causes an inflammatory response resulting in headaches, hives, rashes, swelling, fatigue, abdominal pain, sneezing, mucus production, and so on.

On the flip side, if IgA is overproductive, it will create symptoms by generating a huge immune response to anything foreign, as is seen in autoimmune diseases. When your IgA levels are affected, your body becomes more susceptible to infection. Have you ever been told that you are a strep carrier? I have always questioned this diagnosis because strep A lives in one of your apartments all the time, meaning that you are constantly carrying this virus around. So wouldn't that make everyone a strep carrier? Maybe the person who keeps getting strep has an overgrowth of strep. Or maybe the strep has moved into other areas, like the tonsils, so the person continues to get infected due to a breakdown of the intestinal lining and a decrease in IgA response to strep. Then, when treated with amoxicillin, more probiotics are killed, which allows for more invasions by strep and a further decrease in IgA.

Do you see how this may cause a long-term problem? The common "fix" is to take out your tonsils so that strep cannot infect them anymore. That is all fine and good for the tonsils, but did anyone actually take the strep away? No. It still lives in your gut and has the potential to cause other problems.

Consider that IgA is present not only in your GI tract, but also in your genitourinary and respiratory tracts. It is also present in tears and breast milk. Why wouldn't strep then attack your sinuses? Or your lungs? Or your urinary tract? Why do people with poor gut health often suffer regular yeast or bladder infections? Are these independent of each other? No. They are the same tissue, just in different locations. Consider ulcers: These are "holes" in your mucosal membranes; they are red, irritated areas of tissue. If someone has this irritation in her gastric lining, wouldn't it be logical for that same person to have hemorrhoids? Or mouth ulcers? Or canker sores? If sores and inflammation develop at one end of the "tube," why wouldn't they develop at the other end? When these questions are posed to a patient, I typically find that she does have other symptoms of mucosal irritation but has never drawn the connection between an ulcer in her mouth and an ulcer in her stomach or anus, even though it's all the same tube.

## GERD: The Most Common Offender

While we are discussing ulcerations, we should also discuss one of the most commonly diagnosed GI conditions: gastroesophageal reflux disease, or GERD, which currently affects more than 15 million Americans. Instead of thinking about this as a disease, think of it as a functional change in your physiology. You can't "catch" GERD. It isn't an epidemic that is spread from person to person. There is no cure for it. Most GI doctors state that it is a life-long condition that is improvable with weight loss, but it is not curable. You are welcome to believe that explanation and live on medications for the rest of your life, or you can consider *why* this physiological change may have happened. And there's a great reason why you should do that: Because GERD is a functional response, and not a disease, it is reversible.

Begin by considering the two types of reflux development: excessive acid production and lack of acid production. Yes, a *lack* of acid can actually cause heartburn.[16] In fact, a majority of my patients have a diagnosis of GERD due to a lack of acid production. Despite this, many of them were previously placed on an acid blocker due to the assumption that they were overproducing acid. And while they may no longer experience the feeling of acid burning in their throats, they are now experiencing bloating, malabsorption, intestinal overgrowth, and nutritional deficiencies. Many of them even develop diverticula in their intestines, or colon polyps. And most doctors don't relate these developing symptoms back to the GERD because the symptoms are currently "stable" due to the medications. In fact, a study released in the *Journal of the American Medical Association* stated that those who take acid-reducing drugs have a higher incidence of community-acquired pneumonia due to acid suppression's impact on bacterial flora.[17] If you knew that a drug designed to reduce heartburn might give you pneumonia, would you even think twice about taking it? You would likely at least explore other options for treatment, which may require thinking about acid in a different way. Let's explore how this phenomenon with acid works.

## HOW ACID WORKS IN YOUR BODY

When food lands in your stomach, acid and enzymes are released to break down the food. When you are constantly "running from a bear," you do not release these enzymes and acid due to a decrease in your parasympathetic response. So the food just sits there. The lack of acid production (and therefore digestion) causes the mass of food to push back against your esophageal sphincter, releasing the minimal amount of acid that was produced back into your esophagus.

Because the amount of acid may be minimal, you may not experience traditional heartburn. You may feel like you have a lump in your throat or have a hoarse voice. You may also feel slight discomfort behind your rib cage. The movement of the sphincter is well understood, which is why most doctors correctly state that weight loss and less food in your stomach will help reduce your symptoms. But how about looking at the reason why digestion was slowed enough to cause this laxity in the sphincter? Should the treatment be to minimize the acid even further with an acid blocker? Wouldn't that only worsen the problem in the long term?

## Your Gallbladder: To Keep or Not?

Another common GI situation revolves around your gallbladder, which is an organ responsible for digesting fat. When food lands in your stomach, it releases bile to help break down and absorb nutrients from that food. If digestion is affected due to your stress response, bile will not be regularly released from your gallbladder, which will often result in the development of gallstones. Removal is often suggested, as it is an uncomplicated surgery with minimal recovery time—and odds are good that you know someone who has had this done. However, once your gallbladder is removed, you need to know (because most patients are not told) that your fat absorption will be affected. As a result, many people experience diarrhea or fat streaks in their stools.

In addition, vitamin D deficiency can occur because vitamin D is a fat-soluble vitamin. Many patients experience gas, bloating, and discomfort after eating. They may also start taking fish oil supplements, having heard that this is good for general health, yet they cannot absorb them due to minimal bile production, so the effort is wasted. Their triglycerides will then rise due to a lack of fat absorption.

So if you have had your gallbladder removed, you'll need to consider two things. First, from this point on, you'll need to take digestive enzymes when you eat to help absorb and break down fat. Second, you'll need to consider why your gallbladder was removed in the first place. If it was due to stone development, take a close look at your digestion and stress levels.

It has been well established that the gastrointestinal function and release of bile from the gallbladder is hormonally, behaviorally, and neurologically mediated. This is undisputed. A study released in 1999 stated that GI motility varied based on stress response. Scientists evaluated recent research and found that chronic changes occur within smooth muscle in response to stress. The most frequent response was a delay in emptying the contents of the stomach.[18] Part of this gastric emptying involves your gallbladder, and if your gallbladder is slow due to this stress, it will not release what is needed and stones will form.

In addition, a study published in 2004 showed that stress will suppress gallbladder function, increasing stone development. As you now know, adrenal fatigue causes poor digestion, which results in a sluggish digestive system.[19] This sluggishness results in stone development and gallbladder issues. Bottom line: The adrenal glands play a large role in gallbladder function!

## The Issue of Constipation

Many patients with adrenal fatigue have constipation concerns. When I ask people if they have any concerns about their gastrointestinal function, they usually state that it is fine. Then, upon further questioning, I find that they typically have a bowel movement only every 2 to 3 days! Most people assume that they have normal function if their stools are not hard or like rabbit pellets. But here's the problem with that: Typically, people eat at least three times a day. Think about how much food you consume. (Let's be conservative and say about 5 to 6 cups of food each day, just as an example.) Do you have bowel movements that equate to a good portion of that volume? Think about an infant. When they eat, within about an hour, they have eliminated the waste from that meal. Does your body work like this? Do you really remove all that you eat? If the answer is no, think about all of the toxins your body is accumulating!

Your body removes stool because it is waste; it is literally considered to be garbage. If garbage is accumulating, so are toxins and inflammation. I have found that constipation is caused mostly by endocrine imbalances. A study released in 2013 stated the most common concurrent symptoms of those with chronic constipation were gastrointestinal, endocrine, and psychiatric issues.[20] Knowing what you have learned so far about the connections among adrenal fatigue, GI disorders, and psychiatric effects, it is reasonable to consider all of the above a result of the imbalances in your endocrine system. Your endocrine system also directly affects your thyroid. If your thyroid function is low, constipation will occur. And if your adrenal glands are too busy running from the bear, they will not digest or remove waste. Furthermore, if these stresses are affecting regular bowel function, this causes inflammation and further overgrowth in your intestines. This then causes more stress on your system, decreasing the amount of other hormones your adrenal glands produce. Your body should eliminate what it eats. If you notice that this is not occurring, have a full evaluation not only of GI function, but also of endocrine function to assess your stress response. If this situation has been chronic, you should also consider the toxic load this places on your system and its impact on liver function.

## Your Liver, the Lifesaver

Your liver is an organ in your GI system that plays a critical role in disease development. It is responsible for keeping your system clean and free of toxins. It cleans your blood. To understand how your liver affects gastrointestinal function and toxicity, imagine a receptionist sitting at her desk. She has a variety of tasks to complete each day, such as filing, answering the phone, and greeting people. When she first starts the job, she is very organized and creates a list of things to do, prioritized by their importance. As something is placed on her desk, she decides whether it should be handled immediately or filed for later.

Over time, her boss keeps dumping more and more files on her desk. She finds herself clearing stack after stack as the phone is ringing and people are walking into the office, expecting to be greeted. She quickly has to determine what to do first. If the workload becomes too large, she starts filing more tasks for later in her inbox. Meanwhile, the pile in her inbox grows and grows, leaving her with more work than she can handle.

Think of these stacks of paperwork as the things your liver has to take care of. These include exposure to external toxins, such as smog, food additives, pollen, infected water, drugs, alcohol, other poisonous substances, and drug therapies, as well as internal paperwork such as hormone elimination, bile manufacturing (which helps carry away waste and break down fats during digestion), protein production, cholesterol production, conversion of excess glucose (sugar) into storable forms (and changing it back, when needed), regulation of amino acids, iron storage, and conversion of ammonia to urea for excretion. All this, plus resisting infections by removing bacteria from your bloodstream and regulating blood clotting.

Your liver is *essential* to your body's everyday functions. Because your liver decides the importance of each toxin that it encounters, it commonly puts aside everyday tasks to address the bigger threats. For example, when you enjoy that glass of wine at the end of your day, your liver finds that to be of higher importance than clearing estrogens or iron from your system. When your liver gets too bogged down with additional tasks, your body begins to become toxic and symptoms of toxicity occur. When it can no longer effectively clear the external toxins being introduced, this puts stress on your system. It is a huge bear! Your body then alters GI function, slowing digestion and increasing your toxic load even further.

The increased demand on your liver is a stress itself and can worsen adrenal fatigue. A study published in 2009 evaluated the effects of stress on the development of liver disease and found a positive correlation between stress and a decline in liver health. The researchers found that stress has an inflammatory effect on your liver! They reviewed a number of studies that established a clear link between stress and the development of viral hepatitis. Those with a type 1 personality (think overachievers) had more severe symptoms of hepatitis C. Researchers also found the same clinical association between high stress levels and the development of cirrhosis of the liver.[21] So whether we like it or not, our bodies are affected by stress. We need to recognize this link in order to prevent disease. Your liver takes the brunt of it all. And as your adrenal fatigue worsens, your liver has a harder time keeping up. It is simply part of the vicious cycle of adrenal fatigue!

# NOTHING IS INDEPENDENT

Your gastrointestinal system is not independent of your other systems. Your body thrives on its inputs and outputs. If your body is not processing food, absorbing nutrients, and removing waste effectively, this will promote inflammation and disease development. The reasons why your GI system isn't functioning properly should not be overlooked by your medical doctor. By eliminating the causes of malfunction and healing and supporting the systems necessary to restore regular function, you can reverse your symptoms and prevent further disease.

Treating adrenal fatigue is critical when treating GI disorders, as it is at the core of the development of these conditions. Think back to the onion, mentioned in Chapter 1. We each have a core, and over the years we develop layers of symptoms. The symptoms surrounding your GI system are simply a layer developed over a core of adrenal fatigue that slowed digestion, changed absorption and nutritional status, and caused a flora imbalance. Treating your GI symptoms with herbs and nutrition can be quite simple, but if you do not address the core, or the cause of the issues, your symptoms will inevitably return. To truly heal yourself, it is critical that you do not ignore your endocrine system's powerful effects on your gastrointestinal system.

# MY TURNAROUND
## JENNIFER ENNESSER, AGE: 30

Despite her healthy diet and active lifestyle, Jennifer Ennesser was struggling. "I had digestive problems, weight gain, severe fatigue, brain fog, and memory loss. I have always been active—I was an athlete growing up—but my daily activity started to decline since I was so tired. I also constantly felt nauseated and bloated," she shares. Jennifer was also dealing with a lot of stress. "I had stress at work, my mom was sick with cancer, and my very good friend had just passed away. That wreaked havoc on me both mentally and physically."

Jennifer tried getting help, but nothing worked. "I had gone to several other specialists, an allergist, a GI doctor, and I tried Chinese medicine, but nothing relieved me of my digestive issues," she says. That's when Jennifer decided to turn to naturopathic medicine. "I'm not a huge fan of masking the problem with drugs without really getting to the root of the issue. Naturopathic medicine, for me, was the way to get back to the core, listen to my body, and naturally combat the stressors that affect it," she explains.

When Jennifer first visited Dr. Pingel, she wasn't sure what could be causing all of her discomfort. But it didn't take long to find the culprit. "I was so lucky to find Dr. Pingel. When she diagnosed me with adrenal fatigue, I was surprised. I had never heard of adrenal fatigue and didn't imagine that it could be the cause of my problems." But once Jennifer began taking supplements and following Dr. Pingel's dietary recommendations, she noticed results. "The plan was easy. I lost 21 pounds and went from a size 8/6 to a 4/2! I am back to working out three to four times a week and have a tremendous amount of energy afterward," she states.

With her health under control, Jennifer feels confident she can handle whatever life throws her way. "I very recently lost my mom to cancer and just started a new job. But despite those things, I feel as though I am able to manage the stress better . . . things don't seem so daunting to deal with. I'm much more centered and calm," she shares. "I feel stronger both mentally and physically because of the treatment I received from Dr. Pingel. Now I'm my old energetic self again."

# 8

# IS ADRENAL FATIGUE KEEPING YOU AWAKE?

Sleep is essential; your body cannot heal without it. During sleep, your body recovers from the day's activities, repairs tissues, metabolizes toxins, and regenerates cells. Without sleep, you cannot recover from any health-related issues, yet an estimated 50 to 70 million Americans report having chronic insomnia.[1] And our lack of sleep is causing higher mortality rates now than ever.

## HOW ADRENAL FATIGUE AFFECTS YOUR SLEEP

Let's go back to our forest. You have survived the bear attack. It is getting late and you feel tired, so you find a nice tree to sit down behind and rest. After taking some deep breaths, you close your eyes and start to doze off. Just as you are finally resting, a sound in the bushes startles you. Immediately, your mind begins racing: What was that? Was it a bear? You look around and fail to see anything. The forest is calm and there is no sign of danger, so you close your eyes again. But this time, you can't sleep. Now you're worrying about the bear. What if he is going to jump out and attack you? What if it isn't a bear, but maybe a snake? You look around in anticipation as your heart beats faster. You are exhausted but cannot possibly sleep.

After drifting in and out for small increments of time, you finally fall asleep again a few hours later. You finally find yourself in deep sleep and *bam!*—you hear another rustle. Again, you jump up to find nothing but a calm forest, the moon shining on the water, and stillness around you. But your heart is beating very rapidly now. Checking your watch, you realize it's about 3:00 a.m. Deciding that, in spite of your exhaustion, sleep is not going to happen, you carry on in your travels.

Does this sound familiar? How many times have you woken up in the middle of the night in a quiet bedroom, wondering why you were startled? Do you find yourself tired in the early hours of the morning, but because you cannot sleep you decide to get up anyway? Then, 5 to 6 hours later, you are exhausted and want to take a nap, but you can't due to your schedule, and the cycle starts all over again.

## Using Prescription Sleep Aides

In order to handle our increased economic stresses and busy, multitasking lifestyles, doctors are prescribing more and more sleep aides, which are putting us at higher risk of early death. In fact, a recent study stated that an estimated 6 to 10 percent of all American adults took a hypnotic drug for poor sleep in 2010. The study followed subjects who were prescribed hypnotics (including Ambien and a variety of benzodiazepines) for sleep for $2\frac{1}{2}$ years and compared them to a control group of people who did not take hypnotic medications. As predicted by the researchers, the group that was prescribed hypnotic medications had a substantially higher mortality rate than those not taking medications: Receiving hypnotic prescriptions was associated with a threefold higher incidence of death. (Media reports of celebrity deaths from overdoses of prescribed medication are a very visible example of this heightened mortality.) Even more amazing, during the evaluation process, researchers also noticed that those using hypnotics had higher incidence of cancer development, which could not be attributed to preexisting conditions.[2]

But taking a pill to make yourself sleep only helps with your symptoms—and recklessly, at that. Research has shown that there is a hormonal basis for sleep patterns, meaning that how your hormones are balanced contributes to how well you sleep.[3] Researchers from Pennsylvania State University collected blood from 11 patients with insomnia and 13 people without sleep disturbances every 30 minutes for 24 hours. They measured the levels of the stress hormones ACTH and cortisol and found that average levels of both hormones were approximately four times higher among the insomniacs than the controls. Insomniacs with the worst sleep disturbances secreted the most cortisol, especially in the evening and nighttime hours. This suggests that they are suffering from hormonal changes that cause hyperarousal and prevent sleep.[4] Knowing this, shouldn't we focus on the causes of poor sleep, such as poor hormone regulation via the adrenal glands, rather than treatment that involves sedation with addictive substances?

Let's go back to the forest again. As you are lying down to sleep, you decide to take an Ambien or Xanax to help you sleep through the night. And you do sleep—however, you wake up to a bear attacking you. You did not hear it coming because your senses were dulled and suppressed. Your body tried to warn you, but you did not (and could not) listen. Now your life is in danger. Was it worth the sleep?

# THE INS AND OUTS OF SLEEP

A normal sleep pattern repeats itself on a 24-hour cycle. In adults, sleep should consume one-third, or 8 hours, of our 24-hour cycle. Think of sleep as being divided into two categories based on electroencephalogram (EEG) readings: rapid eye movement (REM) sleep and non-REM sleep. When you fall asleep, you begin with non-REM sleep, which consists of four stages. As your sleep continues, it grows deeper until REM sleep is triggered. One full sleep cycle of non-REM and REM sleep typically lasts about 90 minutes, and a full night's sleep usually consists of five or more cycles. You dream during REM sleep. With each cycle, the REM period grows longer, many times reaching an hour long. Have you ever noticed that you wake up every 1½ to 2 hours? That is a standard sleep cycle.

## The Importance of REM Sleep

The fact is that you need to dream because it means you are accessing your REM sleep, and REM sleep is when your body begins to repair itself. In fact, when I start correcting this situation in those who are chronically fatigued, many complain of dreaming too much. My response to that is, *great!* Remembering odd dreams is a good way to know whether or not you are entering REM sleep throughout the night. Those who wake up thinking about day-to-day matters are likely not accessing REM.

Studies actually show that REM sleep is also related to weight management. REM requires the highest expenditure of energy during your sleep cycle and therefore burns the most calories—4 to 8 percent more than non-REM sleep. In the *Journal of Endocrinological Investigation,* researchers studied the inverse relationship between decreased sleep and increased obesity. They compared metabolic rates during different stages of sleep, the animal's energy expenditure during hibernation, and differences in sleep patterns during different seasons. After evaluating all of these factors they were able to draw a significant conclusion that REM sleep burns calories, making it an active sleep and therefore helpful in maintaining weight.[5]

Another study compared two groups of overweight or obese non-diabetic individuals: those who were insulin sensitive and those who were insulin resistant. They then compared the sleep patterns of these groups to investigate whether irregular insulin secretion had an impact on sleep. The study strongly links the insulin-resistant individuals to shorter sleep duration, supporting the theory that blood sugar regulation is an important factor in sleep.[6] Think back to Chapter 2, where we discussed the relationship between the development of diabetes and adrenal fatigue. If your adrenal glands release cortisol irregularly, it promotes insulin resistance, weight gain, and a prediabetic state. Taking all of this into consideration, you will likely find that if you have irregular cortisol patterns (for example, low in the morning and high at night) you will remain awake at night and fall asleep during the day. When you get less REM sleep, you feel less well rested. Well, these phenomena are related, as they all stem from adrenal gland irregularities. If insulin resistance and irregular cortisol rhythms result from adrenal fatigue, and if REM sleep is dependent on the complete relaxation of your body, then consider how strongly you need to support adrenal gland function in order to give your body the opportunity to repair itself during sleep.

There have been documented links between insomnia, restless leg syndrome, aging, and the development of metabolic syndrome (or type 2 diabetes). This can also lead to PCOS, as it stems from insulin resistance.[7] Insomnia affects your body in many different ways.

## THE DANGERS OF SLEEP AIDES

Treatment comes down to determining how many systems have been affected and then treating each one, in addition to improving adrenal function. In some patients, this is very easy and produces fast results; in others, it may take longer. If the patient is on medications such as Xanax or Ambien, it is even more difficult, as his body's signaling is affected by the suppressive effect of the medications, making it harder to read his body's cues to repair. So while taking these meds, you may think you are in a deep sleep, but really you're not. Sleep aides may cause sleepwalking and perceived sleep, but your body is still in an awake state. Your brain is still awake, as well. Numerous articles state the negative effects of Ambien, including higher incidence of falls and accidents due to sleepwalking, more emergency room visits, daytime drowsiness, lower work performance, daytime driving impairment, and other negative side effects and symptoms.[8]

These studies suggest that medications such as Ambien put your body on autopilot and prevent you from thinking clearly, resulting in a reduced ability to function at work, impaired driving ability, and an inability to focus on details. They produce the appearance of sleep, but what we really need to consider is how deep the sleep is, relative to REM and non-REM sleep. If you were really getting deep REM sleep by using Ambien, accidents and death would not be more likely with use because you would actually be asleep in your bed, not walking around eating in the middle of the night, and you would not feel exhausted when you woke up.

I have a patient whose previous physician had prescribed Ambien many years ago, as the patient was entering menopause, because her hot flashes were keeping her up at night. She told me that her husband would find her in the kitchen in the middle of the night, at the stove, making herself a meal. Sometimes he would find her cleaning the house, and one time in particular she was cleaning wine glasses. When he approached her, she was asleep. She does not recall any of these events and said she thought she was in bed all night. She easily could have burned or cut herself in this state.

She also reported that she kept taking the Ambien because she always felt tired and thought Ambien was keeping her asleep all night. It was not until her husband told her about her late-night activities that she discontinued using it. She now sleeps beautifully, thanks to hormone replacement therapy, and her husband is also thankful; he was worried that she would get in the car and drive in the middle of the night while on Ambien.

## SLEEP AND PSYCHIATRIC DISEASE

Inadequate sleep over time has been shown to increase the risk of obesity, diabetes, heart disease, and psychological disorders. Math skills, logic, and everyday thinking are affected when your body has not had time to rest. It has been proposed that those who lack sleep have a higher incidence of psychiatric disorders. In fact, there is an undisputed link between psychiatric disease development and lower levels of gamma-aminobutyric acid (GABA) receptors in the brain. (GABA is the neurotransmitter that your brain releases to calm your body.)

Taking this back to the bear scenario, when you anticipate encountering a bear, you release the neurotransmitters epinephrine, norepinephrine, and cortisol. These have a stimulant effect. In order to calm ourselves down after the threat passes, we release inhibitory neurotransmitters, the most effective of which is GABA. GABA is synthesized in your brain from a strong excitatory neurotransmitter called glutamate, with the help of the active form of vitamin $B_6$. We have the ability to make and maintain GABA levels. But if your body is constantly overstimulated, it cannot keep up with GABA production.

It is known by the medical community that lower levels of GABA are linked to major depressive and anxiety disorders. And stress, via the "bear," activates sympathetic output and increases activity of your brain that will induce sleep disruption via the hypothalamic-pituitary axis. Benzodiazepines (such as Xanax) and non-benzodiazepines (such as Ambien) are often prescribed for this purpose, as they impact GABA receptors in the brain. These medications were only intended to be used in the short term, for a period of less than 2 weeks. Unfortunately, this is not how they are prescribed.

Long-term use of benzodiazepines results in dependency and withdrawal, daytime drowsiness and dizziness, memory concerns, low blood pressure, and a change in melatonin secretion. And this further *prevents* naturally induced sleep. Even more alarming are the side effects from the use of non-benzodiazepines. They also result in memory impairment, rebound insomnia, and abuse, but even more apparent is a higher risk of death.[9]

Another aspect of these medications, and a basis for the addictive quality of them, is that when you take a medication that mimics the function of GABA your body does not see the need to produce its own GABA. So when the medication is removed from your body, you suffer rebound insomnia. Earlier I stated that GABA is made from glutamate. Consider the impact on glutamate if your body was not prompted to convert it into GABA due to long-term use of these medications. This would leave higher amounts of glutamate in your system.

Glutamate is incredibly excitatory, and it commonly produces anger, frustration, and agitation. When I have screened GABA levels in those who used benzodiazepines for long periods of time, their GABA levels do not seem to rebound. Even years after using these medications, their bodies no longer make GABA. This requires other natural therapies to induce a calming effect, and often these must be used for the rest of their lives. I also find that these patients' glutamate levels are incredibly high, resulting in mood changes. Those who have experienced withdrawal from these medications will recognize how potent glutamate can be, in regard to agitation and anger. These scary side effects to medication use are a good incentive to focus, right from the start, on the causes of insomnia as a basis for treatment.

GABA and other neurotransmitters, such as serotonin, are made from amino acids. Without proper nutrition and signaling from your brain to manufacture these neurotransmitters, your body will decrease the signal to produce, which will cause a deficiency. This results in periods of anxiety and an inability to fall asleep or stay asleep. It can also result in depression, due to the nature of dopamine and serotonin. Serotonin is well known as a neurotransmitter associated with depression because the most common antidepressants affect serotonin receptors. Serotonin and dopamine typically have an inverse relationship, in that as serotonin rises, dopamine falls.

So, think about this situation: You have chronic stress (as in Stages 1 and 2 of adrenal fatigue), meaning that your adrenal glands are releasing large amounts of dopamine in response to the stress. Initially, serotonin levels are a normal level, which would help you sleep and balance your mood. But as dopamine continues to increase, serotonin keeps dropping and you start feeling depressed, experience insomnia, and feel agitated, anxious, and all around unstable. An antidepressant (such as a selective serotonin reuptake inhibitor, or SSRI) is prescribed, which alters the sero-tonin levels available in your brain. As your brain recognizes more serotonin, it wants to decrease the amount of dopamine, but it can't, because dopamine is released during times of stress. So your body gets into a fight with itself over what should be dominant, the dopamine or the serotonin. And this just results in the development of more symp-toms. Your day becomes variable and unpredictable, which makes it hard to function.

Many people are not aware that neurotransmitter levels can actu-ally be tested in your urine. We can assess your levels of epinephrine, norepinephrine, dopamine, serotonin, GABA, glutamate, histamine, glycine, PEA, and so on. Doctors could run these tests prior to prescrib-ing an antidepressant. Adrenal function and neurotransmitter balance could be assessed prior to the initiation of therapy. Wouldn't that be helpful? It would certainly avoid a tug-of-war between your adrenal gland and your brain, which will ultimately worsen your situation or spin out of control and cause other detrimental effects.

## SLEEP AND ATTENTION DEFICIT HYPERACTIVITY DISORDER

Let's also consider the effect of sleep on children with attention deficit hyperactivity disorder (ADHD). They typically struggle to achieve qual-ity sleep. Evaluations of their neurotransmitter levels show imbalances in norepinephrine, epinephrine, and GABA. Consider the impact on these children if sleep were restored: They would have sharper focus, better stress response, and an overall higher quality of life. Studies have started to investigate using melatonin with these children to promote more restful sleep, as it has been proven that with better sleep they show greater focus during the day.[10]

Since melatonin works in response to light and dark, the amount that's secreted varies with the length of the night. The secretion of mel-atonin is affected by numerous biochemical pathways, and therefore a full neuroendocrine workup would be indicated if melatonin levels were low.[11] It is manufactured from the amino acid tryptophan, which is converted into serotonin with the aid of zinc, vitamin C, vitamin $B_6$, and magnesium. From there, serotonin is converted into melatonin with the help of the same cofactors, plus $B_5$.

Note that without adequate levels of serotonin, you cannot make melatonin. Without adequate levels of vitamin C, $B_6$, and $B_5$, plus zinc and magnesium, one cannot make serotonin or melatonin. When your adrenal gland is stimulated in response to the "bear," it uses these same vitamins (C, $B_6$, $B_5$, and $B_{12}$) to assist in response. This pulls these nutrients from these other pathways. It has also been shown that melatonin will feed back on the signal for cortisol release (ACTH),[12] telling your brain to slow its production of cortisol. That means that if your body has enough serotonin to make melatonin, cortisol will be reduced and you will sleep. Without addressing the "bear response," this pathway cannot function, and therefore results in further cortisol release.

# SLEEP AND RESTLESS LEG SYNDROME

Another common component of sleep concerns is restless leg syndrome (RLS). People are concerned that they cannot sleep due to restlessness and are informed by their doctors that they have a condition called RLS. Another pharmaceutical is prescribed, but it does not address the underlying issue. Your muscles use electrolytes and minerals to contract and relax. If your mineral balance is off-kilter, your muscle contraction will be, as well. An old remedy was to eat more bananas for this condition, due to the potassium content of this fruit. However, it is not simply potassium that is involved in this process.

Low or imbalanced levels of sodium, magnesium, iron, potassium, chloride, and other minerals are involved. When your body responds to stress by releasing hormones from your adrenal glands, it also promotes the dumping of potassium via your urine. This results in potassium deficiency. If potassium is low, sodium levels are affected, which has an impact on your body's hydration status. And when your body becomes more dehydrated, it develops an even greater mineral deficiency.

RLS can be easily cured by achieving the appropriate mineral balance. I commonly recommend magnesium supplements in variable amounts to cure this situation. I also support the adrenal glands in order to slow the release of excessive amounts of potassium in response to aldosterone and cortisol. You may be wondering why I wouldn't simply recommend supplementing with potassium. It's because excessive amounts of potassium can be harmful to your heart rhythm. It is crucial that the balance be well monitored because if your system is restored to normal and hydration levels are maintained, RLS will go away without the side effect of heart arrhythmia.

A study released in 2013 evaluated MRI imaging of the brain in patients with RLS and found a strong link between iron levels and RLS development. Those with RLS had lower levels of iron in particular regions of the brain, leading researchers to the conclusion that low iron may have a role in the development of restless leg syndrome.[13] I have found this clinically, as well. It's common for those with lower iron levels to have poorer sleep due to restless legs, feelings of fatigue, weakness in the limbs, and poor memory function. Why? Because iron is responsible for carrying oxygen throughout your body. If iron is scarce, your body chooses to send the oxygen to your organs instead of your limbs. This results in weakness, twitching, and a feeling of restlessness.

One drug conventional doctors commonly use to treat RLS is a dopamine agonist. Now keep in mind that dopamine is a neurotransmitter that opposes serotonin, and it is also released from your adrenal glands in times of stress. A study published in the *Asian Journal of Psychiatry* investigated the prevalence of depression in 112 participants with RLS and determined that about one-third had depression.[14] While the researchers of this study determined that it was a comorbid condition and not directly related, I disagree. If the condition is supposedly treated by affecting dopamine, then why is depression, which is linked with serotonin production, not a factor? Those with adrenal fatigue have low mineral levels, insomnia, anxiety, depression, and other endocrine-related abnormalities. Are these all independent of one another?

The way this medication works is that it increases the amount of dopamine in your system, which will lower the amount of serotonin produced. It has been recognized that those with RLS are at greater risk of psychological issues and lower quality of life.[15] If serotonin levels are low, then melatonin levels will also decrease. Therefore, sleep and neurotransmitter release must play roles in the development of this disorder. And if you couple that with mineral loss and lack of sleep, the condition worsens.

Simply put, RLS is a symptom of an underlying nutritional or neuroendocrine abnormality. It is the result of neurotransmitter imbalances and nutritional deficiencies. The links between both of these conditions and adrenal fatigue are apparent and must be considered.

## YOUR ADRENAL GLANDS RULE YOUR SLEEP

As we have discussed throughout this chapter, your adrenal glands can and should be linked back to the development of sleep disorders. This includes the inability to either fall asleep or stay asleep and the development of sleep disorders relating to attention deficit disorder, depression, anxiety, insulin resistance, and restless leg syndrome. The medical community spends infinite amounts of time and money coming up with new drugs to improve sleep, but with these drugs come unwanted side effects. If your doctors spent as much time evaluating the impact of stress on your body as pharmaceutical companies do developing drugs, the diagnosis of insomnia would be far less common. The significant addiction and side effects that come with "sleep medications" are not something to be ignored.

Sleep is essential for health and affects multiple pathways in your body. Hopefully the medical community will continue to draw associations between all of these biochemical pathways and begin to recognize the importance of focusing on the entire person when treating sleep disorders, instead of simply treating the symptom.

# MY TURNAROUND
## JOHN ZIMMERMAN, AGE: 31

Two years ago, John Zimmerman was both mentally and physically drained. "I really didn't sleep much at all. I had lost interest in about every aspect of my life. I was very stressed and anxious, and I was always exhausted," he admits. "I had been diagnosed with ADHD, severe depression, and insomnia and was on a lot of medication. Other doctors told me I would never get off of the prescription drugs, and they just kept prescribing more drugs."

After his friend suggested he see a naturopathic doctor, John made an appointment with Dr. Pingel, who diagnosed him with adrenal fatigue. "I had never heard of adrenal fatigue before meeting Dr. Pingel. "Soon, I was off my prescription medications. I feel great now. I have more energy. I sleep now. I think a lot clearer. Everything is easier now—exercising, being social," he says. "I eat a lot better now. The majority of my meals are home cooked with clean, natural foods and fruits and vegetables. I take supplements, and I came off the other medication I had been on." For John, the plan was simple but life-changing. "Once I started feeling better, it all came on at once. I had a lot more clarity for once in my life that I hadn't had for 7 or 8 years before then."

Treating his adrenal fatigue helped John in other ways, too. "Once I felt better, I became more active and more sociable. Before, I didn't really exercise at all. Now, I exercise every other day. My weight wasn't really an issue, but I always had a gut when I was on the medication. On Dr. Pingel's plan, I lost 15 pounds," he shares. "I had friends and family concerned about me. She's definitely seen the difference. I didn't want to be that person everyone had to worry about. My mom has definitely seen the difference. I'm much more out-going and social."

With his health under control, John's life is much better. "It's amazing to sleep without medication. I think more clearly and everything is easier," he reveals. "Dr. Pingel was good at educating me and informing me. In comparison to the treatment that I received before, Dr. Pingel's was night and day. This experience has been nothing short of amazing!"

# 9

# ADRENAL FATIGUE: THE NUTRIENT THIEF

In order to achieve true health, your body needs to be able to fully absorb the nutrients in your food. As you've discovered in the last several chapters, your adrenal glands are connected to almost every organ in your body. And as you've also learned, when you have adrenal fatigue, your system goes into constant fight-or-flight mode, triggering numerous changes within your body. All of these changes ultimately affect your ability to absorb nutrients from the foods you eat, resulting in numerous vitamin and mineral deficiencies.

Considering your adrenal glands' role as your body's control center, is it any surprise to learn that these glands also regulate much of your body's nutrients? Your adrenal glands require sufficient nutrients not only to function, but also to control electrolyte and mineral balance. In addition, they manage how your body uses nutrients to regulate your thyroid, sex hormones, neurotransmitters, blood sugar, and blood pressure. Knowing this, you can probably see a connection between nutritional deficiencies and the symptoms and health you may have been experiencing with your adrenal fatigue. In this chapter, you will learn which nutrients are most affected by adrenal fatigue, as well as the side effects that result from these deficiencies.

## THE IMPORTANCE OF NUTRIENTS

Your body relies on numerous biochemical pathways, and each pathway requires specific nutrients in order to perform its role. Just as a manufacturing assembly line needs individual parts arranged in a certain order to produce a final product to sell, your body also requires certain nutrients to function properly. But, unfortunately, the area of nutritional evaluation is often overlooked by doctors.

It is commonly known, for example, that vitamin $B_{12}$ has a role in producing energy, but it is important to also recognize how your body makes and absorbs the B vitamins and how they affect your basic biochemistry. For example, let's look at the neurotransmitter serotonin. Your body must have adequate amounts of both vitamin C and $B_6$ to produce serotonin, a hormone related to your mood, appetite, memory, sleeping habits, and more. Knowing that these nutrients are needed to produce serotonin should play an important role in how a doctor treats someone who feels depressed. If this person has adrenal fatigue, she will likely be deficient in these nutrients. Therefore, treating her adrenal glands and adding more vitamin $B_6$- and C-containing foods to her diet may be a much better (and safer) alternative to using antidepressant drugs, like SSRIs, for therapy. This is why understanding the nutritional impact of adrenal fatigue is critical not only to healing your adrenal glands, but also to resolving your symptoms.

## VITAMINS AND MINERALS 101

Micronutrients are nutrients your body needs in small amounts in order to stay healthy. They come from two sources: vitamins and minerals. Furthermore, all vitamins and minerals are broken down into two main categories: water soluble and fat soluble. This distinction is made because it makes a difference therapeutically. Fat-soluble nutrients are harder to break down and therefore have a higher risk of causing toxicity in your body, whereas excess water-soluble nutrients will simply be eliminated via your urine and pose a low risk of overdose. Water-soluble vitamins include all of the B vitamins, vitamin C, and all minerals, which are too vast to list but include calcium, magnesium, biotin, potassium, boron, and strontium. That only leaves four vitamins (A, D, E, and K), which are the fat-soluble vitamins.

Each pathway in your body utilizes these vitamins and minerals to manufacture a physiological response, such as the release of estrogen or stimulation of your thyroid. You cannot make products, such as hormones, without them, so your body will adapt. If you think of a simple equation, such as $A + B \rightarrow C$, you can relate this to what your body is doing. It takes tyrosine (A) and adds it to iodine (B) to make T4 (thyroid hormone). Now let's say that you don't have enough iodine; what will happen? Well, either your body won't be able to complete the process and will shut down the function of your thyroid or your body will find an alternative route for energy production in place of your thyroid. Maybe it will pull iodine from another pathway (if available) to resume thyroid production, or maybe it will create a new product (D) and start a different route in your body.

Tyrosine is also a starting substance for the formation of epinephrine and norepinephrine, which are also stimulatory, just like thyroid hormone. So if iodine is not available, your body may end up sending tyrosine down this particular pathway to produce an "energetic" effect by making more norepinephrine, which, over time, creates anxiety. Remember, your body is one huge biochemical pathway, full of reactions. It does not want to have tyrosine just lying around. Instead, it wants to be productive. So when this extra norepinephrine is created, it creates a symptom that is stressful to your body because it is not used to having so much of one product and so little of another. This worsens your adrenal fatigue.

# WHICH CAME FIRST: THE DEFICIENCY OR ADRENAL FATIGUE?

People often ask whether nutritional deficiencies occur because of adrenal fatigue or cause adrenal fatigue. The answer is: *both.* If your body can't do what it needs to, it becomes stressed. And if your body has experienced years of constant external stress, it loses nutrients via malabsorption and the overstimulation of pathways that use up leftover nutrients. This is the hamster wheel we spoke of in earlier chapters. Regardless of the cause, the treatment involves replenishing what was lost and providing extra support for the pathways currently being affected.

# THE SYNERGY OF NUTRIENTS

An incredibly important factor in nutrition is the balance of your nutrients. (You may have heard of the need for balance between calcium and magnesium. Many calcium products now also contain magnesium to help ensure this balance.) Nutrients will not work as well without their synergistic partners as they will when you give them in combination. Going back to the example of your thyroid and iodine, once thyroid hormone is created, iodine then combines with selenium, zinc, and vitamin A to use it appropriately. So simply giving iodine to improve thyroid function will not have as much of an impact as giving all four nutrients. Complicated? Yes. It takes a good knowledge of all of the nutrients involved in each pathway to truly understand the synergy involved. But that is where physicians come in. Your doctor can guide you, share research with you, and explain the benefits of each nutrient and how various nutrients work together. Throughout this chapter, we will discuss the synergistic properties of nutrients. And this synergy also plays an important role in healing your adrenal glands through your diet.

# VITAMINS AND MINERALS AFFECTED BY ADRENAL FATIGUE

In this section, we will go through the major vitamins and minerals affected by your adrenal glands. You may have heard media reports on some of these nutrients, such as B vitamins. For example, many people are told that if they are under stress, they should take more B vitamins—and this is true! But there are other nutrient deficiencies that occur with adrenal fatigue, as well. We will review the major nutrient deficiencies associated with adrenal fatigue in the order of their synergistic properties (how well they work together). Because most people seem to understand the role B vitamins play in alleviating stress, we'll start by discussing them.

## B Vitamins

The B vitamins receive much recognition for their connection to your adrenal glands, weight loss, neuropathies, and general wellness. Every time you release cortisol from your adrenal gland, you use up B vitamins. The supply of these vitamins takes a huge hit in a system bogged down with adrenal fatigue, so the symptoms associated with low levels of B vitamins are commonly observed in adrenal fatigue patients. $B_{12}$ is found mainly in animal-based foods, and deficiencies are primarily seen in cultures with low meat consumption. For example, in Chile, where they consume lots of vegetables and little meat, $B_{12}$ deficiencies are quite common. However, $B_{12}$ has a counterpart called folate, which is another B vitamin. Folate is found in vegetables, and in too low amounts it is responsible for fetal neural tube defects, such as spina bifida. Folate deficiency is virtually nonexistent in Chile.[1] This is a primary example of the impact diet can have on disease development, and it is why a varied diet that includes all of the essential minerals is key to preventing and treating adrenal fatigue and subsequent disease development.

## Vitamin B$_{12}$

Low amounts of vitamins B$_{12}$, B$_6$, and folate are responsible for eleva-
tions in homocysteine, a inflammatory marker linked to hypertension
and cardiovascular complications. Although a person's diet may incorporate a large amount of B$_{12}$, the question of the absorption of these
B vitamins must be addressed, as B vitamin deficiency is becoming
very common in America—a country where meat is one of our primary
sources of food. This deficiency is increasingly apparent in the elderly
population. It has been shown that the elderly have the lowest levels of
B$_{12}$, and research has linked this to changes in our intestinal mucosa as
we age, resulting in lower absorbed B$_{12}$, despite intake. This is concerning because researchers are finding higher levels of dementia, cardiovascular complications, and osteoporosis in the B$_{12}$-deficient elderly.
Also, due to the nature of B$_{12}$ and folate and their required balance in
your body, it is concerning that B$_{12}$ levels are low and common processed foods add folic acid (folate), further throwing off the balance.[2] So
when evaluating adrenal fatigue, it is important to not only look at the
need for a particular vitamin, but also at the absorption of that vitamin
and its balance relative to other nutrients.

## Vitamin B$_6$

Vitamin B$_6$ is an essential vitamin also required for adrenal hormones.
It is always something to consider when treating any stage of adrenal
fatigue and requires higher supplementation during Stage 1 to prevent
the progression to Stage 2. B$_6$, or pyridoxine, is a water-soluble vitamin
involved in converting foods into energy; maintaining healthy skin,
teeth, gums, and nerves; forming melatonin and serotonin for mood and
sleep; and balancing menstrual cycles. (It is often used to alleviate
PMS.) In addition, B$_6$ builds and breaks down amino acids, supports
your body's immune system, and—perhaps most importantly—allows
your body to absorb B$_{12}$. That's right: B$_{12}$ depends on B$_6$. And as you may
recall from the previous section, B$_6$, B$_{12}$, and folate are required for
maintaining homocysteine.

Your body also needs them in order to produce hormones, release cortisol, and break down sugar, fats, and proteins. Consider these three to be a team for combating adrenal fatigue fallout. In fact, when I administer $B_{12}$ shots, I almost always add a touch of $B_6$ to the shot, too, so that the body has even better support. $B_{12}$ is also involved in resetting our sleep–wake cycles. When adrenal fatigue causes cortisol to "misfire," it changes your circadian rhythms, usually resulting in poor sleep and poor daytime energy. $B_{12}$ (methylcobalamin) has been shown to improve this rhythm by enhancing your circadian clock's sensitivity to light.[3]

Methylcobalamin was given to nine healthy subjects for 4 weeks. Researchers measured nocturnal melatonin levels after exposure to bright light, in addition to plasma melatonin levels present in a 24-hour period. They found that sleep cycle, as it relates to melatonin, was far more advanced in the $B_{12}$ group than the placebo group.[4] This means that those who were given $B_{12}$ had a more restful sleep than those who did not receive that supplement. So although $B_{12}$ does not have an impact on total melatonin levels or cortisol, it is involved in shifting your cortisol peak, resulting in more energy during the day and better rest at night.

Earlier in the chapter we discussed the biochemical pathways of your body (A + B → C). One of the major functions of $B_6$ is as a coenzyme, which, in terms of our equation here, means it is required for A to turn into C. Place that $B_6$ right over the arrow. A coenzyme cannot operate alone; it must be combined with another substance to work. For example, to turn tryptophan (an amino acid involved in serotonin production) into niacin (another B vitamin), you have to have $B_6$. Niacin is a precursor for the production of adenosine triphosphate (ATP), which is the scientific name for energy. Without $B_6$, you cannot create niacin, and without niacin, you cannot create energy. Niacin is also used as a cholesterol-lowering therapy in conventional medicine. It is believed to raise HDL and slightly lower LDL. But before we assume that the issue is low niacin levels, maybe we should consider that it could be low $B_6$

levels due to adrenal fatigue. That way we could treat that first, allowing your body to make its own niacin.

Niacin has also been shown to enhance sleep in those with adrenal fatigue. A small study of six subjects with normal sleep patterns and two insomniacs were monitored by EEG to evaluate sleep patterns before and after niacin administration. They were given 500 mg twice daily for 1 week, 1,000 mg twice daily for 1 week, and 1,000 mg three times daily for the last week. The two subjects with insomnia experienced significant increases in REM sleep by the third week. Sleep efficiency went from 58.5 percent in week 1 to 79.5 percent in week 3. After withdrawing the niacin therapy, sleep efficiency dropped to 41.5 percent.[5] The study points out that $B_6$ is required in this pathway and perhaps the extreme drop after removal of therapy revolved around the usage of $B_6$ and its involvement in other pathways.

Vitamin $B_6$ is also highly involved in the production of red blood cells, specifically in heme, which is the oxygen-containing component of your red blood cells. Without $B_6$, you cannot make amino acids. Without amino acids, you cannot make protein. For these reasons, I recommend an oral or intramuscular injection of a high dose of $B_6$ to anyone experiencing adrenal fatigue. Interestingly, the FDA's recommended daily amount (RDA) for $B_6$ is somewhere around 1 to 2 mg, based on age and sex.[6] I tend to dose somewhere around 100 to 250 mg in those with adrenal fatigue, which is quite a difference. Why is this so? The RDA doesn't account for your pathways being affected by stress or hormonal irregularities. If you are reading this book, it is likely that you are concerned about some aspect of your health, and I would bet that $B_6$ is involved with that process.

## Vitamin $B_5$

Vitamin $B_5$, or pantothenic acid, also has a major impact on energy production and is a coenzyme for everyday reactions. Like $B_6$, it helps to convert food into energy and to manufacture blood cells. Vitamin $B_5$ helps to keep your GI tract healthy and is critical to the production of hormones by your adrenal glands. It also aids in synthesizing cholesterol and is currently being reviewed as a possible treatment for reducing triglycerides and LDL (bad cholesterol) while raising HDL (good cholesterol) by supporting conversion into coenzyme A, which plays a critical role in the metabolism of fats, proteins, and carbohydrates for energy.

Recent studies have been investigating the use of $B_5$ to manage cholesterol in place of statin use. $B_5$ supplementation was given to 120 patients with low to moderate cardiovascular risk. After 16 weeks, it was shown to lower triglycerides and LDL by 3 to 5 percent more than diet modification alone, which resulted in a 1 percent reduction in overall cardiovascular risk.[7] Other benefits of $B_5$ include skin and wound healing. By the time they reach Stage 2 adrenal fatigue, many patients have started to see the first symptoms of disease development; at that

## B VITAMINS AND THEIR RELATIONSHIP TO STRESS

With B vitamins playing such a pivotal part in adrenal health, it is key that they are in balance! Here is a list of all of the B vitamins and their roles in adrenal function.[8]

- Vitamin $B_1$ (thiamin)—protects adrenal glands, lowers stress-induced cortisol response.
- Vitamin $B_3$ (niacin)—improves sleep quality and quantity, is involved in production of serotonin.
- Vitamin $B_5$ (pantethine/pantothenic acid)—protects adrenal glands, lowers stress-induced cortisol response.
- Vitamin $B_6$ (pyridoxal-5'-phosphate)—cofactor for manufacturing the neurotransmitters GABA, serotonin, and dopamine.
- Vitamin $B_7$ (biotin)—involved in metabolic breakdown of fats, carbohydrates, and proteins.
- Vitamin $B_{12}$ (methylcobalamin)—resets circadian rhythms to improve sleep and normalize cortisol.
- Folate (5-methyltetrahydrofolate)—essential for neurotransmitter formation.

point, the patient should increase her dietary consumption of B$_5$. The RDA of this vitamin is 5 mg for adults, but I commonly prescribe higher amounts (100 mg) for those with significant adrenal fatigue (Stages 2 and 3). That said, you should always consult with a physician before taking more than the recommended amount of any vitamin.

Those with acne have experienced great success with healing face lesions through B$_5$ therapy.[9] The research is scarce, but the wound-healing effects and the impact of B$_5$ on hormone regulation seem to be the major reasons why this therapy has worked. For example, I had a 16-year-old patient who was plagued with horrible acne scars. He had tried Retin-A (a prescriptive and toxic form of vitamin A), antibiotics, and acne extractions, but only 100 mg daily of B$_5$ did wonders for his skin. Now he looks like an entirely different person. The benefits of this vitamin are abundant and eating a whole food, unprocessed diet will let your body better absorb and use this nutritional component.

## Vitamin C

Vitamin C is a water-soluble vitamin needed for numerous biochemical processes in your body. Many common habits and environmental exposures will deplete your vitamin C levels, requiring higher intake if you're regularly exposed to toxins. Those include drinking alcohol and smoking, physical trauma, physiological stress, variations in absorption via your GI tract, and other environmental factors, such as air quality and the toxicity of the individual.[10] Notice that everything I mentioned also plays a role in adrenal fatigue. Vitamin C is an important nutrient to supplement in those with adrenal fatigue; it quickly helps improve symptoms when taken orally, and in many cases, intravenously.

Vitamin C is needed for your adrenal glands to function. Large amounts of it are also excreted via your urine during times of stress. People who have high levels of vitamin C do not show the expected mental and physical signs of stress when subjected to acute psychological challenges. What's more, they bounce back from stressful situations faster than people with low levels of vitamin C in their blood. In one study, German researchers subjected 120 people to a surefire stressor: a public speaking task combined with math problems. Half of those studied were given 1,000 mg of vitamin C. Signs of stress such as elevated levels of the stress hormone cortisol and high blood pressure were significantly greater in those who did not get the vitamin supplement. Those who got vitamin C reported that they felt less stressed when they got the vitamin than they did before supplementation.[11]

Considering that the most common symptom of low vitamin C levels is fatigue,[12] we need to note the relationship between the adrenal glands and stress. The recommended daily amount is only 60 mg, and the study above quoted 1,000 mg for benefit. Unfortunately, 20 to 30 percent of American adults consume less than 60 mg and are considered deficient.[13] Low levels of vitamin C can also cause personality changes, such as depression, and decline in psychomotor performance resulting in reduced alertness and motivation.[14] Some of the other symptoms of vitamin C deficiency include anemia, joint pain, easy bruising, poor immune function, poor hair health, dry skin, and decreased wound healing.[15] Now how many of those symptoms are also symptoms of adrenal fatigue? To ignore the similarity is a mistake!

External sources include fruits and vegetables; citrus has a high concentration. Low vitamin C levels are predominately known for their relationship to the development of the condition called scurvy, but it is so much more involved than that. Vitamin C is involved in the production and synthesis of neurotransmitters, such as dopamine, norepinephrine, and tryptophan—many of the neurotransmitters we have discussed in relationship to the adrenal gland! It is also involved in cellular respiration, carbohydrate metabolism, synthesis of lipids and proteins, breakdown of cholesterol to bile,[16] conversion to active folate, and iron metabolism.

Vitamin C has numerous benefits for your body and is used to treat a variety of disorders and diseases. One of the commonly overlooked aspects of vitamin C is its involvement in our absorption of iron. Administering 200 mg of vitamin C per 30 mg of iron will increase iron absorption in your gut![17] Taking around 500 mg of vitamin C orally each day, in combination with 80 mg zinc, 400 IU vitamin E, and 15 mg beta-carotene, seems to reduce the risk of visual acuity loss in macular degeneration by 27 percent. It also halts the progression of this disease by 25 percent.[18] The administration of vitamin C has been shown to improve the cardiovascular system. Those who have peripheral arterial disease tend to have low levels of vitamin C and higher levels of an inflammatory marker called C-reactive protein.[19] Vitamin C is also beneficial in therapies for cancers, the common cold, gastritis due to *helicobacter pylori*, high blood pressure, reducing lead toxicity, osteoarthritis, physical performance in the elderly, and sunburn![20]

Vitamin C, or ascorbic acid, can be administered orally or intravenously. The concern with oral administration is that vitamin C absorption is related to the amount you take. So the more you take in orally at one time, the less you absorb, which usually results in diarrhea or abdominal discomfort. For those who have significant vitamin C

## THE MYERS' COCKTAIL

The Myers' Cocktail was built off the work of the late John Myers, who used intravenous (IV) nutrient therapy to treat a wide range of clinical diseases. Each doctor may modify the exact formula of this IV cocktail, but it usually contains magnesium, calcium, trace minerals, zinc, B vitamins, and vitamin C. This therapy has been found to be effective against fatigue, migraines, asthma attacks, fibromyalgia and other pain conditions, upper respiratory conditions, chronic sinusitis, seasonal allergic rhinitis, cardiovascular disease, and more!

Many patients with fatigue respond favorably to Myers' infusions, with results lasting from days to months. In one study, 10 patients with chronic fatigue syndrome received a minimum of four treatments, once per week, and more than half showed improvement in symptoms of fatigue.[21] This therapy has been used for many years by nutrition-based physicians as a supplement to diet and exercise to improve overall health and energy. So if you find that you need additional help treating your adrenal fatigue, ask your physician if you're a candidate for the Myers' Cocktail.

requirements, including those with adrenal fatigue and diseases such as cancer and autoimmune conditions, vitamin C is given intravenously, which avoids absorption issues in the GI tract. Commonly given to those with adrenal fatigue as a nutrient tonic called the "Myers' Cocktail" (which includes not only vitamin C but also minerals and B vitamins), this type of therapy can quickly improve the nutrient status of someone with adrenal fatigue and help them restore their health faster than oral supplementation could.

# Calcium, Vitamin D, and Magnesium

This whole idea of synergy is complicated, isn't it? One of the most common examples of synergy revolves around the use of calcium in conjunction with vitamin D and magnesium. So what happens when these nutrients aren't taken together? Well, let's start by taking a closer look at calcium.

## Calcium

Consider the recent news that calcium supplementation can cause cancer and cardiovascular complications. Joseph Mercola, DO, released an article discussing calcium and its relationship to these diseases.[22] He cites research showing that higher bone density due to increased intake of calcium is linked to a higher risk of estrogen-based cancers. He also cites articles that show that calcium supplementation can cause higher levels of plaque deposition in your arteries, and therefore a higher risk of heart attack.

Now, before you toss your calcium supplement, I want to point out that this article strictly evaluated calcium administered alone, without magnesium or vitamin D.[23] It showed that there was a 27 percent increase in heart attack from calcium supplementation alone. The research released on giving calcium in balance with appropriate levels of magnesium and vitamin D found that the combination did not produce harmful effects. What's the takeaway here? Synergy is important! When minerals are not given in balance, they can actually cause more harm than good.

Unfortunately, the idea that calcium was bad for you hit the mainstream media, and many patients started to approach me about calcium supplementation and their worries about cancer and cardiovascular health after being on it for so long. The key to understanding these studies is to take a close look at the supplementation. In the studies, the subjects *only* took calcium supplements. It was not a combination product with other minerals and vitamin D. If you give your body any single mineral without supporting the other minerals in your body, that one mineral will leave deposits in places you don't want it, like your arteries, joints, and cells.

To act upon this synergetic effect and perform the jobs that your body needs it to, calcium requires magnesium and vitamin D. It also needs boron, strontium, manganese, phosphorus, silicon, and vitamin K to build bone. It works synergistically in your body to produce a desired effect. It was not intended to be taken alone, in its elemental form. If you were making a cake that required 2 cups of flour, 1 egg, and 1 cup of sugar, but you added 4 cups of flour instead, how would the cake turn out? Not well. The ingredients for baking are in particular proportions, and so are the compounds that make up your body.

Did you know that calcium is required not only for bone health, but also for muscle contraction, nerve signaling, blood clotting, blood pressure regulation, cell-to-cell communication, and insulin and glucose signaling? Calcium even assists sperm in fertilizing an egg! It is essential to your body. The problem is not with calcium, it is with the exclusive use of it with the assumption that it will build bone all by itself, without the assistance of other minerals and vitamins.

Think back to that bear again. When you are stressed and cortisol is called upon, it changes the way your body uses nutrients. It increases your production of sugar (a process known as gluconeogenesis), which affects a variety of nutrients. The energy required to produce sugar to run from the bear counteracts any energy we would get from breaking down carbohydrates. This energy usage also expends your nutrients, causing deficiencies, abnormal cholesterol levels, and a reduction in amino acids, all of which result in a variety of neurotransmitter issues, such as changes in serotonin, dopamine, epinephrine, and norepinephrine.

Even worse, your body is not built to make and break down sugar at the same time. So in order to conserve energy, it halts the breakdown of dietary sugar while it is creating new energy sources. This results in abnormal glucose and insulin response and creates a feeling of fatigue. Think of it this way: If you were building a house all day long, and then, after finally finishing, you had to take it all apart and start all over again, you would be very tired. You would likely run out of nails, and you'd waste a lot of drywall and wood in the destruction process.

Your body is no different. You need to assemble all of your materials and tools, follow the blueprint, and build from the ground up, in a particular order. You cannot put in a toilet before you have built a bathroom. It won't work right. Your body is a well-built house, with electricity, plumbing, and rooms. There are places where you break things down and places where you build things up. If your body has expended too much energy trying to restructure and build new rooms, it will grow tired. Adrenal fatigue is a process of breaking things down and building new things, all at the expense of your energy. Your body has to be rebuilt, in the correct order, with the correct tools and materials, in order to run with the energy it once had.

When someone has a severe adrenal insufficiency, such as during Stage 3, they do not have a lot of cortisol being released anymore, which puts them in a different situation from those in Stages 1 and 2. As we've discussed, people in Stage 3 tend to have a lot of muscle aches and pains, fibromyalgia, or chronic fatigue. If cortisol output is low in these patients, then they would experience low calcium, promoting stiff muscles.

## Vitamin D

Vitamin D is typically released in your body when your calcium level is low, so when calcium is high (as in this situation of high cortisol output that's common during Stage 1 and sometimes Stage 2), vitamin D production is inhibited. The high levels of calcium will inhibit parathyroid hormone production, which will affect the way that calcium is used or stored in your bones. So an adrenal output of cortisol will ultimately result in high sodium and calcium, but low potassium, magnesium, phosphate, and vitamin D levels. No wonder our bodies feel so out of whack!

Vitamin D is currently a huge area of research, as low levels have been linked to cancer, bone health, poor mood, dementia, sleep, and autoimmune conditions.[24] This nutrient is released to assist with calcium absorption in your gut, so it is key in mineral balance. When calcium is consumed, vitamin D is triggered to assist in bringing calcium into your blood. Without vitamin D, you cannot absorb the calcium from your food, which, as was discussed in the Mercola article, will result in unwanted calcium deposits. As a fat-soluble vitamin, vitamin D affects your nerves and cell health, which are composed of fats. It is often low in cancer patients, autoimmune patients, and those with high cortisol levels, like those in Stage 1 and possibly Stage 2 adrenal fatigue.

The low levels of vitamin D in people with high levels of cortisol can be caused by many factors. If cortisol is elevated, digestion slows, lowering the absorption of dietary vitamins. Vitamin D is also manufactured in your liver, which is bogged down during times of stress. I live in Arizona, where the population has regular sun exposure, so I am constantly questioned on the impact of the sun on vitamin D production. This vitamin is synthesized in your skin from sunlight, but it has to be further changed into its active form by your liver and kidneys. This means that your levels of vitamin D are dependent on more than just sunshine exposure. If sunshine were the only factor, the majority of my patients would have very healthy levels, which I do not find to be the case. Also, considering that the majority of the patients I see have adrenal fatigue or endocrine abnormality, it makes sense that they have lower levels. In these patients, absorption must be a factor, as they likely have poor intestinal health. By supplementing with vitamin D in a sublingual form (as opposed to capsule form), I find that patients absorb it better while they work to reverse the effects of cortisol elevation and restore their bodies' ability to absorb nutrients from food.

Unfortunately, food sources of calcium and vitamin D are often misunderstood. Most people jump directly to dairy products as a primary and "essential" source of these nutrients. But the problem with pasteurized dairy products from cows in America is that cow's milk is overconsumed and highly inflammatory. If you think about it, humans are the only mammals who consume milk past infancy. This is likely the reason why so many of us become lactose intolerant as we get older.

Were you aware that it is possible to get adequate calcium and vitamin D, in addition to other balanced minerals, from plant-based sources? Green, leafy vegetables are fantastic sources of calcium and also contain vitamin K, vitamin C, folate, and natural fiber. And most nut milks have been fortified with more vitamin D than their dairy-based counterparts.

It is actually possible to get every nutrient you need from a plant-based diet, if you know where to obtain each nutrient and you eat the appropriate amount. (You actually don't even need a large amount of these nutrients. The important thing is to have small, balanced amounts.) According to the conventional medical community, dairy is the best source of calcium and vitamin D. But while they state that it is the best source per serving, they don't mention that dairy also contains a lot of fat and has inflammatory properties. In addition, many adults are lactose intolerant. So what are some other (better) options? Look at "Sources of Calcium and Vitamin D in Foods" on page 162 to see a comparison of naturally occurring calcium and vitamin D levels in various foods and dairy products. You may be surprised by what you find!

As you consider taking supplements, keep in mind that your body can make its own vitamin D in your liver and kidneys. You do not need a high amount of supplementation if everything is in balance. Your body wants small trace amounts of all minerals and vitamin D to be absorbed together; it is not as interested in large amounts of any vitamin or mineral all at one time.

## Sources of Calcium and Vitamin D in Foods

| Food, Serving Size | Calcium | Vitamin D |
|---|---|---|
| Almond milk, 1 cup | 451 mg | 2 mg |
| Almonds, 1 cup | 367 mg | 0 |
| Blackstrap molasses, 2 tbsp | 400 mg | 0 |
| Collard greens, 1 cup | 266–357 mg | 0 |
| Kale, 1 cup cooked | 90–179 mg | 0 |
| Milk, 1 cup | 276 mg | 0 mg naturally/100 IU fortified |
| Rhubarb, 1 cup | 105 mg | 0 mg naturally/100 IU fortified |
| Sesame seeds, 1 cup | 1,404 mg | 0 mg |

## Magnesium

Magnesium is a cofactor, or "helper," in more than 300 biochemical reactions in your body. It is required for energy metabolism, hormone binding, muscle contraction, cardiac excitation, and neurotransmitter release. Primarily absorbed in your small intestine, this mineral is excreted from your body via your kidneys. The majority of your stored magnesium is located in your bones. Studies have shown that magnesium has an effect on potassium and sodium levels and is directly involved in producing energy. A deficiency in magnesium leads to an increase in sodium and a decrease in potassium, which affect your hydration, muscle contractions, and energy production.[25] Magnesium plays a critical role in nerve transmission, cardiac rhythm, muscular contraction, blood pressure, and glucose and insulin metabolism.

Additionally, low levels are strongly linked to dementia, restless leg syndrome, and chronic fatigue syndrome.[26]

Magnesium is often used to reduce the symptoms of asthma. In a double blind study, intravenous magnesium was given to 20 patients during asthma attacks. Thirty percent of subjects reached a normal oxygen level when given magnesium, compared to the placebo group. This has made magnesium a popular choice for dealing with bronchial attacks.[27] Magnesium has also been shown to reduce the need of certain medication in 58 percent of study subjects with preeclampsia and eclampsia.[28]

Also, a study assessing the role of electrolyte imbalances in cardiac

## ADRENAL FATIGUE, MINERALS, AND KIDNEY STONES?

When the adrenal hormone aldosterone is released from your adrenal glands, it stimulates the release of potassium via your urine. It also increases the amount of sodium in your body. And when cortisol is released from your adrenal glands, insulin is also released. Insulin closes the potassium channels and opens the calcium channels, leading to a decrease in potassium and an increase in calcium. It also deposits more fat by decreasing fatty acids levels in your bloodstream and storing them.

Because your cells are made from fats, you need fatty acids for proper mineral absorption. Inversely, someone with type 1 diabetes, whose body doesn't produce enough insulin, will have a high potassium level and low stored body fat content. Remember that insulin promotes fat storage, so a type 1 diabetic, who has absent insulin, will have less fat deposition, whereas a type 2 diabetic, who has high insulin levels, will have more fat deposition.

When calcium is increased in this situation, it has an affect on both magnesium and vitamin D due to their synergistic relationship. And when calcium levels are elevated in your bloodstream, say from the release of insulin via cortisol, phosphate levels are then reduced by promoting excretion via your kidneys. Some of the most common kidney stones in humans are calcium- and phosphate-based, which indicates that those with kidney stones may want to consider addressing adrenal function, in addition to diet, as part of their treatment.

arrhythmias found that more than 70 percent of those with ventricular arrhythmias had low magnesium levels. And when researchers administered magnesium it caused a significant decrease in the number of irregular heartbeats. The conclusion was that magnesium would be a good treatment for ventricular arrhythmias.[29]

In relation to adrenal fatigue, magnesium also has a direct affect on excitatory hormone release. This means that when your adrenal glands release norepinephrine and epinephrine, magnesium can actually calm that response.[30] Researchers have known since the late 60s that while calcium will increase the release of epinephrine and norepinephrine from your adrenal glands, magnesium will have the opposite effect. In fact, they discovered that after stimulating the cells with calcium and causing a stimulatory effect, they tried again, adding magnesium to the mix, and the response was blunted. This is a great example of the importance of nutrient synergy and how strongly adrenal output is regulated by mineral balance.[31]

It's interesting that the release of norepinephrine and epinephrine from your adrenal glands promotes a reduction in magnesium by increasing your calcium levels, but that magnesium supplementation reverses this effect, calming your system. This offers a natural alternative to antianxiety medication! The problem is that high levels of calcium stimulate epinephrine and norepinephrine, and cortisol will ultimately stimulate higher levels of calcium via insulin. Calcium and magnesium have an interesting relationship in that they can affect each other in many ways. Simply put, if they are not in perfect balance, each of these nutrients will drastically affect the production and regulation of the other mineral. And when one mineral is affected, numerous others will feel those effects.

## Selenium

Selenium is essential for your body to function properly. Just like a car needs fuel, your body needs selenium. Without it, your thyroid and immune system cannot work properly, leading to fatigue, poor immune status, and toxic overload. Selenium is a very important nutrient involved in numerous chemical reactions within your body. It is an antioxidant and is required for the conversion of the hormone T4 to T3 in your thyroid; it has also been strongly linked to immune function, particularly as it relates to your thyroid gland. Clinical research has shown that taking 200 mcg of selenium daily, in combination with thyroid medication, significantly reduces antibodies for Hashimoto's by 6 to 30 percent after 3 to 12 months of treatment.[32]

In Chapter 6, we discussed the strong link between Hashimoto's thyroiditis and adrenal fatigue. We discussed that adrenal fatigue causes more storage of thyroid hormones, which leads to autoimmune conditions. But it also causes a selenium deficiency that could have an impact on these antibodies. Selenium helps keep HIV from transitioning to AIDS, making it a strong contender in our fight against this disease.[33] In addition, selenium has been shown to reduce the risk of miscarriage and is required for sperm motility. Low levels have been associated with poor mood, cognitive decline, and decreased immune health, while increased intake has been linked to lower cancer risk and improvements in cardiovascular disease.[34] In fact, some research has shown that taking 100 to 200 mcg of a high-selenium yeast daily for 6 months significantly lowers total cholesterol by 8.5 to 9.7 mg/dL.[35]

Selenium has been shown to decrease the toxins contained in mercury, making it a huge component of environmental medicine (a practice where the doctor evaluates the patient's environment, risk of toxic exposure, and causation of disease).[36] I routinely screen nutrient levels in patients and can say with confidence that most of my patients with adrenal fatigue have had low selenium levels. In addition, those patients often experience thyroid disorders, fertility concerns, and poor immune health.

Selenium used to be abundant in our soil, but because of overfarming the same plots of land, the nutrient components in our soil have declined. This explains why selenium deficiency is so common today. In addition, our poor, overworked thyroids are using up every ounce of selenium we have due to constant stress. The toxins we are exposed to on a daily basis simply use up all of our selenium so there is none left to assist in areas where it is needed, resulting in an increase in symptoms. At any rate, most people will benefit from incorporating more selenium into their diets and increasing selenium supplementation.

## Iron

When conventional medicine started investigating the relationship between nutrients and fatigue, iron was one of the first whose importance was recognized. Iron is responsible for delivering oxygen to your tissues via your red blood cells. An insufficient amount of this mineral is commonly thought to be the primary cause of anemia (low red blood cell count, which results in low oxygen transport), and rightfully so. When your blood is low in iron, it affects your red blood cells' ability to carry oxygen to your tissues. Your red blood cells become smaller and carry less oxygen. This is anemia.

Oxygen is required for your body to function normally. And without iron to fix and maintain the flow of oxygen, you'll feel fatigued. Most of the iron in your body, approximately 65 percent, is distributed within your red blood cells. Another 10 percent is located in your muscle fibers and other tissues. The remainder is stored in your liver, macrophages (white blood cells), and bone marrow. Iron is necessary for your body to reproduce red blood cells and perform cellular metabolism and aerobic respiration. It is also involved in the production of neurotransmitters, such as dopamine, norepinephrine, and serotonin. However, iron is not easily excreted by your body, and iron overload can cause problems. High levels of iron can lead to toxicity, a common problem in those with liver sluggishness or liver diseases—both of which are symptoms surrounding later stages of adrenal fatigue

The most common symptom of iron deficiency is fatigue. This occurs because your blood is not carrying oxygen to your cells. If you do not have enough iron to carry the oxygen, your heart has to work harder to pump oxygen to your tissues. Heartbeat irregularities often occur at this point. Other common symptoms include cold hands and feet due to lack of circulation, dizziness, headaches, pale skin, dark circles under your eyes, and chest pain. More common (but less obvious) symptoms are brittle nails, swelling or soreness of your tongue, cracks in the sides of your mouth, frequent infections, restless leg syndrome, insomnia, numbness, and restless arms and body.[37] Many of these symptoms are often attributed to other causes, such as the thyroid, potassium and magnesium deficiencies, and in some cases, severe diseases such as multiple sclerosis. This is one of the reasons I screen iron levels in all of my patients. Most routine screenings by physicians will only include a blood count, which shows anemia but not the precursors to anemia, such as low iron levels. The majority of the symptoms listed here occur due to low iron storage levels (ferritin), and these low iron storage levels are the first sign of developing anemia. By only screening the complete blood count, most physicians will miss a patient's low iron levels and dismiss his or her complaints of fatigue as normal.

Most of your dietary absorption of iron occurs in your duodenum, which is located at the beginning of your small intestine. The absorption can be highly influenced by other dietary factors, such as proton pump inhibitors, antacid medications, a high-fiber diet, calcium, coffee, and tea. The GI infection *Helicobacter pylori* will also affect your absorption of iron.[38] *H. pylori* is common in those with recurring ulcers, GI distress, and a strong history of stress (aka adrenal fatigue). It is no wonder so many people have an iron deficiency. The Centers for Disease Control and Prevention reports that 18 percent of children between the ages of 1 and 5 have anemia. Women between the ages of 19 and 49 make up another 18 percent.[39]

Another important reason to screen iron storage levels is because iron is mainly stored in your liver. When your body is significantly inflamed, as it is during Stage 3 adrenal fatigue, it will store more iron in your liver, leading to liver disease. Iron can also be stored in and around the cells of your heart, and this will affect your cardiovascular function. When I come across a patient with elevated iron storage levels, I know that they either have a genetic mutation causing iron storage (a condition called hemochromatosis) or they have extreme inflammation causing excessive iron storage in the liver. When screening patients for hemochromatosis, I also have them undergo genetic testing and sometimes find that they have a particular gene that makes them carriers of the disease and more likely to be affected by this iron storage. This is important because excessive iron storage can lead to diabetes. Research indicates that excessive iron will accumulate in your pancreas, which will affect your production of insulin, causing insulin resistance or type 2 diabetes. Iron can also be deposited in your joints, causing arthritis.[40] Screening your iron storage levels will provide great insight into possible nutritional therapy because proper treatment will vary depending on the iron content of the foods you eat and whether you follow an anti-inflammatory diet. Knowing your iron levels will let you determine what herbs you might be able to take to support your liver and its function.

## Zinc

Zinc is a nutrient that is commonly known to affect immune function. Zinc also helps different parts of your body communicate with one another. This is why it is a major component of many of your body's enzymes.[41]

This mineral is absorbed via your small intestine, and it is also secreted into your gut. The absorbed zinc is then passed along to your liver before it enters your bloodstream for use in your other tissues. Zinc is involved in protein synthesis and the breakdown of carbohydrates, fats, and nucleic acids. In other words, it has a hand in your ability to lose weight and the production of energy. Involved in virtually every system, zinc has an effect on your hormones and their receptor sites because it either drives or halts conversions. More specifically, zinc is involved in the signaling of the receptor for insulin and preserving pancreatic beta cells, which are required to produce insulin and regulate glycemic control.[42] This protective effect of zinc on your beta cells has prompted more studies on using zinc as a therapy to control blood sugar. In a study released in 2013, researchers evaluated zinc as an alternative therapy for those who suffer from type 2 diabetes and found that zinc improved glycemic control. It was suggested that further studies be performed, as zinc is a promising candidate for treating diabetes in place of traditional medication.[43]

With the adrenal glands' impact on the development of diabetes and immune function, it is not surprising that zinc is a commonly suggested nutrient by health advocates. When you have adrenal fatigue, you use up all of the nutrients required for your "daily operations." And with zinc being involved in so many pathways, it is commonly depleted in those with adrenal fatigue. Aside from the many functions we have discussed, it is also involved in the synthesis of thyroid hormones. And ironically, the synthesis of zinc requires adequate thyroid hormone levels, meaning that in order to produce thyroid hormones you need zinc, but in order to produce zinc, you need those very same thyroid hormones. In a 2013 study, researchers found that a case of alopecia (hair loss) related to hypothyroidism did not experience hair regrowth once the thyroid was stabilized. Amazingly, when they added 50 mg of elemental zinc to the treatment, the hair grew back.[44]

It has been shown that if you are deficient in zinc, you will absorb more zinc from your food, whereas if you already have sufficient amounts, your absorption will be less efficient. Your body knows the impact of perfectly balanced zinc levels and will adjust absorption accordingly (assuming your digestion is not affected by chronic stress). In fact, the balance of intake versus elimination of zinc is a tightly regulated system. Shifts occur quickly in order to keep your zinc levels stable. The typical human consumes 14 to 30 mg/kg of zinc each day, so a 150-pound person should get 1 to 2 grams daily, although balance can be maintained with as little as 10 mg daily.

The requirements for zinc vary greatly depending on your age and nutritional status. Those with adrenal fatigue will have a higher daily requirement than those without. As expected, children, pregnant women, and lactating women will have higher daily requirements due to zinc's impact on growth. In low-income countries, the main food consumed is grains, which contain a low amount of zinc and a high amount of phylate. Phylate can block the zinc absorption from breast milk and other dietary sources.[45] If you are experiencing adrenal fatigue or have symptoms associated with zinc deficiency, then zinc is an essential element you should incorporate into your diet and supplement.

When supplementing with zinc, it is important to evaluate the amount of elemental zinc, rather than entire amount. For example, 200 mg of zinc sulfate contains about 50 mg of elemental zinc. So when someone is told to take 50 mg of zinc, they may mistakenly only take 50 mg of zinc sulfate, which would not be enough. Because of this, I typically prescribe zinc picolinate (another form) because it is more absorbable, making the label dosage more accurate. It also has fewer gastrointestinal side effects. Someone with adrenal fatigue should be taking somewhere between 20 and 50 mg of elemental zinc, depending on the number of symptoms present.

## Glutamine

A deficiency in the amino acid glutamine also plays a role in the development of adrenal fatigue. Glutamine is most known for its ability to build proteins, but it has more subtle roles that are strongly affected by adrenal fatigue. Glutamine is needed for the regeneration of mucosal cells, so it is a required component when you're healing your intestinal walls to solve issues stemming from poor absorption. It also aids in the function of your immune system, is a component of your neurotransmitters, and is required for normal brain function.

Glutamine is typically low in those with adrenal fatigue, because it has been released during adrenal overstimulation, which begins in Stage 1. I use it to heal the intestinal mucosa in patients with leaky gut syndrome and IBS symptoms and to prevent mood changes associated with neurotransmitter imbalance. It is typically taken as a powder because that form is easiest to absorb, but it can also be taken in capsule form. As a muscle builder, it is typically used in high doses of more than 20 grams daily. For the purposes of intestinal healing, the dosage should be much smaller—3 to 5 grams daily. Most people in Stages 2 and 3 of adrenal fatigue have some sort of intestinal change and would benefit greatly from this nutrient.

## Omega-3 Fatty Acids

Last, but certainly not least, is the massive benefit of omega-3 fatty acids. The research is abundant on these nutrients and spans from treatment of depression and bipolar disorder to cardiovascular disease, neurodegenerative disease, and even dermatological conditions. It is no secret that fatty acids are key to our health. Most baby formulas are now being fortified with docosahexaenoic acid (DHA) in an effort to benefit brain growth. Products are marketed with the amounts of eicosapentaenoic acid (EPA) and DHA listed on the packaging. With so much focus on these nutrients, I feel it is important to review their true, researched benefits and how they relate to adrenal malfunction. Omega-3 fatty acids are composed of DHA and EPA, which work very differently in your body. EPA is a potent anti-inflammatory and works similarly to a corticosteroid, but without the side effects. Muscle aches and pains, cardiovascular inflammation, joint pain, or any inflammatory process will benefit from dietary addition of EPA. DHA has a strong effect on prohibiting cholesterol from depositing in your arteries and has a positive neurogenerative effect, prompting its addition to formulas and cereals in children.

There is a third omega in this scenario: omega-6. Omega-6 has an inflammatory component, and red meat contains a lot of it. This is the basis behind the removal of red meats from your diet to treat inflammatory diseases, like autoimmunity and cardiovascular diseases. But red meat needs to be removed from diabetic diet plans, as well, as diabetics commonly have high levels of inflammation, too (see Chapter 2). The typical American diet is composed of more omega-6 fatty acids than omega-3s, and that is of concern to practitioners and dietitians because it promotes further inflammation. This process of inflammation is closely tied to the stages of adrenal fatigue. As I have mentioned throughout this book, the balance of nutrients in your cells is critical for proper functioning. Patients with adrenal fatigue are slowly depleting nutrients and slowing their digestion, which affects their cells. Recall that your cells are primarily made of fat and that without proper absorption and mineral balance, the fat in your cell will decrease further, increasing the malabsorption effect. The more severe your adrenal fatigue, the more fat-deficient you become, which results in a more inflammatory response. This is why people in Stage 3 tend to have fibromyalgia or chronic pain. Those with severe autoimmune conditions, such as rheumatoid arthritis, will benefit greatly from fatty acid intake to control their pain.

A review released in July of 2013 examined the effects of DHA in learning and behavior in school-aged children and found that a variety of research articles showed improvement in cognition and behavior with DHA supplementation.[46] Another study showed that the administration of omega-3 fatty acids conveyed a strong benefit to the regeneration of neurological function in infants with fetal alcohol syndrome.[47]

For the last 20 years, a strong focus has been put on omega-3s and their impact on the cardiovascular system. Omega-3 fatty acids have been shown to reduce triglycerides by helping your body clear triglycerides from your blood and by preventing your body from making triglycerides in the first place. Omega-3s also reduce total cholesterol levels.[48] Research also supports the idea that supplementation with omega-3s will reduce your risk of cardiac death.[49] The strong anti-inflammatory component alone will improve cardiovascular complications (such as hypertension and heartbeat irregularities) and will prevent plaque deposition. The chronic imbalance resulting from adrenal fatigue promotes a higher risk of cardiovascular effects, such as arrhythmias. There is evidence that omega-3 fatty acids will enhance the regular rhythm and function of your heart, therefore reducing sudden death events.[50] This ability to act on your heart rate and the omegas' direct effect on inflammatory markers make a strong case for their use in the treatment of autoimmune conditions, irritable bowel disease, and cancer. One of the more recent findings with omega-3 supplementation is that it has the ability to sensitize your body to insulin and promote weight loss. Yes, consuming more fat can promote weight loss!

When asked what everyone should take for everyday, overall wellness and disease prevention, omega-3 fatty acids are always at the top of my list. Their health benefits are vast and are still being discovered and explored.

As you can tell after reading this chapter, it is essential that you consume vitamins and especially minerals depleted by adrenal fatigue. Without replenishing these depleted nutrients, your body will not achieve and maintain optimal health and you will be at greater risk of developing disease. It is absolutely true that food can heal your body. If nutrients are properly ingested and adequately absorbed, your body will run like a finely tuned machine. For more information on how to get more of these vital nutrients into your diet, see Chapter 11.

# MY TURNAROUND
## MORGAN PORTER, AGE: 23

Morgan Porter had been suffering with health problems for years and never knew the reason why. "I am one of those patients where I was always sick and couldn't figure out what was going on with me. Before I found Dr. Pingel, I had chronic asthma and endometriosis. I was sick eight times a year with sinusitis because of how bad my gut health was," she explains. "I've been to a lot of different specialists. My doctor had thrown her hands up. I was having all sorts of weird symptoms and didn't know what was causing it."

Morgan's mother, who was a patient of Dr. Pingel's, recommended that Morgan see her as well. That's when Dr. Pingel diagnosed her with adrenal fatigue and *H. pylori*, a bacterial infection that occurs in the stomach. "I was in late Stage 1 of adrenal fatigue, heading into Stage 2. I knew I needed to manage my adrenal fatigue and my GI issues. Before, I was constantly prescribed antibiotics for my gut issues. I knew that wasn't getting me the help I needed and I had to look outside the box," she says.

On Dr. Pingel's plan, Morgan treated her adrenal fatigue and her *H. pylori* with supplements and soon began to notice results. "After about 4 months of treatment, I suddenly had this new sense of energy. I was eventually able to restore my gut health, and I was feeling better than I ever felt. I finally was listening to what my body needed," she shares. "Before, I was exhausted and didn't want to do anything, I was eating crappy foods, and I was always tired and sick. I hated to work out because I never felt well. Exercising and eating are much easier now, and I lost 16 pounds. Everyone in my family sees really great changes. The biggest thing is that I finally have my life back!"

Today, Morgan is living a much better and healthier life. "Since seeing Dr. Pingel, my life has done a 180. Now I'm feeling so much better. Once you start on this path, you don't want to go back, because there's such a difference in how you feel. You see the results you've been waiting for." In fact, the naturopathic treatment has had such a positive influence on her that Morgan has decided to become a naturopathic physician herself. "I was going to be a nurse before this, but I've been so inspired by her that I now want to be a naturopath and help people the way Dr. Pingel helped me."

# 10

# IS YOUR MEDICATION KEEPING YOU SICK?

My father had cardiovascular disease. After surviving a heart attack at 40 years old, he was being treated for angina and had a screening angiogram every 6 months by a cardiologist. He took a number of cardiovascular medications to manage and prevent, as he was told, a future cardiovascular event. A few months prior to his death at age 58, he had his usual full workup by the cardiologist: a stress test, electrocardiogram (EKG), and angiogram. His physicians said that everything looked great and that his blood pressure and cholesterol were well controlled by his medications. They told him to simply continue on his medications and come back for his routine follow-up.

Within 3 months, my dad had a massive stroke that obliterated his thalamus, putting him into a vegetative state. As I sat there next to my father, who was noncommunicative, I thought about the assurances his doctors had given him that he was doing everything he could to maintain wellness. I thought about what he was going to miss. I was a 24-year-old college student at the time, which meant he was going to miss my wedding, my children, my career. He was going to miss being a grandparent and retiring with his wife, whom he adored. I thought of our weekly phone call and how much I would miss chatting with him. As I sat there at his bedside, without receiving any reassurance—or even an acknowledgment, when I asked questions—from his doctors, I decided to make a career change. It was at that point that I decided to go into medicine.

I pursued alternative medicine because I could not understand how the conventional model could help people live long and healthy lives if it failed to educate its patients. Maybe this was due to insurance restraints on time and the number of patients being managed, but sitting there in that hospital room, unable to summon a doctor unless my dad went into respiratory failure, I felt like a number—just someone there to fill a room. The nurses were sweet, and I know all of his caregivers meant well. They just did not know the answers I wanted, and they did not want to admit that. I wish they would have had a real conversation with me at that point, rather than simply telling me to watch and wait. Would we have left him on life support for as long as we did if we were told that there was no chance of recovery? Some honesty and human kindness would have been appreciated by all of us who sat by his side for 12 hours a day, waiting for just one sign of life, as we were told it was possible. It wasn't.

A huge part of this picture is that my dad was a lifelong smoker. He ate poorly, drank alcohol, and smoked about a pack of cigarettes every day. I know his doctors had told him to quit smoking. I know they told him to eat better. I know they told him to exercise. But did they inspire him to try? Did they teach him how? Or did they simply medicate him and tell him that as long as his numbers were good, his risk was low? As a physician, I have learned a lot from my patients. I have learned that lifestyle management is the best predictor of longevity and symptoms management, and that it has no negative side effects. My most active senior patients are those who refuse to take medications and instead eat a primarily vegetarian diet, drink lots of water, exercise daily, and avoid excessive toxin exposure.

I often look back and wonder, why didn't just one doctor offer to help him and educate him on what might be missed in life by refusing to modify his lifestyle? My dad tried. I remember him trying diets, the nicotine patch, and walking the dog. I remember how disappointed he was when he failed at those attempts. He had the desire, but no one helped him. No one inspired him. Knowing what I know now, it's clear to me that my father's life could have been saved if just one person had educated him on why he should quit rather than just telling him to do it—if he'd received just a touch of honesty and humility from a caring doctor to convince him to make changes for himself. That is what is missing today in the practice of conventional medicine.

# THE PRINCIPLES OF NATURAL MEDICINE

I feel that it is important at this point to provide a disclaimer: I am not opposed to conventional medicine. I believe in its benefits, but I also feel that it lacks the preventative aspect and the attention to lifestyle that need to be addressed. As an integrative physician, I believe that your body has the ability to heal itself. I do not blame doctors for prescribing medications, because that is what they learned to do. That is our medical model. What disturbs me is the lack of extrapolation of medical knowledge and attention to detail when it comes to our health. The practice of medicine is just that: practice. We learn as we go. We learn from our patients. But treating everyone the same based on a study funded by a pharmaceutical company is not helping us with patient care. As a naturopathic physician, I have sworn an oath, just as any other doctor has, and it is as follows:

1. **RECOGNIZE THE HEALING POWER OF NATURE:** Trust in the body's inherent wisdom to heal itself.
2. **IDENTIFY AND TREAT THE CAUSES:** Look beyond the symptoms to the underlying cause.

3. **FIRST, DO NO HARM:** Utilize the most natural, least invasive, and least toxic therapies.

4. **DOCTOR AS TEACHER:** Educate patients in the steps to achieving and maintaining health.

5. **TREAT THE WHOLE PERSON:** View the body as an integrated whole in all its physical and spiritual dimensions.

6. **PREVENTION:** Focus on overall health, wellness, and disease prevention.

Without educating each patient about ways to stay healthy and looking at each patient individually to determine risks versus benefits of individual therapies, we cannot say that we are doing no harm. This chapter looks further into our pharmaceutical use in America and discusses the most common medications, the risks and benefits of each medication, as well as possible outcomes from the use of those medications.

Remember that all of the major diseases in America have developed from stress-induced adrenal fatigue and are falsely managed by these prescriptions. Also, most people haven't been told how they can avoid being on medication. These medications then cause side effects, which also cause stress on your body, which worsens adrenal fatigue. This chapter is meant to educate you about these medications—not to lecture you about or oppose them. It would be hypocritical of me to say that medications are never of benefit. Of course they are. But many times, they are not. This is the area of medicine that's not being discussed, and it's something that reminds me of my father on a daily basis, especially when I meet a new patient who has not been fully informed about her current medical therapy and the measures she could take to truly reverse her disease.

# THE BUSINESS OF PRESCRIPTION MEDICATION

The Mayo Clinic released a study in 2013 stating that nearly 70 percent of Americans take a prescribed medication and 20 percent take more than five prescribed medications. In fact, $250 billion was spent on prescription medications in 2009. And a large proportion of these medications include antidepressants and opioids.[1] Consider that fact for a moment: The most commonly used medications manage pain or treat depression and anxiety. Knowing what you now know about adrenal fatigue, isn't it reasonable to assume that stress management could have an impact on widespread medication use and save us billions of dollars every year?

Take a look at the classes of pharmaceuticals listed in "Medication in America: An Inside Glance" on page 180, and notice how many times something regarding the nervous system appears. Mental health medications are the third most commonly prescribed class of medication, and that includes meds for conditions like depression and anxiety, yet we also have the central nervous system listed as number six and the nervous system as number ten. I suspect they are including insomnia medications in one of these nervous system classes, and possibly some other stronger relaxants.

## TREATING THE SYMPTOM, NOT THE CAUSE

Most of the nervous system conditions could easily be classified in the mental health group as well, meaning that even a larger percent of our medications come from this category. Insomnia, anxiety, depression, mood swings, obsessive behavior, ADHD: All of these nervous system or mental health conditions can be related back to adrenal fatigue. So if we were to treat mental health issues differently we would drastically reduce the amount of pharmaceuticals we prescribe and use.

Aside from the nervous system disorders, all of the other classes can be linked back to poor adrenal health, as well. We have already discussed how your cardiovascular system is affected by your adrenal glands because they can change your blood pressure and cholesterol, as well as create inflammation. This same inflammation that affects your cardiovascular system will also inflame your joints and muscles, resulting in chronic pain. The excessive weight you gain from the storage of

# MEDICATION IN AMERICA: AN INSIDE GLANCE

Here are the top 10 classes of pharmaceuticals prescribed in the United States as of 2012.[2]

1. Antihypertensives
2. Pain management
3. Mental health
4. Antibacterials
5. Lipid lowering
6. Other central nervous system
7. Antidiabetics
8. Respiratory support
9. Anti-ulcer
10. Nervous system

These are the 25 most commonly prescribed medications in America in 2012.[3]

1. Hydrocodone (pain management)
2. Levothyroxine (hypothyroidism medication)
3. Lisinopril (antihypertensive)
4. Simvastatin (lipid lowering)
5. Metoprolol (antihypertensive)
6. Amlodipine (antihypertensive)
7. Omeprazole (reflux medication)
8. Metformin (antidiabetic)
9. Salbutamol (respiratory support)
10. Atorvastatin (lipid lowering)
11. Azithromycin (antibiotic)
12. Amoxicillin (antibiotic)
13. Alprazolam (sedative)
14. Hydrochlorothiazide (antihypertensive)
15. Zolpidem (sedative)
16. Furosemide (diuretic—cardiovascular)
17. Fluticasone (steroid)
18. Sertraline (antidepressant)
19. Citalopram (antidepressant)
20. Gabapentin (pain management, anti-epileptic)
21. Tramadol (pain management)
22. Oxycodone (pain management)
23. Prednisone (steroid)
24. Warfarin (blood thinner)
25. Ibuprofen (pain management/NSAID)

insulin and the development of diabetes will contribute to your use of diabetic medications and also to physical problems, such as increased pain and more frequent use of anti-inflammatory medications.

Adrenal fatigue will also cause digestion changes (including heart-burn, diarrhea, constipation, and bloating), in addition to lowering thyroid function. Inflammation from long-term adrenal fatigue causes allergy development, worsening asthma, and bouts of bronchitis and pneumonia. It also has an impact on your immune system, causing your body to heal slowly after an illness and sometimes requiring the use of antimicrobials. By managing your stress you will reduce your use of medications. It is that simple.

With 20 percent of Americans taking more than five prescription medications, consider the quantity of side effects that are likely occur. Instead of supporting the natural pathways in your body, these pharmaceuticals alter your biochemistry, causing an adaptation within your body that results in the development of further symptoms and worsening your existing adrenal fatigue. This sends you back to the doctor, where you are likely to receive another prescription, and the cycle continues.

A great example of this is the use of statin drugs to treat high cholesterol. Most people are aware that if you are prescribed a statin drug, you have to have your liver enzymes checked regularly. But do you know why? It's because the major side effect of these drugs is liver damage.[4] Yes, your cholesterol will be lower, but your liver will be compromised. You may also develop significant muscle aches and pains that can be detrimental to your quality of life. But your cholesterol will be low. And statins are typically prescribed to lower your risk of a heart attack because the theory is that the lower your cholesterol is, the less there is to stick to the insides of your arteries. However, anyone who understands the physiology of this, as well as the underlying adrenal fatigue, knows that the walls of your arteries have to be damaged or inflamed for cholesterol to stick to them. So someone with normal cholesterol but poor artery integrity has just as great a chance of a heart attack as someone with high cholesterol and great artery integrity. I have had a number of patients who were prescribed a statin simply because their fathers had high cholesterol, or their siblings, or their mother. The statin was considered to be a preventative measure. A family history of high cholesterol is not enough to warrant prescribing a drug that will ultimately damage your liver and cause further side effects.

Studies continuously investigate ways to reduce risks and lower the side effects of statins, but they keep coming up short. The medical community has not found a way to reduce the risk of a cardiovascular event safely via pharmaceuticals.[5] When a person's cholesterol cannot be managed by a low dose of a statin, it can be more harmful to increase their dose and use statins in combination with other therapies than it would be to let the patient live with high cholesterol.

## THE TRUTH ABOUT ANTIHYPERTENSIVE DRUGS

Hypertensive drugs are designed to lower your blood pressure, and there are many types. Some block sympathetic output (beta-blockers), some block calcium channels (calcium channel blockers, or CCBs), some act as diuretics by altering sodium concentrations in your blood, some block the conversion of a substance that narrows vessels (angiotensin-converting enzyme, or ACE), and others use various other mechanisms. But whatever way they work, they all have the same purpose: to lower your blood pressure.

Interestingly enough, some people respond to one class and not another. This is likely because blood pressure is affected by many different things. If your blood pressure is elevated because of sympathetic output (or the fight-or-flight response), a beta-blocker will work better than a diuretic. If sodium is to blame, a diuretic will work better than a CCB, and so on. By considering the cause of your blood pressure elevation, you can pick the drug that would be best, or you can consider why that change (say a sympathetic output) is occurring and treat the cause. This is where the evaluation of adrenal fatigue comes into play.

## The Side Effects of ACE Inhibitors

ACE inhibitors are the most commonly prescribed medications for hypertension, and one drug in this category, lisinopril, is the third most common prescription in America. Its side effects are incredibly common, and the side effects for ACE inhibitors as a class are significant in number and cause for concern. Considered normal and unproblematic by most physicians, the most common side effects of these drugs are a dry cough and a skin rash. Doctors commonly dismiss these symptoms and manage the situation by adding nonsteroidal anti-inflammatory medications. Other very common side effects include low red blood cell count, low white blood cell count, and high levels of potassium.[6]

Elevated potassium is not a surprising side effect, as this class of drug targets aldosterone, the hormone released from your adrenal glands in response to stimuli requesting an increase in blood pressure. Your adrenal glands are at the source of this blood pressure elevation. So if the number one prescribed drug for hypertension acts on (or targets) your adrenals to lower blood pressure, is it any surprise that your adrenal glands have a direct effect on your blood pressure?

As you may recall, aldosterone is released in order to retain sodium and lose potassium via your kidneys to raise your blood pressure. So if you were to take a drug that blocked this mechanism, what do you think would happen? Your blood pressure would lower, your potassium would increase (causing irregular heartbeat), and your sodium would decrease (causing swelling in different areas of your body).[7] And why don't we heal the adrenal fatigue first and eliminate the cause of the increased aldosterone?

## The Side Effects of Beta-Blockers

Metoprolol, the fifth most commonly prescribed antihypertensive, is in a class known as beta-blockers. Beta-blockers work by blocking sympathetic output. Recall that when your adrenal glands are stimulated by a "bear," they release hormones via your sympathetic nervous system, resulting in heart palpitations and increased blood pressure. Beta-blockers will block that output, once again showing us that our adrenal glands are at the source of elevated blood pressure.

A beta-blocker lowers your heart rate, lowers the force of contraction by your heart, and regulates an abnormal rhythm. There are some known interactions with this type of medication, so it needs to be closely monitored when used with other medications. Beta-blockers are also used to treat migraines, glaucoma, and some hyperthyroid conditions. The Mayo Clinic reports that the most common side effects of beta-blockers are fatigue, cold hands, headache, upset stomach, changes in bowels, and dizziness. Less common but still relevant side effects are shortness of breath, insomnia, lowered sex drive, and depression.

Considering that the most common concerns of patients are typically those listed above, doctors should hesitate to prescribe these medications. In fact, these side effects are viewed so negatively that a very recent study advised doctors to reconsider telling the patients about the side effects, as the possibility of the beta-blocker preventing death by a heart attack is more important than the side effects. The study, published in 2013, said that the side effects were not overly severe, and because the patients have a negative reaction when reading or hearing about the side effects, it might be better for the physician to simply not tell them.[8] This study basically suggests that your physician should lie to you about the side effects, in order to prevent your death. But it is never acceptable for a physician to lie to his patients, and it is unwise to take it at face value that a specific medication can save your life by preventing a specific event from occurring.

While beta-blockers can save someone's life in certain situations, a patient should never take any medication without being notified of the potential side effects and making his or her own informed decision. This goes for any treatment. When speaking to a patient about dietary changes, herbal therapy, nutrition therapy, and lifestyle management, a physician should always inform the patient of the risks and benefits and ask him to decide what he is willing to commit to. You are in control of your own health, and letting a doctor ultimately decide what is or is not important to you is a mistake. If you had the option to treat your underlying adrenal fatigue and not only prevent elevated blood pressure but also an inflammatory disease, gastrointestinal disease, neurological changes, hormone irregularities, and insomnia, which would you choose: taking the drugs with side effects or addressing the adrenal fatigue, the common core of all of these issues?

## The Side Effects of Calcium Channel Blockers

Amlodipine is the sixth most commonly prescribed drug in the United States. It works by blocking the calcium channels in the muscle that causes contractions of your heart. In doing this, it slows your heart rate and lowers your blood pressure. It also reduces your heart's oxygen requirements. My issue with this class of drugs concerns how it affects your calcium levels and how it affects blood flow throughout your body.

Let's consider what oxygen does for your body. You need oxygen for your cells to work. If you lower your heart's oxygen needs, how does this affect the cells in the rest of your body? How does blocking calcium impact the level of calcium in your blood? If calcium is out of balance with other minerals, will it cause calcium deposits in your kidneys, breast tissue, and perhaps arteries? Unopposed calcium will promote plaque deposition in your arteries and cause high blood pressure, heart attack, and stroke.

Let's extrapolate our thinking a little: If a CCB blocks the movement of calcium from your blood into your muscle, then the calcium remains in your blood and it is unopposed, meaning it is not balanced by other minerals, such as magnesium. So then is it unreasonable to investigate the possibility that CCBs, although they lower blood pressure, may actually worsen plaque deposition? A 2013 study published in the *Journal of Vascular Surgery* stated that carotid artery stenosis (stiffening and narrowing of arteries) was not improved despite optimal cardiovascular therapy or the use of medication to stay within a normal range. The study included other pharmaceuticals, in addition to CCBs, but it showed that even when blood pressure and cholesterol are maintained, arteries will continue to narrow and harden.[9]

In addition to a lack of education on the potential side effects of this class of drugs, there are many documented interactions with other medications. You should always thoroughly review the side effects of these and any other drugs before commencing therapy.

We know that adrenal fatigue will lower magnesium levels and raise calcium levels, causing muscle contraction abnormalities such as restless leg syndrome. Now, if your elevated calcium levels also caused muscle contractions in your heart, wouldn't you end up with elevated blood pressure? So those people that respond to CCB therapy may also respond to therapy with magnesium as part of the treatment of adrenal fatigue. Considering the overwhelming side effect profile of these calcium channel blocking drugs, we should consider treating adrenal fatigue before prescribing these pharmaceuticals.

## The Side Effects of Diuretics

The next class of antihypertensive drugs that falls in the top 25 is diuretics. Number 14 is hydrochlorothiazide (HCTZ) and number 16 is furosemide. These are typically the first medications prescribed for patients who are diagnosed as prehypertensive. HCTZ works by dumping minerals, primarily sodium, in an effort to lower blood pressure. Unfortunately, it also eliminates other minerals, and the most common side effects of this drug are low levels of sodium, potassium, chloride, and magnesium. HCTZ also increases levels of calcium and uric acid and causes hyperglycemia (high blood sugar) and elevated cholesterol. These small, very common changes can be incredibly detrimental to the rest of your body. Diabetes development, elevated cholesterol, and major mineral deficiencies are a given with this medication if the side effects aren't closely monitored and supplements aren't given to replace lost minerals. Unfortunately, this is not common practice for more doctors who prescribe HCTZ. As we discussed in earlier chapters, when calcium levels are high in relation to magnesium, bone changes and plaque deposition in your arteries occur. Isn't the point of this medication to *lower* your risk of a heart attack? And what about magnesium? It is a main component of bone and relaxes your mind and muscles, as it's involved in muscle contraction. Sodium, although commonly looked down upon, aids in how our muscle contract. Without sodium, we cannot contract our large muscles! These classes of drugs can cause much more harm than good, and if the cause of the elevated blood pressure is addressed, these do not need to be used.

Furosemide is a type of diuretic called a "loop diuretic," and it affects a different part of your kidneys to achieve a similar result. The side effects are similar to HCTZ's, with a couple of exceptions. Loop diuretics will lower calcium instead of raise it and will typically elevate liver enzymes. While cramping and dizziness are very common, furosemide will affect magnesium and potassium, blood sugar, and uric acid much like HCTZ would. Diuretics in general are typically the first choice of treatment for early hypertension development. But due to the massive nutritional deficiencies associated with these drugs—deficiencies that will promote further disease development—they should be avoided when possible.

Adrenal fatigue causes elevated blood pressure in a variety of ways. First, it can be the result of increased fight-or-flight response. Second, it can change the calcium and magnesium levels in your body. Third, it can alter the function of aldosterone, effecting sodium and potassium balance. When you look back on the classes of hypertensives discussed, they all act upon one of these mechanisms. Let's consider treating adrenal fatigue first, and then assess whether or not a drug is needed before jumping on board with a pharmaceutical that may cause side effects and potentially worsen adrenal fatigue by bogging down your liver.

## THE PROBLEM WITH PAIN: PAIN MANAGEMENT PHARMACEUTICALS

The use of pain management drugs is ranked second only to that of hypertensive medications. That said, take a look back at the list of the top prescribed drugs in America. Number one is hydrocodone, which you may know as Vicodin, Lorcet, or Lortab. Let me say that again, the *number one* drug prescribed in the United States is Vicodin. Number 22 in the entire nation is oxycodone. (Percocet is the most recognized brand.) Both of these drugs are highly addictive and are responsible for numerous deaths and rehab visits each year. According to a 2012 report from the Centers for Disease Control and Prevention, since 2003, there have been more deaths from prescription opioid overdoses than from heroin and cocaine combined. In fact, 9 million people report chronic long-term use of opioids and 5 million report nonprescribed use on a regular basis. Not yet convinced that we, as a nation, are overmedicated? Well, consider this: The average dose of morphine prescribed per person in 1997 was 96 mg. In 2007, it was 700 mg—seven times the amount prescribed only 10 years earlier![10]

Let's look back again at the top 25 prescribed drugs in America. We have Vicodin and oxycodone, as previously mentioned, but also on the list are tramadol, prednisone, and ibuprofen. That means 5 out of the 25 most prescribed drugs in America are involved in pain management. But is it true that so many people are in pain? And if so, why? What are we doing to ourselves to produce such pain?

With about one-third of Americans categorized as obese,[11] it is not surprising that our joints hurt. But instead of taking medication for pain, why not focus on reversing obesity? With diabetes, heart disease, Alzheimer's, and cancer all being closely linked to inflammation,[12] it makes sense that people suffering from these diseases are in pain, so we should look at reversing these diseases to prevent pain rather than simply treating the symptoms and writing them off as side effects.

Also, why are doctors prescribing such addictive mediations for pain rather than looking for alternative options? Acupuncture can do wonders for pain.[13] Diet, lifestyle, and nutrition are also important pain-management tools.[14] In fact, intravenous magnesium is used to treat severe headache pain in hospitals.[15] So why aren't magnesium supplements used as a daily treatment instead of pain medications? Think about what we said on page 186: Diuretics have a massive impact on electrolyte imbalances, resulting in low magnesium. Guess what that gives you? Pain! Using nutrition as a pain reliever would be a healthier option. Additionally, one of the side effects of these medications is death. That's right, death. Are those who take these medications prepared to trade their lives for pain relief?

It's common for pain to initially develop due to the effects of adrenal fatigue, causing increased inflammation, nutritional deficiencies, and excessive weight gain. By taking pain medications, adrenal fatigue is worsened due to the major impact these drugs have on your liver, plus the addictive quality of these meds changes the way you perceive pain. If you are in pain, your body is trying to tell you something. It is drawing attention to a problem. Listen to your body and find the cause, rather than suppressing the pain. If you suppress the pain for too long, you will no longer read the signals your body sends, and that will land you in Stage 3 adrenal fatigue.

## The Mechanism of Blocking Pain

So what do these medications do, exactly? They are opioids, which means they block pain receptors. You've heard of morphine and heroin, both of which are opioids. Oxycodone is the same thing, and Vicodin works the same way, too. It's incredibly unfortunate, but numerous patients have come to me taking not only an opioid, but also Ambien and Xanax, two more depressant medications used for sleep or anxiety that are commonly prescribed without the patient being told how addictive they are. One side effect of opioids is respiratory depression, meaning that your breathing slows or even stops altogether. They also slow your heart rate, with the potential of stopping it altogether. This is not a good combination with a sleep or antianxiety medication. These opioid and depressant medications were made for short-term use, such as after surgeries or major accidents; they were not meant for treating chronic pain.

Simply put, the side effects are not worth it. Evaluate the cause of your pain, not the pain itself. Think again of the oath I shared above that doctors take when we graduate medical school: First, do no harm. Is the ridiculously high use of opioids following that first, and arguably most important, promise?

# KILL! KILL! THE ROLE OF ANTIBIOTICS

The two most commonly prescribed antibiotics in America are amoxicillin and azithromycin, which you may know better as the Z-Pak. There is a time and place for these pharmaceuticals, and when used sparingly, the side effects are minimal. When considering the widespread use of antibiotics, I think back to my internships in pediatrics. I worked with a few different conventional physicians and saw about 10 patients each hour. I would estimate that about 80 percent of those patients walked out of the office with a prescription for an antibiotic, primarily amoxicillin. And I would guess that maybe only 30 percent truly needed it, as most presented with viral symptoms, not bacterial.

This was not always the doctor's fault. Parents would often demand prescriptions for antibiotics for their kids. On numerous occasions, I saw a doctor state that the illness was viral and tell the parent to go home and give the child fluids, let him rest, and wait it out. The parents would go on about how they have to work and would demand a script. I would chat with the doctors afterward about how frustrated they were because they knew the antibiotic would not help and would only harm the patient by lowering his or her immunity due to the damage antibiotics do to good bacteria in the gut. It is for this reason that I educate my parents, and the public, on the risks and benefits of each medication.

In November 2013, the CDC came out with a shocker to many patients: Antibiotics have become resistant to infection and are not a valid therapy. They stated that "Antibiotic resistance is one of the world's most pressing public health threats," and that "Antibiotic overuse increases the development of drug-resistant germs." They went on to say, "More than 50 percent of antibiotics are unnecessarily prescribed in office settings for upper respiratory viruses and up to 50 percent of antibiotic use in hospitals is either unnecessary or inappropriate."[16] This was a huge blow to our medical system, but it's something commonly preached by holistic doctors.

If the "bug" is something that will cause harm to a person, such as severe strep throat that puts a person at risk for further disease development, an antibiotic is absolutely needed. A bad bladder infection can lead to numerous kidney problems and may also require an antibiotic. But a common cold, which is a viral upper respiratory infection, is not grounds for use. Instead, it should be monitored and your body needs to kill the virus on its own, as this promotes better immunity in the future.

## The Harm Caused by Antibiotics

So what's the harm of using the antibiotic? It kills every bacterium in your body. Think back to your GI system and the good bacteria in your gut that help prevent and reverse infectious disease. In someone who does not have adrenal fatigue, an occasional antibiotic will not cause as much harm as in someone who does have adrenal fatigue. With adrenal fatigue, your GI system is slowed and digestion is poor, leading to more inflammatory responses in your system. This weakens your intestinal flora and has a negative impact on your immune system. Those with adrenal fatigue need more help reestablishing the good bugs because they do not have a well-tuned machine for recovery from illness. This is why people with adrenal fatigue are poor healers and take longer to recover from a simple cold. Many will use an antibiotic after they have been sick for 1 to 2 weeks, assuming it is bacterial when it is not.

Remember that the "landlords," or beneficial bacteria, protect your body from invaders and build your immune system. But the overuse of antibiotics is affecting your immune function, which will lead to further immune problems in the future. This is why you should always take a probiotic at a dose of 100 to 200 billion colony-forming units (CFU) per day for 2 weeks following the use of an antibiotic. This probiotic should contain multiple strains of "bugs," such as *lactobacillus*, *bifidobacterium*, and perhaps *Saccharomyces boulardii*. You have an army to protect you and your body needs to build up the same soldiers it loses from antibiotic use. If you do not replenish the good guys in an adrenally fatigued system, you will continue to get sick regularly, or it will take longer and longer each time you need to recover, predisposing you to a drug-resistant bacterial organism. As pointed out by the CDC, this can be life threatening.

## Why You Should Be Taking Probiotics

I mentioned that following an antibiotic, you should take 100 billion to 200 billion CFU a day and that those organisms should be multistrained, meaning that your probiotic should contain a variety of organisms. Let's take a look at the most common over-the-counter probiotics that might be prescribed by your primary physician. Align contains 1 billion CFU of one strain. That means that to follow my recommendation above, you'd need to take 100 to 200 capsules daily following antibiotics. Phillips Colon Health contains a total of 1.5 billion of three bacterial strains. Yogurt, such as Activia, is commonly recommended by doctors as an adjunct therapy during antibiotic use, but it contains two main strains and the amount of CFUs is not labeled.

It would get pretty expensive (not to mention inconvenient and uncomfortable) to take 100 pills a day of these commonly prescribed probiotics, wouldn't it? And if you have adrenal fatigue and a compromised immune system, you would have to take higher amounts on a daily basis. There's good news, though: There are products that are created with 100 billion to 200 billion multistrained organisms per pill. That means you'll take 1 or 2 capsules daily following antibiotics and can take higher amounts of probiotics on a daily basis to repair the damage from adrenal fatigue. It would also help prevent bacterial and viral infections in the future. This is key, considering that most of our bacteria are now resistant to antibiotics.

It is always important to look at the source of the probiotics as well, as most have a milk base. So if you have a milk intolerance or allergy, you'll need to avoid those. Many of the professional products on the market have an apricot base, eliminating this milk issue. If you consume probiotics at the levels I recommend following antibiotics, your flora will be replenished. At just 1 billion a day, however, it is likely that the virus or bacteria you were suffering from will return. And in those with adrenal fatigue, it is likely that another virus or bacteria will attack soon afterward.

# THE DEPENDENCY CYCLE

One of the biggest concerns surrounding the use of sedative medications is their ability to worsen adrenal fatigue. As I mentioned when we discussed pain medications, symptoms are a way for your body to communicate with you, so when you suppress that communication with a medication, it dumbs down your body's response, worsening the situation. If you have a toddler who wants your attention and you keep ignoring him, he will eventually throw a serious tantrum. If your body has the symptom of insomnia and you give it Xanax, you will no longer hear it crying for help. But the problem will still be there, so your body will find another way to get your attention. The best way for your body to make itself heard? Adapt your adrenal response by raising blood pressure, slowing GI function, depressing your mind, causing anxiety, worsening depth of sleep, or—one of the most commonly noticed—depositing weight around your abdomen. That will surely get your attention, right?

## Drugs for Insomnia

Even more concerning is the increasing use of sleep-inducing medications. Zolpidem, or Ambien, is currently the 15th most prescribed drug in the United States, and the side effects are numerous. It is essentially handed out like candy and deemed nonaddictive. Stepping away from the research for just a moment, think of how many people you know who use Ambien to help themselves sleep. How many of these people do you think can actually get to sleep without it? I can tell you simply from a subjective review of my patient base that none of them state that they can sleep without it. In fact, most are surprised when I am able to eliminate the drug and find alternative ways to induce and maintain sleep by treating the adrenal glands to reverse the cause and temporarily using herbs and amino acids to assist in sleep.

While researching the side effects of Ambien, I came across numerous studies detailing the dangers of this drug. According to the Substance Abuse and Mental Health Services Administration, emergency room visits involving adverse reactions to Ambien rose 220 percent between 2005 and 2010—from 6,111 visits to 19,487 visits! And 74 percent of these patients were over 45 years old. The adverse reactions in this report included daytime drowsiness, dizziness, hallucinations, agitation, sleepwalking, and drowsiness while driving. It was also reported that when this drug is combined with other medications, such as antianxiety medications and pain relievers, it is dangerous and even life threatening.[17]

This is alarming because I find that numerous patients have been given prescriptions for both Xanax (an antianxiety medication) and Ambien, and they are told to take them at night to help them sleep. Although I cannot find concrete statistics on how often these drugs are prescribed together, I can speak from experience—and so can you, as you likely know someone with insomnia who is combining these drugs. I hear many stories from patients about sleepwalking after Ambien use. One told me just yesterday that after taking Ambien her husband would often find her cleaning out a drawer or vacuuming the house somewhere around 2 a.m. She does not remember any of it.

Furthermore, the *Journal of Clinical Sleep Medicine* reviewed legal cases in 2011 surrounding a variety of incidents that occurred due to ingestion of Ambien.[18] In each case, the patients reported 3 to 5 hours of amnesia. Yes, you may think you are asleep, but are you really?

## Medication for Anxiety

Alprazolam, which you may know as Xanax, is the 13th most commonly prescribed drug. It is primarily prescribed for anxiety and insomnia, and it is considered addictive. It is commonly prescribed for those with adrenal fatigue because it has been shown to combat the effects of excessive cortisol release, and therefore it calms your body during an anxiety attack related to adrenal fatigue.[19]

The administration of this drug does not go without consequence. It is highly addictive and when used for extended periods of time could alter a person's stage of adrenal fatigue by suppressing the need for cortisol output at that time. Interestingly enough, chronic use of this drug has also been shown to inhibit your body's control of blood sugar via your adrenal glands.[20] This means that using Xanax can actually promote the development of disease, such as insulin resistance related to adrenal fatigue.

In Stage 2, cortisol output is like a roller coaster. This causes outshoots of cortisol at random times throughout the day, resulting in symptoms such as anxiety, low blood pressure, high blood pressure, and low blood sugar at random intervals. However, with Xanax to control the anxiety portion of this situation, your cortisol response is suppressed until the drug wears off, perhaps at bedtime—preventing sleep. Blood sugar will also rise when the Xanax wears off, and blood pressure will regulate to your normal level. This also has an impact on your quality of sleep. Typically this is when another Xanax is taken. This is how an addiction to Xanax develops. If your adrenals are fatigued, they overreact and produce anxiety, but if you hinder that process, they will fire more often, resulting in more stress on your body and less rest, which makes you turn to more medication. This drug is not easy to withdraw from.

## Medication and Your Nervous System

The 18th and 19th most commonly prescribed medications are antidepressants, or SSRIs (selective serotonin reuptake inhibitors). These drugs simply recycle serotonin, the neurotransmitter responsible for feelings of happiness; they do not create it. So if you make a low amount of serotonin and you take one of these medications, your body will simply reuse what you have. Unless you address why your serotonin is low in the first place, your body will never start making enough of it and you will stay on the SSRI indefinitely. Antidepressants have their place in medicine, as many people suffer from extreme depression. People have acute grief that requires serotonin support. But many are also pre-scribed an SSRI because they have fatigue or hot flashes or moments of anxiety. In this respect, let us consider the other possibilities for these symptoms before quickly jumping to an SSRI. Adrenal fatigue is a very common cause of depression, hot flashes, insomnia, and anxiety. By lis-tening to what your body is trying to tell you and addressing that pos-sibility first, you might be able to avoid constantly taking medications and further worsening your adrenal fatigue.

## The Acid Problem: Too Much or Too Little?

Omeprazole, or Prilosec, treats heartburn by suppressing the release of gastric acid. Does it seem odd that the purpose of one of the top drugs is to inhibit a normal digestive process? Are our diets so bad that our digestive systems have now adapted to cause more acid production in an attempt to break things down? Or are we treating the wrong cause of gastroesopageal reflux disease (GERD)?

Prilosec is considered a proton pump inhibitor (PPI), meaning that it blocks a certain mechanism responsible for producing hydrochloric acid (HCl) in your stomach. HCl helps you break down proteins and is essential to your digestive process. Common side effects of Prilosec include headaches or abdominal pain with long-term use, and calcium deficiency, putting patients at higher risk of osteoporosis. A 2013 article published in the *Expert Review of Clinical Pharmacology* evaluated the risks of using proton pump inhibitors and advised practitioners to be more vigilant in their counseling about the long-term use of these phar-maceuticals. The side effects of PPIs included pneumonia, *clostridium difficile* (a serious bacterial infection), osteoporosis, high risk of frac-tures, low platelet count, anemia, iron deficiency, low magnesium, low levels of vitamin $B_{12}$, and nephritis (kidney inflammation).[21] And some of these symptoms occurred after only 3 months of use.

In 2011, The FDA issued a warning regarding the higher risk of fractures and impaired magnesium absorption with PPI use.[22] The reality is that Prilosec is likely being used even more than reported, as it is now available as an over-the-counter medication and these statistics are based on prescriptions only. Anyone with heartburn can walk in and buy Prilosec without receiving proper counseling on its side effects. More caution needs to be taken regarding this class of drugs. As we discussed in Chapter 7, the majority of reflux cases are actually a result of low acid, and adding acid has a better effect than blocking it. These low-acid situations are caused by excessive stress, which slows digestion. If adrenal fatigue is the source of your heartburn, then that situation needs to be addressed before you add medications that will counteract normal digestion. Since HCl is required for normal digestion, we should question the common use of the medication and wonder why our nation is so plagued with heartburn. Stress and diet may be key components here, and the use of medication would decrease if those aspects of adrenal fatigue were addressed.

## THE KEY TO ELIMINATING MEDICATION

Medications are an amazing and lifesaving part of any medical practice. They are essential in many cases and can save many lives. I do advise caution, however, when it comes to long-term use of the medications we have discussed. If a medication is needed for a long period of time, then it is imperative that the patient be evaluated for adrenal fatigue. As we have discussed, all of the most-prescribed medications treat symptoms that can be tied back to the adrenal glands. And with 20 percent of Americans taking five or more medications, you have to consider that all of those symptoms can be related to the same cause. And if the cause is adrenal function, then taking those medications may worsen adrenal fatigue, resulting in further symptom development and side effects.

Often, patients are not well informed about potential side effects and in many cases, especially in the elderly population, the patient does not even know what a particular medication is for. It is important for each therapy, whether it is a drug or natural therapy, to be discussed with the patient so that he or she can understand how it works and what the short- and long-term side effects are. This allows the patient to decide whether he or she is comfortable with the proposed therapy. Lifestyle and diet should always be discussed, too, as changes in these areas often eliminate the need for any medication. Your body instinctively knows how to heal and will do so if you allow it to. In order to remove the obstacle to your cure, you may need to reduce the number of medications you use so that your body can inform you of its needs and you can finally support the healing process.

# MY TURNAROUND
## PAT WAREHAM, AGE: 69

Pat Wareham was retired, but she was busier than ever—and her health was in jeopardy. "I just didn't sleep. I was suffering from exhaustion. I was on Temazepam, which was addictive. I had to increase my dose because I *still* couldn't sleep. I also took Ambien and was on it for 10 years," she confesses. "I also had IBS. I've had it practically my whole life—since about age 16."

Restless nights and exhaustion ruled Pat's life. "There's nothing worse than sleep deprivation. I had been struggling with it for 20 years. I couldn't get through the day without needing to take a nap. By 3 p.m., I was struggling to stay awake. My focus wasn't there," she says. Pat was also concerned she was developing Alzheimer's. "What really scared me was the memory loss. That's what really drove me to see Dr. Pingel. In my brain, I knew what I wanted to say, but it wouldn't come out of my mouth. That scared me," she shares.

Finally, Pat decided enough was enough and that she wanted to take a different approach. "I met Dr. Pingel when she was first starting her practice (her mother and stepfather lived next door to me). She came to speak at an event, and I went to see her right away. I was thrilled to learn that I didn't have Alzheimer's, and I didn't suspect that my problems could all be related to adrenal fatigue," she says. "I decided to stop the medication altogether. I also took the vitamins, and that helped tremendously. I had no residuals from it at all."

"After 3 months of following Dr. Pingel's treatment, I started feeling better. I was elated because I could introduce myself back into society again. By nature, I'm an active person. When I was fatigued, I was clearly inactive. I'm a pretty outgoing person, but when you can't come up with words, it's hard to converse, so you withdraw. Now, things are much better, much different. I volunteer at the hospital, I play bridge, I play mahjong...I have a pretty active social life," she says. "Now my IBS is under control."

With her adrenal fatigue under control, Pat's quality of life is much better. "When you're juggling a family, a husband, and a business, it's hard to discern who comes first. With my lack of sleep, it became even more stressful. It's not like that anymore. Those days of sleep deprivation are few and far between."

# PART II

## THE ADRENAL RESTORATION PLAN

# 11

# THE TOTAL HEALTH NUTRITIONAL PLAN

Food is the fuel you need for your body to run from the bear. Without it, you cannot survive. With a nation full of busy people constantly on the go and the need for food to be ready at a moment's notice, we are all consuming a lot of processed foods, which is lowering our intake of nutritional foods and promoting disease.

## WHY YOU SHOULDN'T FOLLOW THE USDA GUIDELINES

According to the USDA, your diet should be made up of five food groups: fruits, vegetables, grains, protein, and dairy. They recommend that half of your plate be filled with fruits and vegetables: 1 to 2 cups of fruit and 2 to 3 cups of vegetables per day. They also recommend that you eat 6 to 8 ounces of grains per day and specify that at least half of those should be whole grains, with processed grains being acceptable for the remaining half. Proteins—meats, nuts, beans, eggs, and processed soy products—have an average recommended daily amount

(RDA) of 6 to 7 ounces for an adult. The dairy group, consisting of animal-based dairy products and fortified soy milk, has an RDA of 3 cups per day. Finally, they recommend that you eat 5 to 7 teaspoons of fats or oils daily. This includes oils in fish, nuts, and dressings.

So let's take a closer look at the proportions of foods the USDA recommends. We'll start with fruits and veggies, which each range from 1 to 3 cups per day. The cup equivalent of the grains RDA is approximately 6 to 7 cups, depending on the grain, and 3 servings of dairy products are recommended. The protein recommendation equals about two palm-size hunks of meat, or ¼ cup of beans, or ½ ounce of nuts. So by looking at this overview, you can see that they are recommending a diet primarily made up of dairy products and grains, with meat coming in third. That leaves our poor fruits and vegetables in the smallest quantity.

Another important point to note is the distinction made about grains. They recommend that at least half be whole grains—but why are they not recommending *all* whole grains? What is the nutritional value of processed white flour, other than empty calories? And with the recommended 3 to 8 cups daily for adults, this seems to be a lot of empty calories.

In addition, with your fat intake limited to a few teaspoons each day, how are you supposed to keep your cells healthy? Even more interestingly, if you visit the USDA Web site, there's actually a chart called "How Many Can I Have?" that tells you how many empty calories you can consume, based on your age and sex. Really? My response is "none"—especially in a nation loaded with obese adults and a rising obesity rate in children. On the site, females between the ages of 31 and 50 are told to consume 1,800 calories a day, with 160 calories being the limit for empty ones. So how does that work? Quite simply, it doesn't.

## CALORIES VERSUS NUTRIENTS: A NEW WAY OF EVALUATING FOOD

So if following the USDA guidelines isn't working for you, what should you do? I have an answer: Do away with calorie counting. In my son's preschool, they were always serving Goldfish Crackers as a snack. I argued against this because I did not see any nutritional value in this snack. What was he getting from that snack? A serving of Goldfish Crackers is about 200 calories, with a whopping 360 mg of sodium, 5 g of protein, and 28 g of carbohydrates (refined). It also contains colored dye, artificial cheese flavoring, and preservatives. By comparison, ½ cup of whole almonds contains more calories (about 250) but has zero sodium, 692 mg of potassium, and 20 g of protein—not to mention the omega-3 fatty acids, magnesium, calcium, zinc, and selenium almonds contain. A handful of almonds is more nutritionally dense than a serving of Goldfish, so why do we feed our children these processed crackers? What are we teaching them? Calories are far less important than the nutrients contained in the foods we eat. How so? Well, let's look at a perfect example of how certain nutrients can counteract the effects of adrenal fatigue.

According to an article published in *Alternative Medicine Review,* a deficiency in vitamin $B_5$, also known as pantethine, can compromise the function of your adrenal cortex. Furthermore, when pantethine was administered to people under stress, it was found to improve their cortisol secretion in response to stress. This indicates that vitamin $B_5$ is a necessary nutrient to maintain or restore normal adrenal function.[1] Notice that there is no mention of an allotment of calories in relation to adrenal health—the study was solely based on nutrients. And likewise, this is how we will approach the dietary plan to restore your adrenal health.

# YOUR ADRENAL RESTORATION NUTRITIONAL PLAN

I know what you're thinking: If I do away with counting calories, how do I know how much to eat? You simply follow my adrenal restoration nutritional plan, which is a whole foods–based diet that's designed to support your adrenal glands by focusing on the specific nutrients needed during each stage of adrenal fatigue. The overall goal of this

## IS YOUR DIET STRESSING YOU OUT?

The idea of *not* counting calories may sound foreign or strange to you, but research shows that calorie counting is an ineffective way to lose weight and restore health.

A 2010 study tested the hypothesis that diets may fail because they increase stress and cortisol levels, both of which are associated with weight gain. During the study, researchers tested two aspects of dieting: restricting calories and monitoring intake. The 121 women in the study were assigned to one of four groups: (1) those who restricted their calorie intake to 1,200 calories per day and monitored calorie intake in a food diary; (2) those who restricted their calorie intake but did not monitor intake; (3) those who monitored their intake but did not restrict calories; and (4) those who neither monitored nor restricted calorie intake. Cortisol levels were measured at the start and end of the 3-week study. Researchers found that restricting calories was associated with increases in cortisol levels, while monitoring calories increased levels of perceived stress.[2]

So what does this mean? It means that diets—especially those that focus on calorie counting—often fail because they're too stressful! And since stress is the root cause of adrenal fatigue, you can say good-bye to calorie counting for good! How's that for good news?

plan is to allow your body to process and eliminate toxins while also supporting your adrenal glands, liver, and digestion. And to do that, you need to follow a few guidelines.

**STAY HYDRATED.** Every day, you must drink at least half your body weight in ounces of water. (Other drinks don't count toward this total—you must drink at least that much pure water.) This means that a 200-pound person should drink at least 100 ounces daily. People in the later stages of adrenal fatigue are often dehydrated, so this guideline is crucial. And if you're looking for a calorie-free drink, pick water. It goes right into your cells and balances the minerals your adrenal glands need for normal function. You may choose to drink home-brewed herbal tea, as well.

**EAT MORE, NOT LESS.** The number one thing that will worsen your adrenal fatigue is starving your body. Unfortunately, that is what most people do when they are worried about weight gain but lack the motivation to exercise. They seek diet plans that will help them drop weight quickly, which is not the goal of your adrenal glands. When you have adrenal fatigue, your body will actually store fat so that it is available to provide energy. So if you are not feeding your body the nutrients it needs, then your body will store more fat and eat away at your muscles. The goal of dietary therapy in this case is to get you the proper nutrients you need to replenish what you are currently using to get through your day. And this requires you to eat more, not less.

**AVOID PROCESSED FOODS.** Eliminating calorie counting does not give you license to eat 5,000 calories a day. Luckily, you will find that by eliminating processed foods, you will also eliminate a lot of the empty calories in your day—and this supports your weight loss goals in addition to restoring normal adrenal function. Sounds like a win-win situation, right? The beauty of aligning your diet in this way is that it allows you to eat a larger volume of food while having a positive impact on your waistline.

To treat your adrenal fatigue, focus on the nutrients in your food, not the calories. The protein section of the USDA's Web site states that processed soy products are allowed, but as you learned in Chapter 9, processing food removes minerals—the very minerals that your body needs to combat adrenal fatigue. In addition, "diet" foods are not an option because artificial sweeteners, dyes, and additives cause more stress on your body, thereby worsening your adrenal fatigue. So just say no to processed, prepackaged foods.

**FOCUS ON EATING VEGETABLES, FRUITS, WHOLE GRAINS, AND PROTEIN IN A PREDICTABLE PATTERN.** By focusing on whole foods such as these, you'll not only supply your body with the nutrients being depleted by your adrenal fatigue, but you'll also help keep your metabolism high, which aids in weight maintenance or even weight loss. Your diet should be predictable to your body but variable for your palate—meaning that you should eat a variety of fruits and vegetables at regular intervals each day. You should never leave your body wondering when it will next receive nutrition. You have to keep it fed. In fact, during some stages of adrenal fatigue (such as Stages 1 and 2) where digestion is affected, you have to keep a variety of foods circulating so that your body does not develop intolerances to foods due to slowed digestion from poor adrenal output.

Although they aren't an absolute requirement, gluten-free grains are your best option. Your diet should be more focused on alternative grains such as brown or wild rice, quinoa, oats, buckwheat, amaranth, and spelt because they have a higher nutritional and mineral content. In addition, use nut-based flours to provide protein and good fat support. Protein should consist of GMO-free fermented soy (tofu), beans, lentils, nuts, hummus, wild-caught Pacific fish, organic eggs, organic chicken, and wild game meats.

**ELIMINATE DAIRY PRODUCTS.** Wait, what? If you're eliminating dairy products from your diet, how on earth will you get your calcium? Well, if you cover your plate with vegetables, you will have your calcium (see the chart on the next page). And those necessary fats that are so abundant in dairy? You can get them from your daily protein sources.

**DETERMINE YOUR PORTION BREAKDOWN BY YOUR STAGE OF ADRENAL FATIGUE.** Because your body desperately needs certain nutrients to restore the health of your adrenal glands, you're going to focus on eating nutrient-rich foods and vegetables. On average, your meal breakdown will look like this: 50 percent vegetables, 20 percent fruits, 15 percent whole grains, and 15 percent proteins. This means that 70 percent of your plate is filled with the vitamins and minerals required to reverse your adrenal fatigue. For protein, I want you to take a good look at plant-based proteins, such as tofu, nuts, lentils, and other legumes. Twice a week, you can eat wild-caught seafood or lean, organic, hormone-free poultry or meat as part of this group, but in smaller amounts (3 ounces per day).

# FOOD SOURCES FOR YOUR REQUIRED NUTRIENTS

Below you'll find some great food sources for the nutrients you need to replenish during each stage of adrenal fatigue. These lists are by no means exhaustive, but they'll serve as a great jumping-off point.

**BORON**

Almonds

Apricots (dried)

Avocadoes

Beans (especially red kidney)

Brazil nuts

Broccoli

Carrots

Cashews (raw)

Celery

Chickpeas

Grapes (red)

Hazelnuts

Honey

Lentils

Olives

Onions

Peaches

Peanut butter

Pears

Prunes

Raisins

Walnuts

**CALCIUM**

Almonds

Brazil nuts

Broccoli

Chinese cabbage (called pak choi or bok choy)

Dark green leafy vegetables (especially spinach, Swiss chard, beet greens, kale)

Fish (herring, pike, bass, perch, rainbow trout, pollack)

Flaxseed

Green beans

Lettuce (especially green leaf)

Okra (cooked)

Parsley

Rhubarb

Sesame seeds

Tofu

**MAGNESIUM**

Almonds

Cashews

Legumes

Oatmeal

*(continued)*

Spinach

Wheat bran

### MANGANESE

Chili powder

Cocoa powder and dark
chocolate

Flax

Nuts (hazelnuts, pine nuts,
and pecans)

Pumpkin and squash seeds
(roasted)

Sesame seeds and sesame butter
(tahini)

Shellfish

Soybeans (roasted,
edamame)

Spices and herbs (especially
cloves and saffron)

Sunflower seeds

Wheat germ and bran
(especially rice bran and
oat bran)

### OMEGA-3 FATTY ACIDS

Fish (especially salmon, snapper,
tuna, and halibut)

Flaxseed

Shellfish (especially scallops
and shrimp)

Soybeans (whole)

Tofu

Walnuts

### POTASSIUM

Acorn squash (baked)

Apricots (dried)

Avocados

Bananas

Cocoa powder and dark
chocolate

Dark leafy greens (especially
spinach)

Fish (especially salmon)

Herbs (dried, especially parsley,
chervil, coriander, basil, and
dill)

Mushrooms (especially white)

Nuts and seeds (pistachios,
chestnuts, almonds, cashews,
walnuts, squash seeds,
pumpkin seeds, and
sunflower seeds)

Potatoes (baked, with skin)

Rice bran

Soybeans (dry roasted)

Sun-dried tomatoes

White beans

### SELENIUM

Asparagus

Beef

Brazil nuts

Chia seeds

Fish (especially yellowfin tuna)

Lamb

Mushrooms (especially crimini)

Oat bran
Peanut butter
Poultry
Shellfish
Sunflower seeds
Whole grains

**SILICON**

Barley
Oats
Rice

**STRONTIUM**

Leafy green vegetables
(especially spinach and kale)
Legumes
Root vegetables
Seafood
Spices
Whole grains

**VITAMIN B$_5$**

Avocados
Brewer's yeast
Broccoli
Cauliflower
Corn
Eggs
Fish and shellfish
Kale
Legumes (especially lentils and
split peas)

Meat
Sunflower seeds
Sweet potatoes
Tomatoes

**VITAMIN B$_6$**

Bananas
Beef
Brussels sprouts
Chickpeas
Fish (especially salmon
and tuna)
Nuts
Potatoes
Poultry
Raisins
Rice
Spinach
Squash
Tofu

**VITAMIN B$_{12}$**

Beef
Eggs
Fish (especially tuna)
Liver
Lamb
Poultry
Shellfish (especially clams,
lobster, and crab)
Tofu

*(continued)*

## VITAMIN C

Banana peppers

Bell peppers

Black currants

Broccoli

Brussels sprouts

Cabbage (red)

Cantaloupe

Cauliflower

Chives

Clementines

Dark leafy greens (especially kale, mustard greens, watercress)

Guavas

Herbs (fresh, especially thyme and parsley)

Hot chile peppers (red and green)

Kiwi

Lemons

Mangoes

Oranges

Papaya

Pineapples

Strawberries

Tomatoes

Turnip greens

## VITAMIN D

Beef liver

Cod liver oil

Eggs

Fish and shellfish

Mushrooms (especially maitake and shiitake)

Tofu

## VITAMIN K

Asparagus

Broccoli

Brussels sprouts

Cabbage

Carrots

Dark leafy greens

Herbs (dried and fresh, especially dried basil, dried sage, and dried thyme)

Okra

Pickled cucumber

Prunes

Spring onions (scallions)

Sun-dried tomatoes

## ZINC

Almonds

Beans

Beef

Cabbage

Cashews

Oatmeal

Parsley

Peas

Pumpkin seeds

Shellfish

Spinach

# Customizing Your Adrenal Restoration Nutritional Plan

Now, I must state that this diet will not work perfectly for everyone. Everyone is different, so you might need to make modifications based on your personal history and current weight. For example, if you have a horrible chronic candida (yeast) issue, you should cut back on your fruit intake. If you have an allergy to nuts, you will need to find other protein sources. Your blood type may also play a role. People with type O blood tend to need more protein than people with type A, so they may need to focus on how to add more protein, such as by choosing mushrooms as one of their veggies instead of romaine lettuce. There are modifications for everything, but in general, you can reverse disease processes by focusing on what you are putting in your mouth.

This diet will apply to all stages of adrenal fatigue, though in some cases, additional modifications can be made for even more benefit. To get you started, I've provided the breakdown of meals and nutritional requirements for each stage of adrenal fatigue. Note that each meal should serve as a guide for how you can begin to heal your adrenal glands through nutrition. There are three starter meal plans—one for each stage of adrenal fatigue. These plans will also show you how your daily meals will change as you transition from one stage to the next on your path to total health. To determine when you're ready to move on to the next stage of the plan, retake the questionnaire in Chapter 1. I also recommend that you discuss any dietary changes with your doctor beforehand. Each plan contains a combination of original meal ideas that I have found helpful in reversing adrenal fatigue, along with recipes from Part 3 of this book (listed in italics).

## Stage 3 Nutritional Plan

**OVERVIEW:** The goal in Stage 3 is to minimize further stress and rebuild your body. During Stage 3 adrenal fatigue you are likely sedentary due

*(continued on page 216)*

# STAGE 3 NUTRITION PLAN

## DAY 1

**MEAL 1:** *Open-Face Egg Sandwich* (page 312)

**MEAL 2:** ½ cup mix of almonds and peach slices

**MEAL 3:** Mexican Quinoa: quinoa topped with black beans, salsa, corn, bell peppers, sliced avocado, garlic, and onion

**MEAL 4:** *Peach Blueberry Smoothie* (page 336)

**MEAL 5:** *Chicken Peanut Noodle Bowl* (page 325, Stage 3 adaptation)

## DAY 2

**MEAL 1:** Small bowl of fresh granola with nuts, sliced pear or a handful of berries, and plain soy yogurt

**MEAL 2:** *Cucumber Boats* (page 335)

**MEAL 3:** *Mediterranean Chopped Salad* (page 323, Stage 3 adaptation)

**MEAL 4:** 1 cup mix of cashews and raisins

**MEAL 5:** *Chicken Tortilla Soup* (page 333)

## DAY 3

**MEAL 1:** *Savory Oatmeal* (page 313)

**MEAL 2:** *Nutty Celery Sticks*, 2 servings (page 337)

**MEAL 3:** *Kicked-Up Bean Tostadas* (page 322)

**MEAL 4:** 1 cup green juice/smoothie: handful of kale, 1 cucumber, 1 celery stick, 1 large carrot, ½ cup almond milk, and ¼ cup strawberries

**MEAL 5:** Homemade tacos: hard-shell tacos filled with shredded cabbage, shredded carrots, avocado, tomato, black beans, nut-based cheese (such as Parmela), and salsa; serve with small side of fruit

## DAY 4

**MEAL 1:** *Honeydew Cucumber Smoothie* (page 303, Stage 3 adaptation)

**MEAL 2:** 1 cup mixed berries topped with walnuts

**MEAL 3:** Greek Quinoa: quinoa topped with black olives, tomatoes, garlic, red onion, lemon juice, olive oil, and a dash of red wine vinegar; sprinkle with a nut-based cheese

**MEAL 4:** *3-Layer Mexican Dip* (page 336)

**MEAL 5:** *Steamed Vegetables with Red Pepper Sauce* (page 334)

## DAY 5

**MEAL 1:** *Brown Rice Bowl* (page 314)

**MEAL 2:** 1 cup fresh juice of choice

**MEAL 3:** *Mediterranean Chopped Salad* (page 323)

**MEAL 4:** *Peach Blueberry Smoothie* (page 336)

**MEAL 5:** Sauté cauliflower, broccoli, bell pepper, squash, onion, sweet potato, shallots, cabbage, snow peas, carrots, and bok choy in peanut oil or coconut oil; serve over ½ cup quinoa and top with peanut sauce

## DAY 6

**MEAL 1:** *Honeydew Cucumber Smoothie* (page 303, Stage 3 adaptation)

**MEAL 2:** 1 cup raw veggies with hummus

**MEAL 3:** *Moroccan Stuffed Peppers* (page 321, Stage 3 adaptation)

**MEAL 4:** Gluten-free crackers topped with your choice of nut butter, ½ cup berries

**MEAL 5:** *Black Bean Stew* (page 332)

## DAY 7

**MEAL 1:** *Amaranth Vegetable Omelet* (page 311)

**MEAL 2:** 1 cup mixed berries topped with walnuts

**MEAL 3:** *Salmon and Soba Miso Soup* (page 324)

**MEAL 4:** 1 cup fresh juice of choice

**MEAL 5:** Tofu and seasonal veggies sautéed with coconut oil; serve over ½ cup quinoa or brown rice and top with lemon zest, squeeze of lemon, ground pepper, and a splash of balsamic vinegar to extreme exhaustion, and therefore you require a different diet than those in Stage 1. Water is incredibly important, but absorption is often poor due to adrenal fatigue, so it's a good idea to add water-rich veggies that have a high mineral content such as cucumbers, celery, radishes, tomatoes, green peppers, etc. Also, you will find it beneficial to add coconut water to many of your meals to avoid dehydration.

In Stage 3, you often require a greater salt intake, as low blood pressure is typical of this stage. Protein amounts are a little larger in this stage than in others, and you can incorporate animal protein sources, but they must still be lean. As always, it's preferable to get your protein from vegetables, fish, eggs, legumes, or nuts.

**MEAL BREAKOUT:** You'll eat five or six small meals daily. During Stage 3, the focus is on replenishing your nutrients. You need lots of omega-3 fatty acids, minerals, and B vitamins. Stage 3 adrenal fatigue requires more vegetables, as you need to restock your exhausted supply of nutrients. Focus on having at least three different vegetables at each meal, and during this stage, these veggies should make up about 60 percent of your meal. The amount of fruit and grains should be smaller, and they should treated as side dishes. Because it's difficult to digest, it's best to spread your protein intake throughout the day.

**PRIMARY NUTRIENTS REQUIRED IN YOUR DAILY DIET:** Omega-3 fatty acids, vitamin $B_5$, vitamin $B_6$, vitamin $B_{12}$, calcium, vitamin D, manganese, boron, strontium, vitamin K, silicon, and magnesium. (See "Food Sources for Your Required Nutrients" on pages 209–212.)

## Stage 2 Nutritional Plan

**OVERVIEW:** This is the roller coaster stage, so you have to pay special attention to the predictability of your meals. As a result, when you're in Stage 2 you need more and smaller meals in general. Insulin sensitivity is changing, so you need to stay away from excessive carbohydrates. Unlike people in Stage 1, who can have more calorically dense foods, you'll need to pick nonstarchy vegetables.

I encourage Stage 2 patients to avoid gluten, as it can affect insulin

# STAGE 2 NUTRITION PLAN

## DAY 1

**MEAL 1:** *Eggs Pipérade* (page 308)

**MEAL 2:** 1 cup mixed berries topped with chopped almonds

**MEAL 3:** *Mediterranean Chopped Salad* (page 320, Stage 2 adaptation)

**MEAL 4:** 2 cups baby carrots with side of hummus

**MEAL 5:** *Chicken Peanut Noodle Bowl* (page 325, Stage 2 adaptation)

## DAY 2

**MEAL 1:** *Savory Oatmeal* (page 313, Stage 2 adaptation)

**MEAL 2:** 1 cup mix of walnuts and raisins

**MEAL 3:** Quinoa Primavera: quinoa topped with cucumber, cherry tomatoes, broccoli, zucchini, walnuts, and vegan/gluten-free Italian dressing

**MEAL 4:** *Honeydew Cucumber Smoothie* (page 336, Stage 2 adaptation)

**MEAL 5:** *Roasted Root Vegetables* (page 330)

## DAY 3

**MEAL 1:** 1 egg scrambled with 1 teaspoon of ground flaxseeds and a sprinkle of vegan cheese; serve on gluten-free toast with sliced avocado

**MEAL 2:** ½ cup mix of almonds and peach slices

**MEAL 3:** *Zesty Pasta Salad* (page 318, Stage 2 adaptation)

**MEAL 4:** Four rice cakes spread with 2 tablespoons of cashew butter

**MEAL 5:** Tofu and seasonal veggies sautéed with coconut oil, served over ½ cup quinoa or brown rice and topped with lemon zest, squeeze of lemon, ground pepper, and a splash of balsamic vinegar

## DAY 4

**MEAL 1:** *Mexican Breakfast Burrito* (page 307)

**MEAL 2:** *Guacamole Deviled Eggs, 2 servings* (page 335)

**MEAL 3:** *Moroccan Stuffed Peppers* (page 321)

**MEAL 4:** ½ cup walnuts and a sliced orange

**MEAL 5:** *Tomato-Watermelon Gazpacho* (page 331)

*(continued)*

## STAGE 2 NUTRITION PLAN (cont.)

### DAY 5

**MEAL 1:** *Smoky Lentil, Egg, and Mushroom Skillet* (page 309)

**MEAL 2:** Gluten-free crackers topped with your choice of nut butter; serve with ½ cup berries

**MEAL 3:** ½ collard wrap filled with green peppers, carrots, cabbage, avocado, almond butter, and fresh lemon juice; serve with a vegan, organic soup of choice

**MEAL 4:** *Nutty Celery Sticks*, 2 servings (page 337)

**MEAL 5:** *Steamed Vegetables with Red Pepper Sauce* (page 334, Stage 2 adaptation)

### DAY 6

**MEAL 1:** Small bowl of fresh granola with nuts, sliced apple or a handful of berries, and plain soy yogurt with a drizzle of honey

**MEAL 2:** *Peach Blueberry Smoothie* (page 336)

**MEAL 3:** *Asparagus and Shrimp Stir-Fry* (page 319)

**MEAL 4:** 1 cup mix of cashews and raisins

**MEAL 5:** *Broccoli Rabe and Bean Sauté* (page 329)

### DAY 7

**MEAL 1:** *Quinoa and Butternut Breakfast Bowl* (page 310)

**MEAL 2:** *Quick Bean Burrito* (page 335)

**MEAL 3:** Collard wrap filled with green peppers, carrots, cabbage, avocado, almond butter, and fresh lemon juice; serve with a broccoli-based soup

**MEAL 4:** *Smoked Salmon on Cucumber Slices* (page 337)

**MEAL 5:** *Black Bean Stew* (page 327, Stage 2 adaptation)

sensitivity. No muffins, heavy pasta dishes, or sandwiches made with bread (unless it's gluten free). Instead, when choosing grains, I have patients focus on quinoa, brown rice, amaranth, sorghum, teff, millet, oats, wild rice, and buckwheat. Sweet potatoes are a fabulous source of vitamins for Stage 1, but they fall into the starchy vegetable category and so would be better avoided during Stage 2, when people are having issues with insulin.

Protein is important, but consume it primarily in the form of nuts, seeds, high-protein veggies, and tofu. I encourage a more vegan diet during this stage, as animal-based protein is more likely to cause inflammation. Try to stick with meals that are lower in both salt and sugar due to the likelihood of yeast development and higher blood pressure during this stage.

**MEAL BREAKDOWN:** You'll eat five or six small meals daily, and some meals can in fact be large snacks. Each meal should contain at least three different vegetables, which should make up half of your meal. Your fruit should be colorful—think peaches, kiwi, papaya, mango, berries, pomegranate, citrus, cherries, and plums. Apples, pears, and bananas should be limited due to their high sugar levels. Proteins should come from plant sources only.

**PRIMARY NUTRIENTS REQUIRED IN YOUR DAILY DIET:** Vitamin C, zinc, selenium, omega-3 fatty acids, vitamin $B_5$, vitamin $B_6$, vitamin $B_{12}$, and magnesium. (See "Food Sources for Your Required Nutrients" on page 209.)

## Stage 1 Nutritional Plan

**OVERVIEW:** In Stage 1, you have a higher requirement for fast nutrition because you have slowing digestion and need more energy to get through the day. You can eat more natural sugar (fruit) during this stage than the others because fruit will help maintain your blood sugar levels. You can also afford to eat more food than someone in Stage 2 or 3 because you have a more active lifestyle. You can eat sodium without

(continued on page 222)

# STAGE 1 NUTRITION PLAN

## DAY 1

**BREAKFAST:** *Honeydew Cucumber Smoothie* (page 303)

**SNACK:** Two rice cakes spread with 1 tablespoon of cashew butter

**LUNCH:** Fruity Quinoa: quinoa topped with dried apricots, raisins or cranberries, avocado, pine nuts or walnuts, red onion, chickpeas, and raspberry vinaigrette

**SNACK:** *Smoked Salmon on Cucumber Slices* (page 337)

**DINNER:** *Hearty Chili* (page 328)

## DAY 2

**BREAKFAST:** *Tofu Scramble with Peppers and Mushrooms* (page 306)

**SNACK:** Gluten-free crackers topped with your choice of nut butter; serve with ¼ cup berries

**LUNCH:** *Mediterranean Chopped Salad* (page 323, Stage 1 adaptation)

**SNACK:** ½ cup mix of cashews and raisins

**DINNER:** *Roasted Root Vegetables* (page 330, Stage 1 adaptation)

## DAY 3

**BREAKFAST:** *Quinoa and Butternut Breakfast Bowl* (page 310, Stage 1 adaptation)

**SNACK:** Celery sticks filled with almond butter and topped with dried cranberries

**LUNCH:** *Zesty Pasta Salad* (page 318)

**SNACK:** Handful of walnuts and orange slices

**DINNER:** *Chicken Peanut Noodle Bowl* (page 325)

## DAY 4

**BREAKFAST:** Small bowl of fresh granola with nuts, ½ banana or a handful of berries, and plain soy yogurt with a drizzle of honey; serve with a side of 2 eggs scrambled with green peppers and onions

**SNACK:** 1 cup baby carrots with hummus

**LUNCH:** *Rustic Lentil Soup* (page 316) and side salad with honey-lemon dressing

**SNACK:** Handful of almonds and peach slices

**DINNER:** *Quinoa Tabbouleh* (page 326)

## DAY 5

**BREAKFAST:** *Sweet Potato Hash* (page 305)

**SNACK:** ½ cup mixed berries topped with chopped almonds

**LUNCH:** Collard wrap filled with green peppers, carrots, cabbage, avocado, almond butter, and fresh lemon juice; serve with a broccoli-based soup

**SNACK:** *Guacamole Deviled Eggs* (page 335)

**DINNER:** *Grilled Tuna and Mango Salad* (page 327)

## DAY 6

**BREAKFAST:** 1 egg scrambled with 1 teaspoon of ground flaxseeds and vegan cheese; serve on gluten-free bread with avocado slices

**SNACK:** *Chocolate Lover's Trail Mix* (page 337)

**LUNCH:** *Grilled Portobello and Hummus Stacks* (page 315)

**SNACK:** Gluten-free crackers topped with your choice of nut butter

**DINNER:** Homemade hard-shell tacos filled with shredded cabbage, shredded carrots, avocado, tomato, black beans, nut-based cheese (such as Parmela), and salsa

## DAY 7

**BREAKFAST:** *Honeydew Cucumber Smoothie* (page 304)

**SNACK:** ½ cup mix of walnuts and raisins

**LUNCH:** *Speedy Salmon Wrap* (page 317)

**SNACK:** *Fresh Fruit Salad Cup* (page 336)

**DINNER:** Tofu and seasonal veggies sautéed with coconut oil; serve over 1 cup quinoa or brown rice and top with lemon zest, squeeze of lemon, ground pepper, and a splash of balsamic vinegar much negative impact because you probably have low blood pressure.

In Stage 1, you also benefit more from liquid-based foods, such as soups and smoothies, because of your suppressed digestion. Your B vitamin requirement is likely higher because you are constantly using up your supply. If you can supply nutrients in higher than average amounts during this stage, you can prevent the development of Stage 2 adrenal fatigue.

**MEAL BREAKDOWN:** You'll eat three main meals and two snacks daily. Breakfast should be a substantial meal and have more nutritional value than both lunch and dinner, meaning it may be your largest meal of the day. Each meal should contain at least three different vegetables, which should make up half of the meal. Your fruit should be colorful—think peaches, kiwi, papaya, mango, berries, pomegranate, citrus, cherries, and plums. Apples, pears, and bananas should be limited due to their high sugar levels. In general, snacks should be small and should contain both a source of protein and a carbohydrate.

**PRIMARY NUTRIENTS REQUIRED IN YOUR DAILY DIET:** Vitamin $B_5$, vitamin $B_6$, vitamin $B_{12}$, potassium, magnesium, and omega-3 fatty acids. (See "Food Sources for Your Required Nutrients" on page 209.)

# MY TURNAROUND
## TEAL TERRELL, AGE: 35

Several years ago, Teal Terrell struggled with pain every day. "I had severe joint pain and was extremely tired. One day I would have terrible anxiety and heart palpitations, and the next day I would be exhausted and couldn't get out of bed. My feet and hands were so bad I could barely walk or hold a coffee mug," she reveals. "After having an emergency c-section with my second child, I never felt right. I knew that something else was going on, but I just kept going through each day hoping that tomorrow I would feel like myself again, until one day when I could barely get out of bed."

That's when Teal was diagnosed. "I had all kinds of testing done, including RA, MS . . . every autoimmune disease. I was diagnosed with Hashimoto's thyroiditis and was told by my MD that Synthroid was my only option. When asked if he would be willing to check my adrenals, his response was, 'Why would I do that? You have a thyroid issue.' I knew that would be the last time I was in his office," she shares. "At 35 years old, I was determined that I wasn't going to live the rest of my life feeling this way. So I began my journey and started researching everything I could on Hashimoto's, which led me to discovering adrenal fatigue. Then, I found Dr. Pingel, who specializes in treating adrenal fatigue and thyroid issues."

Following Dr. Pingel's plan, Teal modified her diet and began taking supplements. "I was always a healthy eater, but I am more aware now of how certain foods (dairy, gluten) can create inflammation in the body, so I try to limit my daily intake of them. I have been able to add gluten back into my diet again, as long as I monitor how much of it I have," she says. "Within a month of the treatment plan, I started to notice a difference. I was walking easier, had more energy, and the daily ups and downs were starting to regulate a bit. My joint pain was starting to decrease as well. By August 2013, I was showing no signs of the Hashimoto's marker in my blood work, and I was off my medication."

Today, Teal is living a happier, healthier life. "Everything, from making dinner and taking care of my kids, to working as a therapist, spending quality time with my husband, and maintaining the house, is so much easier. My friends and family notice that I have more energy and am smiling more now," she says. "I can finally be me again."

# 12

# HEALING WITH NATURE'S PHARMACY

When it comes to adrenal fatigue, herbal therapies play a huge role in treatment. The key to the effectiveness of using these herbs relies in the blend that is chosen. For example, rhodiola, an herb commonly used in the treatment of adrenal fatigue and known for its effects on depression and generalized fatigue, works much better when combined with other herbs than it does when used all by itself. This is because herbal therapies are synergistic and should be used as such.

Nutritional therapies, such as amino acids and fatty acids, are another important aspect of treatment. Treating adrenal fatigue is an art, not a science, in that each patient is different and therefore each treatment will affect each person differently. In this chapter, we will review some of the most common natural therapies used to treat and reverse adrenal fatigue and explore the research surrounding their many effects on your body. And by utilizing Nature's pharmacy, you will be able to avoid using pharmaceuticals and support the repair and healing of this amazing gland.

# HERBS FOR COMBATING ADRENAL FATIGUE

There are numerous herbs used to heal the adrenal glands, all with different characteristics and indications. Finding the perfect blend can be tricky. All of these herbs are available in liquid (tincture) and capsule preparations. I prefer the liquids because it's easy to create a customized blend based on an individual's needs, but capsules will also produce the desired effect.

With the aid of a doctor who is familiar with herbal therapies, you can determine the perfect blend for your body, which depends on your stage of fatigue as well as your diet and any other medical conditions you may currently be facing. In this section, we will discuss the most common herbs used to treat adrenal fatigue and its symptoms.

## Beneficial for All Stages

The following herbs and amino acids are beneficial for all stages of adrenal fatigue. While each stage may require a different amount or concentration of these herbs, all support the health of your adrenal glands.

### L-Theanine

This amino acid is found in green tea and in some mushrooms. When used in conjunction with other therapies, L-theanine has a significant impact on sleep, mood, and anxiety.[1] L-theanine is a precursor to the production of serotonin and gamma-aminobutyric acid (GABA), making it a great substitute for antidepressants and anti-anxiety medications. In fact, it has historically been used as a relaxant due to these properties. It has been shown to produce a tranquil state, making it a great sleep aide that doesn't have the side effects of traditional sedatives.[2] It is mild and gives your body the tools it requires to produce what is needed. It will improve your mental state and is great when used in combination with other herbs for adrenal fatigue.

## Lavender

An herb that I use regularly due to its amazing synergistic effects, lavender is fantastic for treating Stage 1 adrenal fatigue because it calms you, induces rest, reduces nervousness, improves headaches, reduces gastrointestinal bloating and infection, reduces nausea and loss of appetite, and smells heavenly.[3] In a 2012 trial, 129 headaches were treated with lavender oil that was placed under the participants' noses and inhaled. Of those treated, 92 responded completely or partially, compared to only 32 out of 68 in the placebo group.[4] Many people, particularly those in Stage 1 or 2 adrenal fatigue, use lavender oil under their noses or on their pillows to help with sleep. Some inhale it, which has been shown to help treat insomnia, pain, migraines, and agitation related to dementia. One study found that dementia-related agitative behaviors were significantly reduced when lavender was used as an inhalant. This study's authors deduced that lavender is a strong alternative to antipsychotic medication in these patients.[5]

A small preliminary study on healthy young adults reported less morning sleepiness when a piece of gauze soaked in lavender oil was left on the subjects' bedside tables overnight for 5 nights.[6] Research also shows that inhaled lavender can be used by itself as a treatment for mild insomnia.[7] It has also been proven to improve psychological well-being: Research has shown that adding 3 ml of a 20 percent lavender oil and 80 percent grapeseed oil mixture to daily baths produces significant improvements in mood.[8]

Many studies are evaluating the use of lavender as a substitute for the highly addictive benzodiazepines used to treat anxiety. Two studies, both completed in 2010, showed that lavender was comparable to lorazepam when used to reduce anxiety.[9] In fact, these studies have prompted physicians to use lavender to help patients deal with the symptoms of benzodiazepine withdrawal. Lavender reduces anxiety for those in Stage 2 adrenal fatigue and lifts the moods of those in Stage 3. It may be used regularly and is relatively safe, with minimal side effects. When used externally in large amounts, it may cause a burning sensation, so there are some restrictions. When using it topically, combine it with other oils or use small amounts at a time to reduce this side effect.

## Passiflora

This is another sedative herb that is used to reduce anxiety, decrease pain, improve nervousness, reduce palpitations due to anxiety, lower blood pressure, correct cardiac rhythm abnormalities, and assist with opioid withdrawal.[10] It has been researched quite a bit in regard to general anxiety disorder and adjustment disorder. One study released in 2001 found that a daily dose of 45 drops of liquid passiflora extract was comparable in effect to 30 mg of oxazepam, a benzodiazepine used to treat anxiety disorder.[11] Another study showed that at 90 mg a day, the symptoms of nonspecific anxiety are comparable to mexazolam, another popular drug for anxiety.[12]

I call passiflora the "antiworry" herb because in herbal medicine, it is typically indicated for those who worry a lot or wake at night with worries. When used topically, it helps with burns, inflammation, and hemorrhoids.[13] The majority of passiflora research studying the herb's anti-anxiety effects focused on a combination product that included passiflora and a variety of other sedative herbs. Sample sizes were small, and there are few studies with statistical evidence concerning the use of passiflora for anxiety reduction. But I encourage you to pay attention to the studies that show a decrease in anxiety when this herb is combined with other herbs. Recall that herbs work best in synergy, not by themselves. Passiflora is no exception. I find it to be a fabulous addition to tinctures made for sleep, reduction in sympathetic output, and general anxiety disorder. My patients see a great benefit when I add it to their existing protocols. Because it is not as strong as its primary herbal counterpart, valerian, it can be used during virtually any stage of adrenal fatigue and reduces the anxiety and fear associated with elevated cortisol output. This herb is relatively safe to use, except during pregnancy.

## Rhodiola

Used in traditional Chinese medicine (TCM) for over 1,000 years, this herb grows in mountain regions throughout the Arctic, Europe, and Asia. It has been proven beneficial in improving mood and depression, and also in treating opioid addiction.[14] The key to rhodiola's effectiveness is its ability to mediate serotonin and dopamine levels, similar to monoamine oxidase inhibitors (MAOIs) used for treatment of depression (which are hardly used by physicians anymore due to the vast side effects of these drugs).

Rhodiola is an adaptogen, meaning it can cause adaptation in your body. Now think about this: In order to manage the constant stress of running from that bear, your body adapted to its surroundings. Instead of handling the stress of the bear as you did previously, now you have anxiety over it, plus insomnia. It was adaptation that caused the development of these symptoms, and therefore another adaptation is required to repair your system. Rhodiola is fantastic at repair and reversal! In either liquid or capsule form, rhodiola is used to increase energy and mental capacity. As an adaptogen, it assists your body in adapting to and resisting stress, whether that stress is physical, emotional, or chemical.

Rhodiola has been shown to improve sexual function, athletic performance, depression, and anxiety. It is also used to treat heart rhythm irregularities, cancer, tuberculosis, and diabetes, and it will prevent infections such as the common cold, flu, and other viral illnesses.[15] Although research is still underway, many recent studies have examined its effects on bladder cancer, improvement of athletic performance by reducing time to exhaustion, and improving mental clarity and mental fatigue.[16] It has also been shown to reduce generalized anxiety disorder after only 10 weeks of therapy.[17] Rhodiola was shown to have a positive effect on mild to moderate depression symptoms after only 6 weeks of once-daily dosing.[18] This herb fits in well with depression therapy as it has a direct effect on your neurotransmitters without the side effects of traditional medication. In addition, it has been proven beneficial in treating the endocrine system by lowering cortisol, thereby reducing anxiety.[19]

Most people know rhodiola as an herb that reduces fatigue. And considering the major impact fatigue has in America, this herb is one to be strongly considered in most therapeutic protocols when treating adrenal fatigue. Rhodiola has been shown to benefit the two different types of fatigue: fatigue created by physical activity and fatigue created by sleep deprivation. A study completed in 2012 examined electronic databases of studies surrounding rhodiola's effect on fatigue and found that rhodiola improved mental fatigue as well as physical fatigue from exercise.[20] And in a 2009 trial, 60 subjects with stress-related fatigue were given either a product containing rhodiola or a placebo twice a day for 4 weeks. The rhodiola group experienced improved concentration, which was attributed to decreased stress-related fatigue, and significant decreases in salivary cortisol compared to the placebo group.[21]

It is also a powerful antioxidant and beneficial in cancer prevention.[22] Another very interesting finding is that this herb has the ability to reduce binge-related eating disorders. In a 2010 study conducted on rats, researchers found that binge eating is related to stressful situations, and due to rhodiola's massive impact on stress management within the body, use of this herb abolished binge eating episodes entirely. In addition, the researchers also confirmed a lower cortisol release during the binge episode, proving its effect on blunting excessive cortisol output.[23]

This herb is incredibly safe, as there are no known interactions with other drugs, and it has not been shown to have any adverse effects during its clinical trials.[24] It calms those in Stage 1 and prevents further symptoms from developing. It lowers anxiety and depression for those in Stage 2, and it prevents further adaptation by your immune system, which typically occurs right before Stage 3. Rhodiola also combats fatigue and allows for better adaption to stress-related activities during all stages. In Stage 3, it prevents cancer from developing, thwarts immune depression, and supports energy. As a synergistic herb, it works best when blended with other herbs like glycyrrhiza, ginseng, schisandra, astragalus, and ashwagandha. It can be taken in capsule or liquid form, and dosage amounts should be discussed with your physician.

# Herbs Beneficial for Different Stages of Adrenal Fatigue

The following herbs have benefits specific to different stages of adrenal fatigue and are listed in order from Stage 1 to Stage 3. Note that some of these herbs may include beneficial properties that span two stages.

## Schisandra Berry

One of my favorite herbs is the schisandra berry. The reason I love this berry is that it has properties that aid in mental clarity but does not contain the stimulatory effect found in other herbs that support the adrenal glands. Schisandra is a fantastic herb for those in Stage 1 adrenal fatigue because it increases focus yet has the ability to calm the strong output of your adrenal glands. Research boasts that this berry resists disease and stress, increases energy, improves cellular functions, aids in liver protection, prevents premature aging, improves premenstrual syndrome, stimulates immune function, speeds recovery after surgery, reduces blood sugar and blood pressure, prevents motion sickness, reduces cholesterol, and improves insomnia. Many patients take it solely for memory loss reversal.[25]

Schisandra, commonly known as *Wu Wei Zi*, is a climbing vine found throughout easternmost Russia, Korea, Japan, and northeastern China. The name means "five taste fruit." According to traditional Chinese medicine (TCM), it was named for its sour, bitter, sweet, spicy, and salty tastes. All of these "tastes" in TCM correspond to the five elements: wood, fire, earth, metal, and water. It is a well-balanced, multifunctional plant. The components found in the berry regenerate liver cells and prevent liver injury.[26] In addition, research has shown that schisandra is helpful in reversing hepatitis. The effects on human metabolism make it a strong therapy for HIV,[27] inhibition of platelet aggregation (which results in lower inflammation),[28] and the reduction of tumors.

Researchers at Johns Hopkins University isolated lignans from the berry to determine the effect on colorectal cancer cells and found that the berry was capable of killing these cells.[29] I commonly add schisandra to herbal tonics that are taken at night, in conjunction with sedative herbs, for patients in Stage 1 adrenal fatigue. The berry is calming and allows your body to rejuvenate and heal during sleep. Patients commonly report feeling calmer when they awaken. Although it is beneficial at every stage, Stage 1 patients will benefit most from the addition of this herb.

## Valerian

Most helpful in Stage 2 (when insomnia is the worst), valerian is commonly used for insomnia, anxiety-related restlessness, mood disorders, attention deficit hyperactivity disorder (ADHD), epilepsy, and even to treat hot flashes.[30] It works similarly to GABA, promoting calmness by increasing your levels of natural GABA and decreasing your sympathetic output.

Research shows that taking valerian orally will reduce the time it takes to fall asleep by 14 to 17 minutes and will double your chances of improved sleep quality. The optimal dose to reap these benefits is 400 to 900 mg of valerian extract up to 2 hours before bedtime.[31] Considering valerian's significant impact on adrenal fatigue and the levels of neurotransmitters, such as GABA, in your brain, it makes sense to incorporate valerian into the treatment of those who are experiencing insomnia due to adrenal fatigue.

It has also been suggested that valerian affects the amino acid 5-hydroxytryptophan (5-HTP), the precursor to serotonin, which may help reduce nighttime hot flashes and induce deep sleep.[32] You can use it in conjunction with other herbs, such as lavender, schisandra, and passiflora. Because valerian has sedative properties, there are some known interactions: You should use caution when consuming alcohol and other GABA agonists (such as Xanax), as valerian will increase their effects. Valerian has also been shown to strengthen the effects of anesthesia, so be sure to tell your doctor that you're taking valerian before you are scheduled to have a surgical procedure.[33]

While valerian is best used during Stage 2, when insomnia is significant, it also has value for those in Stage 1 because it lowers sympathetic output. People in Stage 3 may find that it makes them feel fatigued; however, many of my patients report improvement in pain after taking this herb. Although it is not formally documented, I find that valerian works better as a liquid herbal preparation. I also find it works much better when used with other herbs than it does by itself. The error made by most people is that they buy valerian capsules at a health food store, take them for a while, find they do not work, and give up. Perhaps the capsules are not as well absorbed or perhaps the patient requires a more balanced formulation of herbs. The benefits of this herb are enough to warrant giving it another try—this time with the guidance of a doctor or herbalist who can help you find the appropriate blend to use.

## Phosphatidylserine (PS)

One of the most common ways I treat Stage 1 and early Stage 2 adrenal fatigue is with the fatty acid phosphatidylserine. Originally, it was used to treat Alzheimer's and other forms of dementia, and it has been shown to improve attention, alertness, verbal fluency, and memory in Alzheimer's patients.[34] In a 1993 study, researchers evaluated cognitive decline in the elderly and the effects of the administration of 300 mg of PS daily for 6 months. Statistically significant improvements both in behavioral and cognitive function were noted, and it was also found to be well tolerated.[35] Another study supported these findings, stating that at 100 mg daily, there was a significant improvement in daily tasks.[36] Phosphatidylserine was originally derived from bovine tissue, but now it is commonly extracted from cabbage and soy. The plant-based supplement has been shown to be just as effective and eliminates the risk of infection from a bovine product.[37]

Phosphatidylserine is a fat-soluble phospholipid that is naturally made in humans. It is required for neuronal function, such as cell-to-cell communication, which explains the theory behind why it works for dementia: They believe it improves neuron function. Alzheimer's patients also tend to have an abnormal release of acetylcholine, a neurotransmitter that improves focus. It has been thought that PS actually affects levels of acetylcholine, serotonin, dopamine, and norepinephrine, balancing their levels and restoring neuronal function.[38] This impact on dementia has prompted more research into the effects of phosphatidylserine on cortisol release.

The impact of this nutrient on stress response has been investigated for numerous years. In a study released more than 10 years ago, subjects given 300 mg of phosphatidylserine admitted to feeling less stressed and having better moods.[39] Prior to that, a study in Italy found that when they administered PS to healthy men during exercise, their cortisol response was blunted, resulting in less cortisol release due to stress.[40] Another Italian study confirmed that administration of phosphatidylserine will indeed blunt cortisol response and counteract the stress-induced activation of the hypothalamo-pituitary-adrenal axis in men.[41]

Research continues to explore this effect, and numerous nutraceutical companies have created supplements that include this phospholipid to reduce cortisol levels—and rightfully so. I can tell you from my experience as a clinician that those in Stage 1 or early Stage 2 adrenal fatigue will see significant results with the use of this substance. In fact, I prescribe a particular supplement that includes PS plus two herbs and L-theanine and it is, without a doubt, my best seller. Why? Because it works. I see it when the patient comes in. Someone who used to appear exhausted, overworked, and depleted will arrive joyous, relaxed, and well rested. Their blood work confirms this effect by showing reduced cortisol levels. I have seen patients drastically reduce their stress impact with this therapy. Of course, there are always exceptions to the rule and a few do not notice these changes. Maybe they have begun to enter Stage 3; maybe their livers are bogged down or other nutritional factors need to be considered. But overall, this particular substance plays a leading role in my practice because of its ability to reduce the stress impact of day-to-day life.

## Ginseng

Primarily used as an adaptogen (or to modify the body's response to stress from the adrenal glands), ginseng may also be used as a tonic for upper respiratory infections. Research shows that 200 mg twice daily over a 3- to 4-month period during flu season modestly decreases the developing symptoms of upper respiratory infections.[42] Think back to how adrenal fatigue affects your immune system. In Stage 2, you start to develop illnesses during times of rest and have trouble recovering. Isn't it interesting that an herb like ginseng, which is known primarily as a treatment for stress, also reduces the symptoms of illness?

In a double-blind study, scientists added ginseng root extract to a multivitamin and noted improved parameters in subjects exposed to the stress of a high amount of physical and mental activity. This suggests that the combination of ginseng and multivitamins conveys an anti-stress effect.[43]

Ginseng also improves stamina, stimulates your immune system, and has even been shown to lower blood glucose levels after eating, making it a good treatment option for diabetes.[44] This also makes it a great herb to use during Stage 2 adrenal fatigue, when insulin desensitization is beginning to occur. There is research stating that ginseng has estrogenic activity, and as a result, there are concerns about its potential to induce estrogen-based cancers. However, there is an equal amount of research showing that ginseng improves quality of life, reduces cancer cell growth, and is valuable overall in the treatment of cancer. Further studies are being performed at this point, so there is no definite conclusion.[45]

An important aspect to consider when using ginseng is that it may cause adverse reactions. If overused, it can cause high blood pressure, nervousness, and insomnia. I have yet to see these symptoms in my clinical use, but they have been reported. There are also some drug interactions that need to be considered when using ginseng in even moderate doses, so this is not an herb to take without consulting your doctor.

## Glycyrrhiza — no — high blood pressure

One of the best-tasting herbs used in adrenal fatigue therapy is the beautiful licorice plant, glycyrrhiza. This herb strongly benefits your gastrointestinal system, with research showing a positive effect on the healing of stress-induced ulcers.[46] With adrenal fatigue causing a strong impact on GI function, glycyrrhiza is often chosen to address both GI healing and adrenal support. In a study released in 2004, researchers combined glycyrrhiza with a number of other herbs and made an elixir for the treatment of dyspepsia (indigestion). It was shown to reduce dyspepsia symptoms by 43 percent in 8 weeks.[47]

Now remember that people with adrenal fatigue commonly experience GI distress, including indigestion, heartburn, gastric ulcers, and abdominal discomfort. Glycyrrhiza is a great treatment for ulcers, chronic gastritis, and dyspepsia, and it can reduce acid reflux, cramping, nausea, and vomiting.[48] It raises low potassium (which you may recall is also a symptom of adrenal fatigue), and it has an impact on menstrual cycles by affecting estrogen and testosterone receptor activity.[49] This herb also raises blood pressure, which makes it a great option for those who have low adrenal function and low blood pressure, as is common during Stages 2 and 3 of adrenal fatigue.

If you have very low blood pressure (around 90/60) and feel dizzy, tired, and unfocused, simply adding licorice can raise your blood pressure by 10 to 20 points and provide relief from these symptoms. But if you have high blood pressure, use caution.[50] There is preliminary evidence that glycyrrhiza can help treat hepatitis, but the trial sizes were too small to draw any significant conclusions. That said, this treatment would make sense, as the active components of this herb protect your liver and has antiviral action. I suggest it to patients to treat colds and flus, as well as chronic illnesses such as the Epstein-Barr virus.

Licorice can have a drastic positive impact on adrenal fatigue if used at the appropriate time. I do not recommend it during Stage 1 due to its blood pressure–elevating effects. Use during Stage 2 is highly variable depending on gastrointestinal function, blood pressure, and immune function. This herb is not recommended for smokers and those with high blood pressure. I'd recommend seeking a doctor's advice before taking it during Stage 2 due to the possibility of hypertension.

This herb is best used in combination with other herbs during Stage 3 adrenal fatigue, as it will actually stimulate adrenal gland function and benefit the adrenal glands of those who have used corticosteroids for a long time, such as people with autoimmune conditions who have been taking large doses of anti-inflammatory and steroid pharmaceuticals. You should consult your doctor before choosing to use licorice due to its reactions and interactions with some medications.[51]

It's worth noting that most licorice flavorings are not actually licorice. Instead, they are anise, which tastes like black licorice. Anise is a beautiful herb and is often used to calm the stomach, but it does not have the same components as glycyrrhiza. Don't be mistaken and buy the wrong herb!

## Ashwagandha (also known as *Withania somnifera*)

no-thyroid

Like rhodiola, ashwagandha is considered an adaptogen and has a positive impact on your body's ability to handle stress. However, it also has a very strong impact on your immune system, as an anti-inflammatory, on menstrual disorders, and on fibromyalgia, and it improves cognitive function.[52] This well-rounded herb treats not only your adrenal glands, but also the symptoms arising from adrenal fatigue. It is a gentle herbal tonic and can calm an overactive nervous system. Ashwaganda gently lowers blood pressure, calms anxiety, reduces fever and pain, lowers inflammation, and has an antioxidant effect.[53] It has also been shown to suppress stress-induced increases of dopamine receptors and the output of cortisol.[54] In addition, its anti-anxiety effects are believed to be the result of its binding to the GABA receptor, which makes it a nice alternative to using benzodiazepines, such as Xanax.[55]

One of the most unique aspects of this particular adaptogen is its strong effect on the immune system, making it a good herb for those in end Stage 2 and Stage 3 adrenal fatigue, when the immune system usually begins to be affected. It is shown to induce white blood cell activity, causing these cells to attack invading microbes.[56] In fact, it is commonly used in conjunction with cancer therapies, such as chemotherapy, to avoid the decrease in white blood cells commonly caused by chemotherapy. I have seen firsthand this herb's significant effect on the immune system and blood cells. I have a patient who has battled low platelet, red blood cell, and white blood cell counts. We are using a few therapies, one of which is ashwagandha. I noticed a dramatic difference in her white blood cell and platelet counts after we added ashwagandha to her regimen. There is also evidence that it enhances thyroid secretion,[57] so it is considered to have a mild interaction with thyroid medications. Be sure to tell your doctor if you are taking this herb in conjunction with levothyroxine or another thyroid hormone.[58] This is a great herb to use during Stage 3 adrenal fatigue, although it can be beneficial in all stages.

# THE NATURAL APPROACH TO ADRENAL FATIGUE THERAPY

When treating adrenal fatigue, it is important that your doctor evaluate and understand the blood tests relating to your diagnosis. It is easy to say, "Use valerian for sleep," but without knowing what stage you are in and what other conditions and medications you are currently taking, the effect of that herb may may not be beneficial to you. Using herbs to treat a symptom rather than the cause of that symptom is no better than using pharmaceuticals. The herbs should be used to address the reason the symptom is occurring and restore the normal functioning of the system. When used in this manner, herbal and nutritional therapies are well tolerated. The practice of botanical medicine is an art, and it is important to have a doctor or herbalist on your side to help you come up with the perfect blend of herbs to treat your adrenal fatigue. With the proper support, you can reverse adrenal fatigue and its symptoms.

# MY TURNAROUND
## DEBBIE, AGE: 61*

Even after Debbie's breast cancer was in remission, the effect of the radiation therapy was still taking its toll. "My body had worn down quite a bit due to the stress I was under, and also radiation is extremely hard on the body," she explains. "The first year after radiation, my bone density decreased due to osteopenia. And my white blood count had gone down from the cancer and from taking medication."

Several months after being in remission, Debbie began looking for a naturopathic physician. "Naturopaths not only address what's wrong with you, but they also help with supporting medicine. For example, one of the things I really liked about Dr. Pingel is when she ordered blood tests, she checked everything. A prior doctor said I had a thyroid condition, but nothing was wrong with my thyroid."

After diagnosing Debbie with Stage 2 adrenal fatigue, which was triggered from the stress of having cancer, Dr. Pingel placed her on several different supplements. "One supplement helps with my strength. I also take vitamin D because my vitamin D levels were quite low before the breast cancer, and I also take a vitamin $B_{12}$ shot," she shares. "Now, my blood work has been looking good."

A few months after she started following Dr. Pingel's plan, Debbie began to see results. "I used to have anxiety attacks/panic attacks quite frequently, and now I can't even remember the last time I had one of those. My stress levels are much better. I'm much more relaxed and centered," she says.

In addition to finally conquering her stress, Debbie's white blood cell count is now normal. She says that by treating her adrenal fatigue, she no longer has osteopenia. "I just feel a lot stronger physically. I also exercise 4 days a week—twice a week on the treadmill and twice a week with weight-bearing exercises," she states. "It's all a matter of getting back on the right track after going through something so serious. My wrists now have better bone density, and my oncologist recently said, 'Whatever you're doing, keep doing it!'"

*The patient's name has been changed to protect the patient's identity.

# 13

# YOUR ADRENAL EXERCISE PRESCRIPTION

Exercise is incredibly important not only for our health, but also for our stress levels. Think back to our ancestors, who moved all day long, walking, lifting things, carrying babies, building shelters, and hunting food. Our bodies were simply built to move. Exercise is critical for healing, as it is a mechanism to transport oxygen to your cells and release tight muscles. But the type of exercise needed for overall health does vary by person, and there are a wide variety of options available. You just have to know where to start.

## WHY AREN'T WE MOVING?

Here's the simple truth: We aren't exercising. According to the Centers for Disease Control and Prevention, in 2011 only 20 percent of Americans met the minimum requirement of approximately 2.5 hours per week of cardiovascular exercise and twice-weekly strength training.[1] That means that 80 percent of us are not meeting this minimum requirement. Honestly, that is only a commitment of 3 to 4 hours a week total, and 80 percent of us are not doing it.

The CDC also recommends that children ages 6 to 17 get 1 hour of physical activity each day. But in 2011, only 29 percent of high school students reported hitting that guideline. And 14 percent reported not having any physical activity in the 7 days prior to when they were surveyed. And remember physical education (P.E.) class? It was reported in 2011 that only 27 percent of females and 34 percent of males attended a daily P.E. class. But in 2010, over one-third of all children and adolescents were overweight or obese. And since 1980, this number has grown by 18 percent.[2]

Why don't we exercise? Are we so stressed-out that once we get home we just sit, instead of moving? Are we so exhausted that the thought of physical labor is daunting—even though we know it's good for us?

Simply stated, the benefits of exercise are vast. Exercise carries oxygen to your brain and builds strong bones and muscles. In fact, it is your single best defense against bone loss, such as osteopenia and osteoporosis.[3] And during pregnancy, it helps the expectant mother avoid developing diabetes. In a study released in 2013, researchers looked at the effects of regular exercise on pregnant women beginning in gestational weeks 6 through 8. The women exercised at a moderate intensity 3 days a week throughout their entire pregnancy. This group showed a statistically lower frequency of gestational diabetes and macrosomia (large birth weight) than those who did not exercise.[4]

Most of us know that we need to exercise, but we just don't. Or we do minimal exercise and expect major weight loss. The standard guideline for exercise in popular diet programs, such as Weight Watchers, is 30 minutes a day of aerobic activity, such as brisk walking. Although this will positively impact oxygen flow and heart function, for most, this is not enough to promote weight loss. Exercising for 30 minutes each day translates to burning 150 to 200 calories per session. It takes around 3,500 calories to burn a pound.

The International Association for the Study of Obesity recommends 45 to 60 minutes daily of moderate cardiovascular activity in order to avoid further weight gain. Note that this does not promote weight loss, it just keeps you from gaining additional weight. Patients constantly ask why they aren't losing weight. Let's say someone is 50 pounds overweight when she commits to a healthy diet. She walks the dog 5 days a week for 20 minutes every day. The problem is that this is simply not enough. If you are of a healthy weight, you can get away with less exercise. Just keep moving and you'll maintain your weight. But if you are overweight or obese, you will have to work harder to develop the body you desire and reap the true health benefits of exercise.

## ADRENAL FATIGUE AND EXERCISE

Adrenal fatigue promotes lack of motivation, physical and mental fatigue, excess weight gain, and hormonal irregularities. As part of your overall wellness, these issues have to be addressed, but simply taking supplements and eating a whole foods–based diet will not fully reverse symptoms in everyone with adrenal fatigue. You have to maintain a healthy weight in order to completely free yourself of physical pain, excess weight, and fatigue. For example, I recently had a patient who had joint pain, shortness of breath, excessive weight gain, fatigue, and depression. She recalled that the last time she did not feel that way was when she was exercising 5 or more days a week for an hour at a time. She recalled feeling fantastic and strong and having great energy. She told me that she knows how to get better and that it involves exercising plus diet, but she is not willing to live that lifestyle anymore. Her adrenal fatigue has put her into a depression, and she no longer has the motivation to be well. How can I help her, then? There is no magic pill for weight loss or health. It is a commitment. Just as people commit themselves to worship in religion, you must commit yourself to a change in your life—and the great news is that it's never too late!

Researchers used 8 years of follow-up data on 3,454 initially disease-free men and women (with an average age of 63.7 at the start of the

8 years) who participated in the English Longitudinal Study of Ageing. They compared self-reported physical activity levels at baseline with the development of major chronic diseases, depressive symptoms, and physical or cognitive impairment during follow-up (lack of which was defined as "healthy ageing"). Almost one-fifth, 19.3 percent, made it to the last follow-up evaluation without developing any of those conditions. Compared with participants who had been inactive at the outset, those who reported moderate or vigorous activity at least once a week were, on average, 2.67 and 3.53 times as likely, respectively, to have experienced healthy ageing, even after adjusting for age, sex, smoking, alcohol consumption, marital status, and wealth. Even better news: Those who had become more physically active during the study had a higher likelihood of experiencing healthy ageing than those who hadn't, showing that exercise at any age is beneficial.[5]

## Exercise During Stage 1

Here is how the cycle begins: In Stage 1 of adrenal fatigue, you are on the go and typically maintain your weight easily. You skip meals and immediately lose a few pounds. Weight comes off easily, and if you get to the gym, great. If not, it's no big deal. This stage is critical because if you have not already established an exercise routine, it will be hard to muster up the motivation to start one once you enter Stage 2. If you have already entered into a routine, you typically will not gain as much weight during Stage 2 as you would otherwise. As a result, I highly encourage patients in Stage 1 to establish a set routine and take time every day to let off a little steam with some sort of cardiovascular or endurance exercise. You have the energy at this point, so use it.

Running, biking, endurance walking, dance classes, and boot camps are all great activities to start during Stage 1. But I do throw out one bit of caution: Do not overexercise. Allow yourself to recover, because 30 to 60 minutes of intense exercise every day is plenty. Extreme exercise causes your adrenal glands to work harder and therefore slows recovery and can set you up for worsening adrenal fatigue in the future. I have many patients in this stage who have so much energy that they work out intensely every day for 2 to 3 hours. If they have a high stress level, this much exercise may push the body too far and promote progression to Stage 2. Therefore, it's beneficial to practice yoga, ballet, tai chi, or Pilates during this stage because they calm the mind and strengthen the body. And science has proven it: A 2012 review revealed that 25 of 35 trials addressing the effects of yoga on anxiety and stress noted a significant decrease in stress and/or anxiety symptoms when a yoga regimen was implemented.[6]

Also, in a 2005 study published in the *Medical Science Monitor*, 24 women who were self-described as "emotionally distressed" took two 90-minute yoga classes each week for 3 months. When compared to a control group who did not exercise during the study period, those in the yoga group reported improvements in perceived stress, depression, anxiety, energy, fatigue, and well-being. In addition, their depression scores improved by 50 percent, anxiety scores by 30 percent, and overall well-being scores by 65 percent. Furthermore, their initial complaints of headaches, back pain, and poor sleep quality resolved more so than they did for those in the control group.[7]

Look at your environment and find time to meditate or relax each day. If you plan on doing intense exercise, follow it up with 30 minutes of stretching, yoga, or meditation to bring your body out of the fight-or-flight response. You will get better results (achieve overall wellness) and keep yourself from moving into Stage 2 adrenal fatigue. Your body likes balance, and at this stage, you have the motivation to do anything. Many people do yoga one day and intense exercise another, but I encourage you to do them on the same day. Rev yourself up, and then bring yourself down. This helps you train your body to calm itself down after a stressful or intense event.

## Exercise During Stage 2

In Stage 2, your body weight will begin to slowly increase—maybe a pound here or 3 pounds there. So you may decide to ramp up the exercise and restrict your diet, but you see no change. You do, however, notice that your abdomen and hips are a bit flabbier. In addition, you feel tired and lack the energy to work out like you used to. You may exercise regularly for a few weeks, but then life takes over and you commit to other activities, putting exercise last on your ever-growing to-do list.

The change is frustrating, as you have always been able to maintain a steady weight. Perhaps it can be attributed to age, you think. Ultimately, you give in to foods you know you should not eat because you feel defeated by not seeing results from your efforts—not to mention that your clothes are not fitting your body any longer. Many of my patients get pregnant during this time and find that after pregnancy, they cannot commit to getting their weight back down to where it was before.

In Stage 2, you have to work so much harder than you did in Stage 1. You now have to establish changes in biochemistry so that you can begin to heal the damage that has been done by excessive stress. This often happens when a woman is going through perimenopause, so all of the changes are blamed on "hormones." You cannot cheat during this stage, so don't even think about sneaking in that extra piece of bread or snacking on potato chips. You have reached a point where your body is often afraid of another bear and therefore wants excessive fuel so it can run. As a result, extra calories you consume will be stored.

I commonly hear this from patients: "I used to be able to have a snack at night and work it off the next day, but now I can't." And they're right: They can't. This is a very delicate phase and one where most people start to look for drastic diets to lose that extra 10 pounds. But doing that would be a mistake. You are no longer in Stage 1, where weight will fall off with minimal effort. So do not stress your body even more by starving it or giving it more hormones to metabolize. Don't eat processed diet foods that are hard for your body to digest. Avoid this urge and accept that your body is under stress, and that stress has to be removed in order for your efforts to be recognized.

Refrain from "yo-yo dieting," or you will stay in this stage for quite some time. Those in Stage 2 need predictability and significant discipline. Unfortunately, weight loss is a little more difficult during this stage. Most patients will not lose weight in the first 3 months of working at it; then they will drop a few pounds and hold that weight for another 2 to 3 months before losing more. And most of these patients are easily working out 5 days each week for an hour or more. At this stage, you do not lose a certain number of pounds per week. Why? Because your body has to let go of the fear of the bear in order to lose weight. While you may not see the number immediately drop on the scale, remember that your biochemistry is changing and setting you up for a complete body restoration when your adrenal glands are healed. Your patience will be rewarded in the end. Instead of gaining and losing weight regularly, you will slowly lose the weight and keep it off for life.

The emotional aspect of this stage is also very difficult. Dwelling on your lack of weight loss will only promote more fat storage. Remember the connection between your mind and body: If you think there is a bear lurking nearby, your body will react as if there is one and will ultimately deposit more fat. You have to accept where you are, commit to a supplement and lifestyle regimen, and trust that the weight will come off once your stress levels are under control. Most people in Stage 2 cannot do this and get stuck on a "hamster wheel" of weight gain (or stability at a weight they're unhappy with), and they grow depressed.

At this stage, you have to work harder at the mind-body aspect of healing. In addition to doing more cardiovascular exercise than usual, you have to balance that with relaxation, meditation, and core strength exercises. You have to let go of the things in your life that cause you stress. Consistency is key, so get up and exercise, regardless of the lack of perceived results. Trust me, it will come back and benefit you in the end. How? Well, a 2008 review revealed that the adrenal hormones epinephrine and norepinephrine have been shown to increase by up to 20 times during exercise, and this adrenaline rush provides those in Stage 2 adrenal fatigue with a surge of energy.[8] This exercise will also start to "reset" your adrenal function and will help you let go of excess weight once your stress response is healed.

It's amazing to watch someone who can emotionally do this. I watch the evolution of someone who looks tired, depressed, slightly over-weight, and blue turn into someone who stands tall and smiles with brightened skin. Their weight is not the first thing brought up in con-versation, but instead they comment on their energy, better hormone regularity, and improved skin, hair, nails, and overall mood. At this point, most Stage 2 patients say that they accept their weight for what it is because they feel great and are able to exercise daily and eat good, nutritious food. That's the point at which these people actually start los-ing weight! But if you fight it and are stuck on the hamster wheel, you will not get out. You will simply progress into Stage 3 adrenal fatigue.

## Exercise During Stage 3

Those in Stage 3 have very slow metabolisms due to the stimulatory effect of cortisol and its direct impact on thyroid function. They are typically extremely fatigued and unmotivated. Obesity sets in around this time, and most patients are simply too tired to exercise. They are far more sedentary than those in Stage 2 and have concerns about joint pain that they cite as the reason why they cannot exercise. Emotionally, this is a very difficult time and more emotional support is needed, either from a professional or via yoga or meditation. The patient I men-tioned earlier, who had no desire to commit to diet or lifestyle changes (even though she knew diet and lifestyle were the sources of her health concerns), is a great example of someone struggling with Stage 3. She simply cannot get up and do it due to emotional depression. And this is a common occurrence for those in Stage 3. Therefore, I highly recom-mend a personal trainer and emotional coaching during this stage.

Many times, the depression that has occurred by Stage 3 promotes a feeling of low self-worth, which prevents the patient from achieving success in weight loss and general healing of his or her adrenal glands. But research has shown that exercise can help combat these feelings. In one study, researchers divided 156 men and women with depression into three different groups. The first group took part in an aerobic exercise program, the second took antidepressants, and the third did both. After 16 weeks, approximately 60 to 70 percent of the subjects in all three groups could no longer be classed as having major depression. But a follow-up study revealed that the effects of exercise lasted longer than the effects of antidepressants. When the researchers followed up with 133 of the original patients 6 months after the first study ended, they found that those who continued to exercise after the study, regardless of their original assigned study group, were less likely to relapse into depression.[9]

Depending on the amount of weight you need to lose and the extent of disease development, exercise may be difficult and perhaps even painful, but it must still be completed daily in order to reverse the damage done to your adrenal glands and decrease your weight. Many people have such low adrenal function by this point that simply walking causes exhaustion. I recommend that those in Stage 3 adrenal fatigue consult with their physicians before starting an unsupervised new exercise program. In addition, it would be beneficial to consult with both a nutritionist and a trainer who can work with your doctor to help you achieve success. Consider bringing the suggested exercise plans in this chapter to your physician for review and consultation.

The primary concern is that when you exercise, you release excitatory hormones from your adrenal glands, such as norepinephrine and epinephrine. If your adrenal glands are underproducing, you will experience more fatigue and worsening adrenal fatigue if you jump in too quickly. It is important to build adrenal function first and slowly increase more intense exercise. Yes, this may delay your weight loss, but when your body is repaired, your weight loss goals will be met at a much faster pace. This means that people in this category need to have patience.

Remember: Each person is different. We all come from different backgrounds, with different genes. We all have different health goals, so each of us needs a different plan for exercise. Recognizing your stage of adrenal fatigue will assist you in starting a plan and finding the experts to support you. My best words of encouragement are that you are worth this effort. Don't let anything limit you. It is your health and well-being at stake here, and nothing is more important than that.

# Getting Started with a Routine

I know what you're thinking: It is difficult to start a new exercise routine—especially when you are exhausted and experiencing the symptoms of adrenal fatigue. And those with further complications, such as diabetes, obesity, and heart conditions, may think it's impossible to get into a regular routine. But here is one thing to always keep in mind: No matter who you are or what your health background is, everyone starts at the same place—the beginning.

To begin, you need to define your goal. It is much easier to focus on achieving a goal through exercise than it is to just randomly work out. Investigate why you want to get well. For example, perhaps you want to get well so that you can see your grandson graduate from college, or maybe you want to be well so that you can tour Europe on foot with your husband in your 80s. Whatever your goal may be, take a moment to consider it. Now write it down and make it concrete. Once you establish this goal, be realistic about what you will have to do to accomplish it.

Bryan Huseby, a personal trainer and former athlete who assisted in designing the exercise program you will use as part of your treatment, provided a great visualization exercise to help you establish your goals. Imagine yourself now, with your current symptoms. Now look forward to 5, 10, and 15 years from now and imagine how those symptoms and diseases will progress. Is that where you want to be in 5 years? How about 15 years? What will your quality of life be? To set your goal, you need to consider whether it fits into the acronym SMART: Make it specific, measureable, achievable, result-oriented, and time-based.

## Achieving Your Goal

In order to achieve your goals, you'll need to make an honest assessment of where you currently are, both physically and mentally. Accept this as your starting point, and document it. You'll have to start slowly and build on your current condition. You may have been an active athlete in the past, but your body will not be able to jump right back in where it left off because it takes time to get back to that level of fitness. I used to be a dancer, spending numerous hours per day stretching, dancing, and working on making my body lean and flexible. I stopped dancing while I was getting married, having kids, and attending medical school, and although my weight remained the same, my flexibility decreased.

Mineral deficiencies came along as a side effect of adrenal fatigue, and that made my muscles tighter. When I "jumped" back into ballet and jazz after 10 years off, I found that my body was not capable of getting into the positions I needed it to look graceful and beautiful in dance. It was very frustrating, but I had to realize that my body was out of practice. I used my determination to fuel my practice. Now, with each month that goes by, I find myself more flexible than before, and my goal is to someday be as flexible as I once was.

Taking an honest assessment of my posture was important. Have you found yourself saying something like, "I would like to exercise, but my knees hurt"? If you have gained weight over the years or excessive stress has caused you to slouch in your chair or raise your shoulders, your body may have changed its alignment, resulting in poor posture. When you begin to exercise, your weight is distributed poorly, causing pain. A rotation in your spine or ribs could cause depression into your organs, such as your heart, lungs, liver, or spleen, resulting in decreased blood flow and poor oxygen transport. Take these points into consideration when you begin exercising again. Have your posture assessed and baseline blood tests run by your doctor, and take a note of your emotional status. All of these areas will change as you begin to exercise, and you should continue to monitor them as you progress.

# THE ADRENAL FATIGUE WORKOUT PROGRAM

We created the following exercise routines with two things in mind: You need a workout program that you can follow consistently, in spite of your adrenal fatigue and lower energy levels, and your workout needs to calm you, not add additional stress. I always recommend getting clearance from your physician before beginning a new exercise routine,

# SEVEN SECRETS TO SUCCESSFUL EXERCISE

As someone who has experienced adrenal fatigue, I can give you some personal suggestions and tips that I have found to be helpful when beginning an exercise routine.

1. **PICK THE TIME OF DAY WHEN YOU HAVE THE MOST ENERGY.** Devote that time to your exercise. That way, if you become tired or fatigued later in the day, you can rest without having to worry about exerting more energy.

2. **EXERCISE ON A CONSISTENT SCHEDULE.** Set the time, and do it. Do not allow yourself to reschedule unless you are very sick that day. Schedule it just like you would a business meeting and don't be afraid to tell people that you are unavailable if they try to schedule another meeting during that time. Make it a priority, like you do for everything else you tackle.

3. **KEEP YOUR EXERCISE CLOTHES IN YOUR CAR.** This helps, because if you stop at home on your way to the gym, you will often find other things to do and skip exercise entirely. Be prepared!

4. **PICK SOMETHING YOU ENJOY DOING.** If you need a cardiovascular routine, it does not have to be on a stationary bike or a treadmill. Dance, hike, ride your bike outside, run, join a soccer league—do whatever gets you excited to be there.

5. **BE REALISTIC ABOUT HOW FREQUENTLY YOU WILL EXERCISE.** If you can really only commit to an exercise routine twice weekly, then do not set yourself up for failure by attempting to exercise 5 days each week. I always set a minimum of 2 days, with a set schedule that does not get broken. Then I have two backup days in case something happens. If my schedule allows it, I can add those alternate days on top of my original 2 workout days. I find that, on average, I exercise 3 days each week with this routine. When I set my goal at 4 times weekly, I found myself constantly cancelling and feeling bad about it, and then quitting. Be realistic and set goals you can meet.

6. **GET SUPPORT.** If you are someone who cannot commit to being somewhere on your own, hire a trainer or find a friend to work out with you.

7. **STAY POSITIVE.** Last and most importantly, do not beat up on yourself if you cannot hit the fitness goal you set initially. Keep trying. Know that you can do this, you just have to believe in yourself. Anything is possible.

and I'd also advise you to consider finding a personal fitness trainer.

The following progressive 8-week routines are a fusion of tai chi, yoga, Pilates, and functional fitness. These sample programs are designed to be a guideline for how to improve your overall health and vitality while combating your adrenal fatigue. We begin with the sequence for Stage 3 adrenal fatigue (which will be less stressful on your body) and work our way to the Stage 1 sequence (which is the most demanding workout).

After completing the Stage 3 tai chi conditioning, your body will have the strength and vitality it needs to move into Stage 2. Those exercises will further enhance your strength, flexibility, and stamina for day-to-day activities, or perhaps even inspire you to try new ones. By the end of the Stage 2 program you will be prepared to move on to the Stage 1 workout.

Regardless of whether you are starting at Stage 1 or transitioning into Stage 1 from the previous stages, you will be able to participate in a much wider variety of exercise at that point, including full forms of tai chi, group and individual exercise programs, and even yoga. While this routine is designed to help a person heal from Stage 2 and move into Stage 1, the Stage 1 routine leaves more room for you to explore your interests by determining what you enjoy doing and what your goals are and aligning the two. Although identifying your goals and aligning them with activities that you enjoy are also necessary aspects of Stage 3 and Stage 2, people at these stages may not be able to do what they enjoy or may not have the energy to know what physical activities they like to do.

Your journey toward optimal health and vitality begins with tai chi warmup exercises, though they are actually much more than that. While the primary intention of the tai chi exercises is to loosen up your joints and improve energy circulation, they also promote peace of mind.

## The Adrenal Fatigue Workout Sequence

In the beginning, you may find that only 5 to 10 minutes a day are necessary (based on your current energy and health levels) to begin improving your current health. Later, it will require more time (up to 60 minutes) as your body will need greater demands placed upon it to achieve an improved state of health. You may want to start exercising two or three times each week, assess your progress and your energy levels, and increase your frequency as you're ready. You don't want to further stress your adrenals by moving on to the next exercise routine while you're still recovering from the last one. Ideally, you should work toward the goal of exercising 6 days a week, reserving 1 day for rest. Just remember to take each routine at your own pace and customize it as needed to reduce your risk of injury.

## Guidelines for Exercising with Adrenal Fatigue

Everyone has a different skill level and you should move into these routines slowly, gradually improving as you continue to practice these moves. The basics of breathing, posture, and movement are key to rebuilding your body, taking it back to its natural state, and avoiding injury. Note that correct posture is essential in order to avoid injury, and it enhances your ability to utilize a joint's full range of motion. Please be mindful of how your body feels in the posture described below. If it is painful or uncomfortable, focus on practicing just your posture, to ease yourself back into proper alignment. Once you are comfortable with good posture, move forward with the exercises.

### Breathing

Simply breathing—which takes considerable muscle engagement—can be imbalanced at any stage but will particularly affect anyone with severe adrenal fatigue. Many people learn to hold their breath as a coping response. This negative habit can then lead to further adrenal malfunction. With the imbalance between the parasympathetic and sympathetic nervous systems that typically accompanies the adrenal stress response, it is very important to restore proper breathing patterns.

General rule starting out: Do not force your breathing sequence— simply try to focus on slow and smooth inhales (about 3 seconds) and exhales (also about 3 seconds) that come from your abdomen rather than your chest cavity alone. Try not to hold your breath when you're feeling more stressed, particularly when you're performing exercises, as this can overwhelm a system that's not in a position to handle the added stress. In the beginning, you may need to practice your breathing daily to correct your current breathing patterns. Additional breathing considerations and exercises are also provided in the next chapter and can offer considerable health benefits when implemented daily.

## Posture

Stand or sit tall, with your weight distributed equally between both feet and hip bones.

Keep your shoulders relaxed and your chin slightly tucked. (Try keeping the top of your head flat, like you're carrying a glass of water on it.)

Gently contract your stomach up and in, like you would if you were pulling on a tight pair of pants.

When standing, keep your feet parallel and shoulder-width apart. Bend your knees slightly. By keeping your feet parallel, you will begin activating and strengthening your inner thigh muscles to stabilize your hips and knees.

## Movement

As you perform these movements, you may find your abdomen wanting to relax forward, but I encourage you to continue holding your core tight as often as you can remember to. If you stay aware of lifting the arches of your feet upward as you contract your thighs, glutes, groin, and navel (core), it will help you maintain proper posture.

# Stage 3 Protocol

**WARMUP:** Walk comfortably for 5 minutes. This will get your circulation going, providing greater oxygen and nutrients to the muscles needed to perform the exercises. You can start by walking inside your home, and you can use any assistive device (such as a walker or cane) that you may need for balance and safety purposes. Once you feel stronger, you can move your walk outside, where you'll reap additional benefits from the fresh air and sunshine.

**EXERCISES:** These moves are restorative and help keep your system calm while still increasing circulation, distributing nutrients to your organs, and removing waste from your tissues. This offers your body a chance to recharge both energetically and physically, leading to the secondary effect of increased overall strength. For the full program, including reps, see "Your Stage 3 Routine" on page 258.

### Vertical Tai Chi Circles

Begin in a good standing position, arms relaxed down with wrists crossed in front of your body and palms facing in. Inhale as you raise your arms out to your sides. Continue lifting your arms until they are extended above your head, wrists crossed and palms facing forward. Exhale and lower your arms back to your starting position or, if you are able, bend your knees and squat down as you exhale. Pause for 3 to 5 seconds. Inhale, squeezing your leg and core muscles, and return to the standing position with your arms overhead. This is one complete repetition.

### Horizontal Tai Chi Circles

Begin in a good standing position, arms relaxed down with wrists crossed in front of your body and palms facing in. Inhale as you raise your arms up and out laterally until they are extended above your head with wrist crossed. Your palms will naturally end up facing forward. Exhale and slowly shift your weight toward your right hip and foot; bend your right knee slightly, as if to squat, keeping your left knee straight. Allow your arms to extend out to shoulder level with palms down to balance yourself. Inhale, squeezing your leg and core muscles, and raise your arms back above your head as you return to the previous position. Repeat the movement, now toward your left side and back up. Continue alternating from one side to the other with good form. One squat to each side is considered one full repetition.

## Restorative Yoga Sequence

### Supported Child's Pose

Kneel on a cushioned floor or bed and stack two bed pillows length-wise in front of you. Gently allow your upper body to lean forward and rest on the pillows with your arms reaching out on the floor, supporting you. Sit back on your heels to create a slight stretch in your arms and thighs. Maintain proper breathing as you hold this position.

### Assisted Bridge Pose

Lie on your back with your knees bent and feet shoulder-width apart on the floor. Squeeze your glutes and lift your hips up 2 to 3 inches off the floor. Place a rolled-up towel or folded pillow under your pelvis to support you in this lifted position. (If you feel discomfort in your spine, lower your pelvis until you are comfortable.) Extend your arms out straight on the floor, slightly away from your body, palms up. Keep your stomach pulled up and in and your glutes tensed, maintain proper breathing, and hold this position.

### Legs Up on a Chair Pose

Lie on your back with your feet propped up on a chair, knees and hips bent at 90-degree angles. Extend your arms out on the floor at shoulder level with your palms up. Gently pull your stomach up and in, flattening the small of your back into the floor. Maintain proper breathing as you hold this position.

### Supported Goddess Pose

Lie on your back with your knees bent and feet together on the floor. Pull your stomach up and in and flatten the small of your back into the floor. Allow your knees to gently fall outward and away from each other. Place rolled towels or pillows under each knee to keep them from hanging unsupported in the air. Extend your arms out straight on the floor, slightly out away from your body, with palms up. Maintain proper breathing as you hold this position.

# Cooldown

## Mindfulness Walking

This is more than just walking and looking around. As you walk, pay attention to your feet, ankles, knees, hips, torso, spine, and shoulders to get a general sense of your movements. Through simple observation you may automatically begin making slight adjustments to your body.

After walking for a few moments and noticing your experience, begin to "tune in." Consciously keep your shoulders down and relaxed, lift your head, straighten your spine, and allow your arms to relax. With each step, feel your legs lifting from your hip and knees. Lift your foot so that when you step down, the heel of your foot makes contact with the ground first, and roll from your heel to your toes. Concentrate on your big toe and your second toe as your foot continues to roll forward, and press with those two toes. If you usually drag your feet or your heels, don't—now is the time to correct this. If you walk upright and actually use your legs to properly place your feet, your health will quickly improve and you will not only look more attractive and energized, you will also feel that way.

When you're able, consider doing this walk outside, as studies have shown that simply walking outside (especially in nature) is a great way to destress and boost your immune system. This simple activity lowers your pulse rate, blood pressure, and stress hormones, while increasing your white blood cell count.[10] As you continue to practice mindful walking, look at things that are far away; listen, smell, and breathe in your surroundings and soon walking won't be something that you have to do, it will become something that you can't wait to do.

# Your Stage 3 Routine

## WEEKS 1 & 2

**WARMUP:** Comfortable walk for 5 minutes

**EXERCISES**

| | MOVEMENT | HOLD TIME | REPS | SETS | REST TIME (BETWEEN SETS) |
|---|---|---|---|---|---|
| Tai Chi Circles | Horizontal Circles | 3–5 seconds | 5 | 1 | 1–2 minutes |
| | Vertical Circles | 3–5 seconds | 5 | 1 | 1–2 minutes |
| Restorative Yoga | Supported Child's Pose | 1–2 minutes | 1 | 1 | 0–1 minutes |
| | Assisted Bridge Pose | 1–2 minutes | 1 | 1 | 0–1 minutes |
| | Leg Up on a Chair Pose | 1–2 minutes | 1 | 1 | 0–1 minutes |
| | Supported Goddess Pose | 1–2 minutes | 1 | 1 | 0–1 minutes |

**COOLDOWN:** Mindfulness Walking for 5 minutes

## WEEKS 3 & 4

**WARMUP:** Comfortable walk for 5 minutes

**EXERCISES**

| | MOVEMENT | HOLD TIME | REPS | SETS | REST TIME (BETWEEN SETS) |
|---|---|---|---|---|---|
| Tai Chi Circles | Vertical Circles | 3–5 seconds | 5-7 | 1–2 | 1–2 minutes |
| | Horizontal Circles | 3–5 seconds | 5-7 | 1–2 | 1–2 minutes |
| Restorative Yoga | Supported Child's Pose | 1–2 minutes | 1 | 1 | 0–1 minutes |
| | Assisted Bridge Pose | 1–2 minutes | 1 | 1 | 0–1 minutes |
| | Leg Up on a Chair Pose | 1–2 minutes | 1 | 1 | 0–1 minutes |
| | Supported Goddess Pose | 1–2 minutes | 1 | 1 | 0–1 minutes |

**COOLDOWN:** Mindfulness Walking for 5 minutes

# WEEKS 5 & 6

**WARMUP:** Comfortable walk for 5–10 minutes

## EXERCISES

| | MOVEMENT | HOLD TIME | REPS | SETS | REST TIME (BETWEEN SETS) |
|---|---|---|---|---|---|
| Tai Chi Circles | Vertical Circles | 3–5 seconds | 7–10 | 2 | 1–2 minutes |
| | Horizontal Circles | 3–5 seconds | 7–10 | 2 | 1–2 minutes |
| Restorative Yoga | Supported Child's Pose | 1–2 minutes | 1 | 1 | 0–1 minutes |
| | Assisted Bridge Pose | 1–2 minutes | 1 | 1 | 0–1 minutes |
| | Leg Up on a Chair Pose | 1–2 minutes | 1 | 1 | 0–1 minutes |
| | Supported Goddess Pose | 1–2 minutes | 1 | 1 | 0–1 minutes |

**COOLDOWN:** Mindfulness Walking for 5–10 minutes

# WEEKS 7 & 8

**WARMUP:** Comfortable walk for 10 minutes
## EXERCISES

| | MOVEMENT | HOLD TIME | REPS | SETS | REST TIME (BETWEEN SETS) |
|---|---|---|---|---|---|
| Tai Chi Circles | Vertical Circles | 3–5 seconds | 10-15 | 2–3 | 1–2 minutes |
| | Horizontal Circles | 3–5 seconds | 10-15 | 2–3 | 1–2 minutes |
| Restorative Yoga | Supported Child's Pose | 1–2 minutes | 1 | 1 | 0–1 minutes |
| | Assisted Bridge Pose | 1–2 minutes | 1 | 1 | 0–1 minutes |
| | Leg Up on a Chair Pose | 1–2 minutes | 1 | 1 | 0–1 minutes |
| | Supported Goddess Pose | 1–2 minutes | 1 | 1 | 0–1 minutes |

**COOLDOWN:** Mindfulness Walking for 10 minutes

## Stage 2 Protocol

**WARMUP:** Walk at a brisk but comfortable pace to enhance circulation and prepare your muscles for the upcoming workout. You can start by walking inside if you prefer, but as you gain strength, you can begin to walk outside.

**EXERCISES:** These exercises will help you develop a foundation of strength, stability, and flexibility, thus enhancing your overall mobility and body composition and balancing your physiological stress response. You can split up these workouts and focus on one area daily to give your muscles more recovery time. These are basic body-weight exercises that you can perform pretty much anywhere, though some of them use an exercise band and ball to allow for additional movements. For the full program, including reps, see "Your Stage 2 Routine" on page 266.

## Upper Body

### Modified Pushups (Close Hands)

Lie facedown with your hands next to each other under your chest and your elbows close to your sides. Keep your shoulders down and away from your ears and bend your knees, lifting your feet toward the ceiling. Keeping your back straight, lift your body up with your hands. Slowly lower back down, keeping your spine straight at all times.

### Modified Pushups (Neutral Hands)

Lie facedown with your hands next to your shoulders, your fingertips pointing forward, and your elbows close to your sides. Keep your shoulders down and away from your ears and bend your knees, lifting your feet toward the ceiling. Keeping your back straight, lift your body up with your hands. Slowly lower back down, keeping your spine straight at all times.

### Standing Momentum Arm Raises (Front and Sides)

Stand with good posture. Raise your arms to shoulder level in front of you, making sure your shoulders stay down. Lower your arms halfway down, then raise them back up to shoulder level. Finally, lower down to start position. This is one repetition. Repeat the same exercise, but this time with your arms out to your sides.

### Ts

Lie facedown with your arms out at shoulder level, making a T. (You can place a small rolled-up towel under your forehead to keep your neck in alignment.) Pull your stomach up and in, rotate your pelvis back (flattening out the small of your back), and tuck your glutes under. Keep your shoulders down and lift your arms up toward the ceiling; hold at the top for 3 to 5 seconds, then return to the starting position.

### Ys

Lie facedown with your arms over your head and extended to form a Y with your body. (You can place a small rolled-up towel under your forehead to keep your neck in alignment.) Pull your stomach up and in, rotate your pelvis back (flattening out the small of your back), and tuck your glutes under. Keep your shoulders down and lift your arms up toward the ceiling; hold at the top for 3 to 5 seconds, then return to the starting position.

### Quarter Dog

Kneel on the floor with your toes tucked under. Bend your upper body forward and reach with your arms, placing your weight on your elbows and forearms. Shift your weight over your shoulders while you straighten your knees and extend your hips up toward the ceiling. Keep your shoulders back and away from your ears, and try to intensify the stretch by lifting further forward on your toes. Hold for 15 to 30 seconds, working up to 1 to 2 minutes.

## Lower Body

### Bridges (with March)

Lie on your back with your knees bent and in line with your feet and hips. Squeeze your glutes and lift your hips up off the floor. Hold for 10 seconds, then lower back down and repeat.

If you are comfortable doing Bridge, increase the difficulty by adding marching in place. (Try to keep your hips from dropping while you're stepping.). Repeat.

### Side-Lying Leg Raise

Lie on your left side with both legs fully extended. Turn your toes so they point slightly upward and raise your right leg straight up toward the ceiling. Do not allow your hips to rotate backwards. Pause at the top, then slowly lower your leg.

### Single Leg Chair Lifts

Lie on your back with your left knee bent at 90 degrees and your heel resting on a chair. Lift your right leg straight up in the air, pull your stomach up and in, and then lift your hips a few inches off the floor, putting your weight onto your left heel. Hold this position for 5 seconds then return to the starting position.

### Standing Lunges

Stand with good posture. Step forward with one leg, bending your knee so it is directly above your toes and keeping your hips in line with your foot and knee. You can rest your arms on your hips or raise them up and out at shoulder level for balance. Start with smaller steps and minimal squatting. Squeeze your glutes, contract your quadriceps, and push back upward through your heel as you return to the starting position. Repeat with your other leg. Alternate lunging with each foot, trying to keep your chest up as you perform the movement.

## Chair Pose

Stand tall with your feet and thighs together in good posture. Lift your arms out in front of you at shoulder level (you can challenge yourself as you gain strength and raise your arms further overhead), reaching forward continuously to provide counterbalance throughout the movement. Squeeze your thighs together and, leading with your glutes, sit back as if you were sitting in a chair. Don't allow your back to arch. Go down only as far as you can while maintaining good posture and hold for 15 to 30 seconds. Squeeze your glutes and push back up through your heels. Repeat.

# Core

### Assisted Front Plank

Lie facedown on the floor. Get into pushup position, with your weight on your forearms and your knees. (You can place a pillow under them for support if needed.) Keep your body straight, with your neck aligned with your spine, shoulders down and away from your ears, stomach held up and in, and glutes and thigh muscles squeezed tight. Hold for 10 to 30 seconds to start with and slowly build up to 1 to 2 minutes.

Once you can do that, you can advance to extending your legs straight out and together with your weight on your feet.

### Assisted Side Plank

Lie on your left side with your legs together and knees bent at about 90 degrees. Lift your body up onto your left elbow and forearm, keeping your spine straight. Keep your shoulder down, stomach up and in, and glutes squeezed while you hold for 10 to 30 seconds. Repeat before switching sides.

### Prone Multifidi

Lie facedown with your arms extended above your head. (Use a rolled-up hand towel under your forehead to keep your neck straight.) Pull your stomach up and in, rotating your pelvis back to flatten out the small of your back. Lift your left leg and right arm a couple of inches off the floor and hold for 3 seconds. Do not allow your shoulder to hike up toward your ear. Return to the starting position and lift your right leg and left arm. Hold for 3 seconds and return to the starting position. This is one rep.

When you're stronger, you can perform this exercise on your hands and knees, lifting your arms and legs to align with your body.

### Eccentric Crunches

Sit on the floor and place a rolled-up bath towel or folded bed pillow on the floor perpendicular to your spine to create an arch to crunch over. Lie back over the towel or pillow with your knees bent and feet on the floor. Pull your stomach up and in, rotating your pelvis back while you crunch your upper body a few inches off the floor. Your hands can support your neck, but do not pull upward on it. Slowly relax back down and repeat.

## Cardiovascular

### Intervals

The goal here is to develop muscle endurance, which becomes compromised during the adaptations your body experiences when you're in adrenal fatigue. Cardio particularly benefits your heart and vascular system and limits cortisol overproduction.

Start by walking at a comfortable pace for 3 minutes, then alternate that pace with a greater intensity walk or jog that you can maintain for 2 minutes (work phase). Repeat this alternating pattern three more times to start, which will equal 20 minutes total. Err on the side of lower intensity to start with, to allow yourself to assess how you feel the next day. Light soreness is okay, but if you feel completely wiped or unable to repeat this exercise the next day, you need to pull back and make your work intervals easier.

# Cooldown

## Vertical and Horizontal Tai Chi Circles and Restorative Yoga Sequence

You can continue to perform the exercises on pages 255–257, slowly increasing their difficulty as your body allows. You can do this by squatting deeper with each movement or increasing the time you hold each squat position. Again, these movements should be performed in a slow and controlled manner with constant attention on proper breathing to encourage restoring energy and circulation.

## Mindfulness Walking

Perform as described in Stage 3 (page 257).

# Your Stage 2 Routine

━━━━━━━━━━━━━━ WEEKS 1 & 2 ━━━━━━━━━━━━━━

**WARMUP:** Fast walk for 5–10 minutes
**EXERCISES**

| | MOVEMENT | HOLD TIME | REPS | SETS | REST TIME (BETWEEN SETS) |
|---|---|---|---|---|---|
| **Upper Body** | Modified Pushups (Close Hands) | n/a | 10–15 | 1–2 | 1–2 minutes |
| | Modified Pushups (Neutral Hands) | n/a | 10–15 | 1–2 | 1–2 minutes |
| | Standing Momentum Arm Raises (Front) | n/a | 10–15 | 1–2 | 1–2 minutes |
| | Standing Momentum Arm Raises (Sides) | n/a | 10–15 | 1–2 | 1–2 minutes |
| | Ts | n/a | 10–15 | 1–2 | 1–2 minutes |
| | Ys | n/a | 10–15 | 1–2 | 1–2 minutes |
| | Quarter Dog | 15–30 seconds | 1 | 1–2 | 1–2 minutes |
| **Lower Body** | Bridges (with March) | 10 seconds | 10–15 | 1–2 | 1–2 minutes |
| | Side-Lying Leg Raises | n/a | 10–15 | 1–2 | 1–2 minutes |
| | Single Leg Chair Lifts | 5 seconds | 10–15 | 1–2 | 1–2 minutes |
| | Standing Lunges | n/a | 10 steps each side | 1–2 | 1–2 minutes |
| | Chair Pose | 15–30 seconds | 1 | 1–2 | 1–2 minutes |
| **Core** | Assisted Front Plank | 10–30 seconds | 1 | 1–2 | 1–2 minutes |
| | Assisted Side Plank | 10–30 seconds | 1 | 1–2 | 1–2 minutes |
| | Prone Multifidi | 3 seconds | 10–15 | 1–2 | 1–2 minutes |
| | Eccentric crunches | n/a | 10–15 | 1–2 | 1–2 minutes |

**CARDIOVASCULAR:** Intervals (3 minutes at recovery pace alternated with 2 minutes at work pace); repeat 4 times

**COOLDOWN**

| | MOVEMENT | HOLD TIME | REPS | SETS | REST TIME (BETWEEN SETS) |
|---|---|---|---|---|---|
| **Tai Chi Circles** | Vertical Circles | 3–5 seconds | 10–15 | 2–3 | 1–2 minutes |
| | Horizontal Circles | 3–5 seconds | 10–15 | 2–3 | 1–2 minutes |

| | MOVEMENT | HOLD TIME | REPS | SETS | REST TIME (BETWEEN SETS) |
|---|---|---|---|---|---|
| Restorative Yoga | Supported Child's Pose | 1–2 minutes | 1 | 1 | 0–1 minutes |
| | Assisted Bridge Pose | 1–2 minutes | 1 | 1 | 0–1 minutes |
| | Leg Up on a Chair Pose | 1–2 minutes | 1 | 1 | 0–1 minutes |
| | Supported Goddess Pose | 1–2 minutes | 1 | 1 | 0–1 minutes |

Mindfulness Walking for 10 minutes

## WEEKS 3 & 4

**WARMUP:** Fast walk for 5–10 minutes

**EXERCISES**

| | MOVEMENT | HOLD TIME | REPS | SETS | REST TIME (BETWEEN SETS) |
|---|---|---|---|---|---|
| Upper Body | Modified Pushups (Close Hands) | n/a | 10–15 | 2 | 1–2 minutes |
| | Modified Pushups (Neutral Hands) | n/a | 10–15 | 2 | 1–2 minutes |
| | Standing Momentum Arm Raises (Front) | n/a | 10–15 | 2 | 1–2 minutes |
| | Standing Momentum Arm Raises (Sides) | n/a | 10–15 | 2 | 1–2 minutes |
| | Ts | n/a | 10–15 | 2 | 1–2 minutes |
| | Ys | n/a | 10–15 | 2 | 1–2 minutes |
| | Quarter Dog | 15–30 seconds | 1 | 2 | 1–2 minutes |
| Lower Body | Bridges (with March) | 10 seconds | 10–15 | 2 | 1–2 minutes |
| | Side-Lying Leg Raises | n/a | 10–15 | 2 | 1–2 minutes |
| | Single Leg Chair Lifts | 5 seconds | 10–15 | 2 | 1–2 minutes |
| | Standing Lunges | n/a | 10 steps each side | 2 | 1–2 minutes |
| | Chair Pose | 15–30 seconds | 1 | 2 | 1–2 minutes |
| Core | Assisted Front Plank | 10–30 seconds | 1 | 2 | 1–2 minutes |
| | Assisted Side Plank | 10–30 seconds | 1 | 2 | 1–2 minutes |
| | Prone Multifidi | 3 seconds | 10–15 | 2 | 1–2 minutes |
| | Eccentric Crunches | n/a | 10–15 | 2 | 1–2 minutes |

**CARDIOVASCULAR:** Intervals (3 minutes at recovery pace alternated with 2 minutes at work pace); repeat 4 times

**COOLDOWN:** Repeat Cooldown from Stage 2, Weeks 1 & 2.

# WEEKS 5 & 6

**WARMUP:** Fast walk for 5–10 minutes

## EXERCISES

| | MOVEMENT | HOLD TIME | REPS | SETS | REST TIME (BETWEEN SETS) |
|---|---|---|---|---|---|
| **Upper Body** | Modified Pushups (Close Hands) | n/a | 15–20 | 2 | 1–2 minutes |
| | Modified Pushups (Neutral Hands) | n/a | 15–20 | 2 | 1–2 minutes |
| | Standing Momentum Arm Raises (Front) | n/a | 15–20 | 2 | 1–2 minutes |
| | Standing Momentum Arm Raises (Sides) | n/a | 15–20 | 2 | 1–2 minutes |
| | Ts | n/a | 15–20 | 2 | 1–2 minutes |
| | Ys | n/a | 15–20 | 2 | 1–2 minutes |
| | Quarter Dog | 30–45 seconds | 1 | 2 | 1–2 minutes |
| **Lower Body** | Bridges (with March) | 10 seconds | 15–20 | 2 | 1–2 minutes |
| | Side-Lying Leg Raises | n/a | 15–20 | 2 | 1–2 minutes |
| | Single Leg Chair Lifts | 5 seconds | 15–20 | 2 | 1–2 minutes |
| | Standing Lunges | n/a | 15 steps each side | 2 | 1–2 minutes |
| | Chair Pose | 30–45 seconds | 1 | 2 | 1–2 minutes |
| **Core** | Assisted Front Plank | 30–45 seconds | 1 | 2 | 1–2 minutes |
| | Assisted Side Plank | 30–45 seconds | 1 | 2 | 1–2 minutes |
| | Prone Multifidi | 3 seconds | 15–20 | 2 | 1–2 minutes |
| | Eccentric Crunches | n/a | 15–20 | 2 | 1–2 minutes |

**CARDIOVASCULAR:** Intervals (3 minutes at recovery pace alternated with 2 minutes at work pace); repeat 5 times

**COOLDOWN:** Repeat Cooldown from Stage 2, Weeks 1 & 2.

# WEEKS 7 & 8

**WARMUP:** Fast walk for 5–10 minutes

## EXERCISES

| | MOVEMENT | HOLD TIME | REPS | SETS | REST TIME (BETWEEN SETS) |
|---|---|---|---|---|---|
| **Upper Body** | Modified Pushups Close Hands) | n/a | 15–20 | 2–3 | 1–2 minutes |
| | Modified Pushups (Neutral Hands) | n/a | 15–20 | 2–3 | 1–2 minutes |
| | Standing Momentum Arm Raises (Front) | n/a | 15–20 | 2–3 | 1–2 minutes |
| | Standing Momentum Arm Raises (Sides) | n/a | 15–20 | 2–3 | 1–2 minutes |
| | Ts | n/a | 15–20 | 2–3 | 1–2 minutes |
| | Ys | n/a | 15–20 | 2–3 | 1–2 minutes |
| | Quarter Dog | 30–45 seconds | 1 | 2–3 | 1–2 minutes |
| **Lower Body** | Bridges (with March) | 10 seconds | 15–20 | 2–3 | 1–2 minutes |
| | Side-Lying Leg Raises | n/a | 15–20 | 2–3 | 1–2 minutes |
| | Single Leg Chair Lifts | 5 seconds | 15–20 | 2–3 | 1–2 minutes |
| | Standing Lunges | n/a | 15 steps each side | 2–3 | 1–2 minutes |
| | Chair pose | 30–45 seconds | 1 | 2–3 | 1–2 minutes |
| **Core** | Assisted Front Plank | 30–45 seconds | 1 | 2–3 | 1–2 minutes |
| | Assisted Side Plank | 30–45 seconds | 1 | 2–3 | 1–2 minutes |
| | Prone Multifidi | 3 seconds | 15–20 | 2–3 | 1–2 minutes |
| | Eccentric Crunches | n/a | 15–20 | 2–3 | 1–2 minutes |

**CARDIOVASCULAR:** Intervals (3 minutes at recovery pace alternated with 2 minutes at work pace); repeat 5 times

**COOLDOWN:** Repeat Cooldown from Stage 2, Weeks 1 & 2.

# Stage 1 Protocol

**WARMUP:** Walk quickly or take an easy jog to enhance circulation and prepare your muscles for the upcoming workout.

**EXERCISES:** These exercises maintain good strength, mobility, and body composition and encourage better overall health and resistance to daily stressors on your body. These exercises are a progression from the Stage 2 protocol. Depending on your fitness level at this point, you may need further guidance from a trainer or to start working out at a gym to continue your progress and implement new exercises incorporating other machines or equipment. For the full program, including reps, see "Your Stage 1 Routine" on page 276.

## Upper Body

### Pushups (Close Hands)

Lie facedown with your hands next to each other under your chest and your elbows close to your sides. Keep your shoulders down and away from your ears and your legs fully extended. Keeping your back straight, lift your body up with your hands. Slowly lower back down, keeping your spine straight at all times.

If you can easily do this exercise, you can progress to doing pushups with your lower legs and feet on an exercise ball.

### Pushups (Neutral Hands)

Lie facedown with your hands next to your shoulders, your fingertips pointing forward, and your elbows close to your sides. Keep your shoulders down and away from your ears and your legs fully extended. Keeping your back straight, lift your body up with your hands. Slowly lower back down, keeping your spine straight at all times.

If you can easily do this exercise, you can progress to doing pushups with your lower legs and feet on an exercise ball.

## Standing Momentum Arm Raises (Front and Sides) with Weight

Stand with good posture. Holding either 1- or 2-pound dumbbells or kettlebells, raise your arms to shoulder level in front of you, making sure your shoulders stay down. Lower your arms halfway down, then raise them back up to shoulder level. Finally, lower down to start position. This is one repetition. Repeat the same exercise, but this time with your arms out to your sides.

## Ts Over the Ball

Lie facedown on top of an exercise ball (to increase your range of motion) with your arms out at shoulder level, making a T. (You can anchor your feet along a wall, if needed.) Pull your stomach up and in, rotate your pelvis back (flattening out the small of your back), and tuck your glutes under. Keep your shoulders down and lift your arms up toward the ceiling; hold at the top for 3 to 5 seconds, then return to the starting position.

You can add 1- to 2-pound weights to further intensify the exercise.

## Ys Over the Ball

Lie facedown on top of an exercise ball (to increase your range of motion) with your arms over your head and extended to form a Y with your body. (You can anchor your feet along a wall, if needed.) Pull your stomach up and in, rotate your pelvis back, and tuck your glutes under. Keep your shoulders down and lift your arms up toward the ceiling; hold at the top for 3 to 5 seconds, then return to the starting position.

You can add 1- or 2-pound weights to further intensify the exercise.

## Downward Dog

Kneel on the floor with your toes tucked under. Bend your upper body forward and reach with your arms, placing your weight on your hands, with your arms straight. Shift your weight over your shoulders while you straighten your knees and extend your hips up toward the ceiling. Keep your shoulders back and away from your ears, and try to intensify the stretch by lifting further forward on your toes. Hold for 15 to 30 seconds, working up to 1 to 2 minutes.

## Lower Body

### Reverse Bridge with March on Bench or Ball

Lie with your back on a bench (or an ottoman, if you don't have a bench) or an exercise ball. Position the bench or ball beneath your shoulder blades, with your legs out, knees bent, and feet in line with your hips. Contract your glutes and thighs to lift your hips, then march your feet up and down, making sure your hips stay level throughout and your steps are light.

### Standing Terror Bands

Loop an exercise band low around your ankles, and squat down with good posture. Keep your feet facing forward as you step to one side, keeping tension on the band at all times. Try to keep your chest up and do not drag your feet. Lift your other foot to step to that same side, still keeping tension on the band. Perform 10 to 15 steps down in one direction. Then, while facing the same direction, lead with the opposite leg and take 10 to 15 steps to return to your starting position.

### Glute/Hamstring Ball Curls

Lie on your back with your feet resting on an exercise ball and legs fully extended. Lift up your hips and curl your lower legs inward, making sure your hips stay elevated. Extend back out to return to the starting position. Do 2 sets of 10 to 15 repetitions.

If this feels easy, try performing one-leg curls. (Just lift the resting leg toward the ceiling.)

## Walking Lunges

Stand with good posture. Step forward with one leg, bending your knee so it is directly above your toes and keeping your hips in line with your foot and knee. You can rest your arms on your hips or raise them up and out at shoulder level for balance. Start with smaller steps and minimal squatting. Squeeze your glutes, contract your quadriceps, and bring your back leg forward to rest next to your front leg. From that position, step that same "back" leg out into your next lunge. As your balance permits, omit the resting step and try to take your back leg all the way through to the next lunge. Push back upward through your heel as you return to the starting position. This is one set.

When you can do this with ease, you can add small hand weights to further intensify the exercise.

## Single Leg Chair Pose

Standing with good posture, bring your right foot up and place it against the inside of your left thigh, slightly above your knee. Keep your right knee bent out to your right side. Lift your arms up to shoulder level and reach out to help you balance throughout the pose. Squeeze your left gluteus muscle and squat down, leading with your glutes. Hold this position for 15 to 30 seconds, working up to 1 to 2 minutes.

# Core

## Front Plank

Lie facedown on the floor. Get into pushup position, keeping your legs fully extended, with your weight on your forearms and your toes. Keep your body straight, with your neck aligned with your spine, shoulders down and away from your ears, stomach held up and in, and glutes and thigh muscles squeezed tight. Hold for 10 to 30 seconds to start with and slowly build up to 1 to 2 minutes.

When this is comfortable, you can add alternating straight leg lifts while you are holding, or try bending one knee in toward your chest and holding it up for the duration of the exercise.

## Side Plank

Lie on your left side with your legs together and fully extended. Lift your body up onto your left elbow and forearm, keeping your spine straight and your weight lifted up on the side of your bottom foot. Keep your shoulder down, stomach up and in, and glutes squeezed while you hold for 10 to 30 seconds, working up to 1 to 2 minutes. Repeat before switching sides.

When this is comfortable, you can raise and lower your top leg as you hold this position to intensify the exercise.

## Ball Eccentric Crunches

Sit on an exercise ball, then roll onto your back by walking your feet out in front of you. The ball should rest in the middle of your shoulder blades. Pull your stomach up and in and tilt your pelvis so your glutes are tucked under and your hips are lifted. Arch your back slightly to extend your upper body into a gentle stretch, then contract your abs and raise your torso to just past horizontal. You can support your neck with your hands, but be careful not to pull on it. Slowly lower to the starting position and repeat.

## Oblique Crunches

Lie on your back with your knees bent and your arms extended along your sides. Tilt your pelvis to flatten your lower back into the floor, and then contract your abs to bring your body a few inches off the floor. Your hands can support your neck, but do not pull upward on it. Reach one arm down toward the same side ankle (side crunch), return to your starting position, and then reach toward the opposite side. Return to your starting position without relaxing your body down to the floor.

## Cardiovascular Intervals

You can progress from Stage 2 and continue to support and develop your cardiovascular health by increasing your recovery phase to a comfortable jog (rather than a walk) and increasing the pace or duration of your work phase. If you're ready, you can also alter your workout to maintain a continuous pace, or you can go for a longer total time. The goal is to get in 30 minutes of moderately high intense cardiovascular exercise most days of the week.

You may also want to consider some other activities that can offer great cardiovascular development, including swimming, cycling, and hiking, plus classes such as dance, aerobics, or kickboxing. Maybe you have a goal of running a marathon or participating in a triathlon. There are plenty of trainers and coaches that can provide you with further guidance at this point. This is a great time to explore different activities and find what you enjoy most. Finding something you genuinely enjoy gives you the best chance of consistently engaging in these exercises throughout your lifetime.

## Cooldown

### Vertical and Horizontal Tai Chi Circles and Restorative Yoga Sequence
Perform as described in Stage 3 (pages 255–257).

### Mindful Walking
Perform as described in Stage 3 (page 257).

# Your Stage 1 Routine

=== WEEKS 1 & 2 ===

**WARMUP:** Fast walk for 5–10 minutes

**EXERCISES**

| | MOVEMENT | HOLD TIME | REPS | SETS | REST TIME (BETWEEN SETS) |
|---|---|---|---|---|---|
| **Upper Body** | Pushups (Close Hands) | n/a | 10–15 | 2 | 1–2 minutes |
| | Pushups (Neutral Hands) | n/a | 10–15 | 2 | 1–2 minutes |
| | Standing Momentum Arm Raises (Front) | n/a | 10–15, with weights | 2 | 1–2 minutes |
| | Standing Momentum Arm Raises (Sides) | n/a | 10–15, with weights | 2 | 1–2 minutes |
| | Ts over the ball | n/a | 10–15 | 2 | 1–2 minutes |
| | Ys over the ball | n/a | 10–15 | 2 | 1–2 minutes |
| | Downward Dog | 15–30 seconds | 1 | 2 | 1–2 minutes |
| **Lower Body** | Reverse Bridge with March on Bench or Ball | n/a | 10–15 steps each side | 2 | 1–2 minutes |
| | Standing Terror Bands | n/a | 10–15 each way | 2 | 1–2 minutes |
| | Glute/Hamstring Ball Curls | n/a | 10–15 | 2 | 1–2 minutes |
| | Walking Lunges | n/a | 10 steps each way | 2 | 1–2 minutes |
| | Single Leg Chair Pose | 15–30 seconds | 1 | 2 | 1–2 minutes |
| **Core** | Front Plank | 10–30 seconds | 1 | 2 | 1–2 minutes |
| | Side Plank | 10–30 seconds | 1 | 2 | 1–2 minutes |
| | Ball Eccentric Crunches | n/a | 10–15 | 2 | 1–2 minutes |
| | Oblique Crunches | n/a | 10 each side | 2 | 1–2 minutes |

**CARDIOVASCULAR:** Intervals (3 minutes at recovery pace alternated with 2 minutes at work pace); repeat 5 times

**COOLDOWN**

| | MOVEMENT | HOLD TIME | REPS | SETS | REST TIME (BETWEEN SETS) |
|---|---|---|---|---|---|
| **Tai Chi Circles** | Vertical Circles | 3–5 seconds | 10–15 | 2–3 | 1–2 minutes |
| | Horizontal Circles | 3–5 seconds | 10–15 | 2–3 | 1–2 minutes |

| | MOVEMENT | HOLD TIME | REPS | SETS | REST TIME (BETWEEN SETS) |
|---|---|---|---|---|---|
| Restorative Yoga | Supported Child's Pose | 1–2 minutes | 1 | 1 | 0–1 minutes |
| | Assisted Bridge Pose | 1–2 minutes | 1 | 1 | 0–1 minutes |
| | Leg Up on a Chair Pose | 1–2 minutes | 1 | 1 | 0–1 minutes |
| | Supported Goddess Pose | 1–2 minutes | 1 | 1 | 0–1 minutes |

Mindfulness Walking for 10 minutes

# WEEKS 3 & 4

**WARMUP:** Fast walk for 5–10 minutes
**EXERCISES**

| | MOVEMENT | HOLD TIME | REPS | SETS | REST TIME (BETWEEN SETS) |
|---|---|---|---|---|---|
| Upper Body | Pushups (Close Hands) | n/a | 10–15 | 2–3 | 1–2 minutes |
| | Pushups (Neutral Hands) | n/a | 10–15 | 2–3 | 1–2 minutes |
| | Standing Momentum Arm Raises (Front) | n/a | 10–15, with weights | 2–3 | 1–2 minutes |
| | Standing Momentum Arm Raises (Sides) | n/a | 10–15, with weights | 2–3 | 1–2 minutes |
| | Ts over the ball | n/a | 10–15 | 2–3 | 1–2 minutes |
| | Ys over the ball | n/a | 10–15 | 2–3 | 1–2 minutes |
| | Downward Dog | 15–30 seconds | 1 | 2–3 | 1–2 minutes |
| Lower Body | Reverse Bridges with March | n/a | 10–15 steps each side | 2–3 | 1–2 minutes |
| | Standing Terror Bands | n/a | 10–15 each way | 2–3 | 1–2 minutes |
| | Glute/Hamstring Ball Curls | n/a | 10–15 | 2–3 | 1–2 minutes |
| | Walking Lunges | n/a | 10 steps each way | 2–3 | 1–2 minutes |
| | Single Leg Chair Pose | 15–30 seconds | 1 | 2–3 | 1–2 minutes |
| Core | Front Plank | 10–30 seconds | 1 | 2–3 | 1–2 minutes |
| | Side Plank | 10–30 seconds | 1 | 2–3 | 1–2 minutes |
| | Ball Eccentric Crunches | n/a | 10–15 | 2–3 | 1–2 minutes |
| | Oblique Crunches | n/a | 10 each side | 2–3 | 1–2 minutes |

**CARDIOVASCULAR:** Intervals (3 minutes at recovery pace alternated with 2 minutes at work pace); repeat 5 times

**COOLDOWN:** Repeat Cooldown from Stage 1, Weeks 1 & 2.

# WEEKS 5 & 6

**WARMUP:** Fast walk for 5–10 minutes

**EXERCISES**

| | MOVEMENT | HOLD TIME | REPS | SETS | REST TIME (BETWEEN SETS) |
|---|---|---|---|---|---|
| Upper Body | Pushups (Close Hands) | n/a | 15–20 | 2–3 | 1–2 minutes |
| | Pushups (Neutral Hands) | n/a | 15–20 | 2–3 | 1–2 minutes |
| | Standing Momentum Arm Raises (Front) | n/a | 15, with weights | 2–3 | 1–2 minutes |
| | Standing Momentum Arm Raises (Sides) | n/a | 15, with weights | 2–3 | 1–2 minutes |
| | Ts over the ball | n/a | 15–20 | 2–3 | 1–2 minutes |
| | Ys over the ball | n/a | 15–20 | 2–3 | 1–2 minutes |
| | Downward Dog | 30–45 seconds | 1 | 2–3 | 1–2 minutes |
| Lower Body | Reverse Bridges with March | n/a | 15–20 steps each side | 2–3 | 1–2 minutes |
| | Standing Terror Bands | n/a | 15–20 each way | 2–3 | 1–2 minutes |
| | Glute/Hamstring Ball Curls | n/a | 15–20 | 2–3 | 1–2 minutes |
| | Walking Lunges | n/a | 15 steps each way | 2–3 | 1–2 minutes |
| | Single Leg Chair Pose | 30–45 seconds | 1 | 2–3 | 1–2 minutes |
| Core | Front Plank | 30–45 seconds | 1 | 2–3 | 1–2 minutes |
| | Side Plank | 30–45 seconds | 1 | 2–3 | 1–2 minutes |
| | Ball Eccentric Crunches | n/a | 15–20 | 2–3 | 1–2 minutes |
| | Oblique Crunches | n/a | 15 each side | 2–3 | 1–2 minutes |

**CARDIOVASCULAR:** Intervals (3 minutes at recovery pace alternated with 2 minutes at work pace); repeat 5 times

**COOLDOWN:** Repeat Cooldown from Stage 1, Weeks 1 & 2.

# WEEKS 7 & 8

**WARMUP:** Fast walk for 5–10 minutes

**EXERCISES**

| | MOVEMENT | HOLD TIME | REPS | SETS | REST TIME (BETWEEN SETS) |
|---|---|---|---|---|---|
| **Upper Body** | Pushups (Close Hands) | n/a | 15–20 | 3 | 1–2 minutes |
| | Pushups (Neutral Hands) | n/a | 15–20 | 3 | 1–2 minutes |
| | Standing Momentum Arm Raises (Front) | n/a | 15, with weights | 3 | 1–2 minutes |
| | Standing Momentum Arm Raises (Sides) | n/a | 15, with weights | 3 | 1–2 minutes |
| | Ts over the ball | n/a | 15–20 | 3 | 1–2 minutes |
| | Ys over the ball | n/a | 15–20 | 3 | 1–2 minutes |
| | Downward Dog | 30–45 seconds | 1 | 3 | 1–2 minutes |
| **Lower Body** | Reverse Bridges with March | n/a | 15–20 steps each side | 3 | 1–2 minutes |
| | Standing Terror Bands | n/a | 15–20 each way | 3 | 1–2 minutes |
| | Glute/Hamstring Ball Curls | n/a | 15–20 | 3 | 1–2 minutes |
| | Walking Lunges | n/a | 15 steps each way | 3 | 1–2 minutes |
| | Single Leg Chair Pose | 30–45 seconds | 1 | 3 | 1–2 minutes |
| **Core** | Front Plank | 30–45 seconds | 1 | 3 | 1–2 minutes |
| | Side Plank | 30–45 seconds | 1 | 3 | 1–2 minutes |
| | Ball Eccentric Crunches | n/a | 15–20 | 3 | 1–2 minutes |
| | Oblique Crunches | n/a | 15 each side | 3 | 1–2 minutes |

**CARDIOVASCULAR:** Intervals (3 minutes at recovery pace alternated with 2 minutes at work pace); repeat 5 times

**COOLDOWN:** Repeat Cooldown from Stage 1, Weeks 1 & 2.

# MY TURNAROUND
## SHERI PREDEBON, AGE: 44

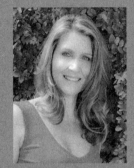

"I had trouble focusing on things and felt really fatigued. I was picking fights with my husband; I was just raging and emotional and upset. It felt like it was PMS times 100. I couldn't control it and I knew I had to change something."

That was Sheri Predebon's life before she knew she had adrenal fatigue. She had struggled with symptoms for years but was never properly diagnosed.

It wasn't until a friend referred her to Dr. Pingel that Sheri finally got some answers. "I had no idea that my body was dominant in estrogen, which was caused by polycystic ovarian syndrome. Dr. Pingel explained how different foods and chemicals can increase the amount of estrogen in your body and how that relates to adrenal fatigue," Sheri states.

By following Dr. Pingel's all-natural plan, Sheri got her life back on track. "Before, I was eating a lot of meat and dairy and drinking gallons of diet cola," she admits. "But after going on this plan, I began eating more greens and more whole foods. I also became a certified nutritionist to educate myself and become very aware of what I was putting in my body."

Today, Sheri's life couldn't be more different. "Before, I had no energy and couldn't get up in the morning, so I wasn't exercising." These days, she has more energy and even regularly competes in fitness competitions. To further her treatment, Sheri decided it was time to reduce the stress in her life. "On a scale of 1 to 10, my stress was at a 9 due to my demanding job and adrenal fatigue. Now I'm working as a consultant, and I make my own hours and my own schedule. My stress is really low now, and life could not be better."

After treating her adrenal fatigue, Sheri has had no sign of her original symptoms in years. "Before, I was always fighting for energy and didn't understand why. My energy and mood are so much better now," she says. Sheri helps guide others who are experiencing health issues due to adrenal fatigue. "I tell my clients to get lots of sleep, eat whole foods, and try to get in to see a naturopathic physician. It's a lifestyle change when you're looking to heal something like your adrenal glands, but it's worth it."

# 14

# THE MIND-BODY CONNECTION

The emotional aspect of healing is often overlooked by conventional doctors, as it is seen as something strictly handled by psychiatrists and counselors. This is a mistake. Recovery is not simply about taking supplements and making dietary changes; it is a whole lifestyle change. And to properly heal adrenal fatigue, you have to deal with your stress in order to stop the physical manifestations of that stress. This means that you have to make time to let your body reach a parasympathetic (or calm) state. If you don't, you will continue to face the same obstacles.

I find that, among my patients, there are different types of personalities when it comes to dealing with both symptoms and therapy. There are the people who are constantly mentioning their shortcomings and looking for a quick fix, and then there are those who accept their condition and move forward with an open mind and heart. Which one are you?

If I told you that in order to get rid of your pain you had to follow a specific diet regimen, take a specific set of supplements, and make the lifestyle changes I recommend, would you commit wholeheartedly? Or would you get bogged down by life and sneak small, harmful items into your diet, skip your workouts, and forget your supplements? Would you turn off your e-mail or cell phone? Could you tell someone no? Would you have the discipline and the ability to deal with the pain on a daily basis while you commit to the healing process? Or would you lean on pain management pills and slip up on your regimen? I am not trying to point out your missteps, as everyone will stumble now and then, but in order to get well, you need to know how committed you really are.

It can be difficult for a patient to commit to a natural lifestyle, especially after many years of eating processed foods, taking medications, and dealing with depression. It is even more difficult if you are overweight or obese and experiencing pain. When I tell you to walk or do yoga, you may say, "I can't, it hurts." So you either find a way to make the activity happen, maybe by starting with physical therapy or working with a trainer who can help you overcome your body's limitations, or you simply don't commit. The choice is up to you. But why not go for it? Ask yourself why you've quit something. Is it truly a physical limitation, or might it be an emotional limitation?

## THE COMMITMENT SACRIFICE

I love bread—I really do. It's great. I love it toasted, on sandwiches, dipped in sauces, everything. But I can't eat it if I want to be well because it will always result in my body feeling fatigued, or it will promote illness. Trust me, there are times that I have a small bite, just to savor that one moment, but I pay for it later. I made a choice many years ago to commit to my health, so I deny myself bread because I am worth that investment. After all, it is just bread!

There are plenty of other wonderful things that I can enjoy in place of it.

This is not about what you can or can't eat, what diet you need to follow, or how to lose weight quickly—this is about keeping your cells happy. Without them, you cannot live. If your adrenal glands are fatigued, you will notice symptoms. By healing your adrenal glands, you're healing the way your cells communicate and opening the door not to decent health, but to optimum health.

I have a patient who has diabetes, high cholesterol, high blood pressure, and an enlarged prostate. He was explaining to me how he went to the movies and ate a huge bag of buttered popcorn, drank a diet soda, and ate candy. Then he went on to explain how when he gets up in the morning he is dizzy and cannot feel his feet when they touch the floor. He often skips breakfast, stays up late eating chips and bread, and is exhausted in the morning. He even stopped playing golf because his knees hurt too much. I asked him this question: Do you want to die?

When I asked him this, he said that he does not want to live his life constantly sacrificing the things he enjoys. He wants to enjoy every day, and eating those things makes him happy. Well, at least he was honest.

But the problem with his answer is that nothing is sacrificed when you're exercising and eating well. There are so many wonderful, delicious foods out there that also provide abundant energy and the opportunity for you to have a full, healthy, active life. Although he did not come right out and admit it point-blank, this gentleman is behaving like he doesn't want to live a long life. He does not have the self-esteem to commit to what would give him more time with the wife he adores and the family who loves him. Think about your children. What about your grandchildren? And what about your spouse? What are their goals for you and for their lives? What do you want to do with your life?

## THE THREE STEPS TO EMOTIONAL HEALING

One of the most difficult things for people to do is face their emotional demons. You probably don't want to face the worst parts of yourself, but it is essential that you do so. Remember that your mind and body are connected, and if your brain is holding on to something, your body will manifest it. Finding a way to let go is critical to this process of adrenal restoration.

**STEP 1: DEVELOP COMPLETE LOVE FOR YOURSELF.** If you do not have it, find it. Ask yourself why you don't think you are worthy of a healthy life. This step is critical and if you have not accomplished it yet, you cannot complete the next step very easily. During this step, many of my patients start therapy with a counselor. I have quite a few that start neurofeedback, which analyzes brain wave patterns to help people train their brains to function more efficiently, to explore what might be holding them back from accomplishing this step. Consider placing notes around the house to remind yourself of your strengths. Remind yourself why you fell in love with your spouse and why he or she fell in love with you. Look at yourself through the eyes of your children, who adore you. It is your time to heal—your time to recover—so take it. This step may take some time, but that is all right because it leads you to success. Don't be afraid of it; don't run from it. Just commit yourself to it.

**STEP 2: STOP MAKING EXCUSES FOR YOUR AILMENTS.** It's time to take control of your body. After all, your mind and body are connected. A great example of this connection occurs during natural childbirth. How is it that you can dismiss the pain with your commitment to your baby? I have had two natural childbirths, and man, they were painful. But that was okay, because that pain was for the good of my baby. Your body and brain, via your adrenal system and the release of adrenaline, have the ability to turn pain signals on and off. For example, I was able to recognize the pain and make a decision not to focus on it but to focus on my baby, instead. Think of when you hear about a traumatic event and the people who rise up to take care of others despite their own pain and injuries (like after a car accident, for example). They made a choice not to focus on their pain.

You can make that same choice now. You can't play golf because your knee hurts? Well, find another sport to play. Or see a physical therapist for your knee. Don't let that ailment stop you from enjoying life. Over the years, I have learned a few techniques for changing my focus from negative to positive. One is to sit down every night and make a list of 10 positive things from the day. Can't think of that many? Look closer. For example, you may think you had a bad day because you were running 20 minutes late for work. Turn it around by writing down that you were grateful to have 20 more minutes with your family this morning. In every bad thing, there is good. Focus on looking for that goodness every night before you go to bed. And when you wake up in the morning, make your life positive. Tell yourself that you will have a good day, without pain and without limitation. At first, this will be very difficult. You will find yourself turning negative and focusing on what you cannot do rather than on what you can. But in time, your focus will change—and so will your health. And after all, you are worth this change.

**STEP 3: COMMIT TO YOUR NEW LIFESTYLE.** This is the final step—you need to really commit. But here's the thing: You won't fully commit until you love yourself and stop making excuses. Do you eat potato chips every night at midnight? If so, stop buying them. Don't give yourself that option. Instead, cut up carrots and leave them in the fridge. Or put almonds in your potato chip bag. When you make the choice to commit (notice I said when *you*, not your doctor, make the choice), go through your entire house and clean out any foods that do not qualify as acceptable on your new plan. Yes, this is wasting money. Accept that. Maybe you can donate the food to a local shelter, but it can't be in your house. Set some rules for the house that no processed food is allowed. This is *your* life, *your* home, *your* health. How do you want to live? The bottom line is, as humans, we won't starve. Eventually you will eat an apple or an orange, some kale, or a bowl of brussels sprouts. If it's all you have, you will eat it and will honestly like it once your taste buds stop craving the processed foods of the past.

As we discussed in the previous chapter, exercise is also critical for good health. We were built to walk all day long and lift heavy objects. We are mobile. However, we choose to sit and get fat. Exercise can be painful, and it is hard work. I go to Pilates every week, and I always dread going. I am tired, I've worked all day, and I have kids at home waiting for me, but I go because I have committed to doing what my body needs to stay well. And I moan and whine when I push myself. I find excuses not to go, but I talk myself into going anyway. No one said this was easy. It is about making that mental change. It's about commitment.

## TOOLS FOR SUCCESS: GOING AGAINST THE NORM

Now that you've learned the three steps to emotional healing, how do you take yourself away from the hustle and bustle of society and actually make them happen? Many people don't even realize the stress they endure on a day-to-day basis. We spend our days responding to everything that occurs right in that instant, rather than taking a more calm and productive approach. We assume that the faster something gets done, the better. But what if you changed your focus and actually got more done while remaining calm?

I once read a book that described how to get 8 hours of work done in 4. Can you imagine that? Do you want to know how they did it? They did not respond to everything at the exact moment it occurred. So let's take a look at what your life may look like now, where you handle everything in the moment it arises, and compare it with a less-stressful way.

Imagine that you're sitting at a computer drafting an e-mail. The phone rings, so you stop writing the e-mail to answer the phone. The person on the phone asks you to make a copy of a document, so you hang up and start copying it. The e-mail is left waiting. As you are copying the document, a coworker walks by and starts to chat socially. In the midst of that conversation, your phone rings again, so you excuse yourself from the conversation and answer the phone. It's your son, and he needs you to tell him where his blue jacket is. You hang up and go back to the document you were copying.

Once you're finished, you drop off the document and head back to your office. On the way, the receptionist stops you, tells you about a problem with how another account is being handled, and asks your opinion of the situation. You share your opinion, taking on the responsibility to resolve the situation, and you let her know that you'll give her a copy of a document you'll create to help her through this concern. When you walk into your office to look for that document, your phone rings and you are called to a lunch meeting. Wow. Is it lunchtime already? Out you go to the meeting, and when you return to your office, you begin to read your e-mails—all 50 of them. You start with the most recent and work your way backward. That's when you remember the e-mail you started earlier. You'd better get that done.

So you've started working on that e-mail again when your best friend texts you about something fun she did the night before. She tells you to check Facebook for the pictures. As a result, you log on to Facebook and find yourself reading about everyone else's lives. Someone mentions a great place they went to for dinner, and you Google it. It sounds nice, so you make a reservation for Friday night. That's when your phone rings; it's your son asking what you're having for dinner. Oh, no—you forgot about dinner. You call for takeout and get back to your e-mail. You finally finish the e-mail you started in the morning and see that you have 10 new e-mails. As you read through them—as well as the e-mails you never got to from this morning—you discover that there is an urgent situation that requires your attention. They e-mailed you at noon, while you were at lunch. So you respond to the e-mail and promise to take care of it right away.

By this point, it's 5:15 p.m. and you have to get home. You get in the car, and while you're driving home, you call the client in need. When you arrive home, you greet your family and boot up your computer to finish going through your e-mail. After deciding to put some of the less-urgent e-mails on hold for tomorrow, it is time to eat dinner with your family. You eat, put the kids to bed, and go watch your favorite show. Right before bed, you check your e-mail again: You have 5 new messages and you decide to answer them right then. Your phone has 10 texts from various people who are just saying hello, and you respond to those, as well. Now it's 10:00 p.m. and you are exhausted. You fall asleep thinking about the e-mails you did not answer and wake up the next day to do it all again. Is this a life? How much of that could have been avoided?

Now let's look at an alternative situation: Imagine that you wake up on time and enjoy breakfast with your family. You head to the office and block out 1 hour to answer and respond to all e-mails. You let calls go to voicemail and even turn off the ringer. You then set an autoreply to let people know that you will check and respond to all e-mails between 9:00 and 10:00 a.m. and then again between 2:00 and 3:00 p.m. You check your voicemail and respond to any business-related calls. Social calls are reserved for a later time or until after all of your morning work is completed. All e-mails and voicemails are returned and completed in the order of receipt—no jumping from one to another.

In this scenario, you finish each task as you go, in order of request. You put a sign on your door and you leave a voicemail message letting people know that your door will be open for questions, daily concerns, etc., between the hours of 10:30 and 11:00 a.m. and right after lunch. Hmm. It's quiet. It's 9:45 a.m. and all of your e-mails have been answered. There is no one calling you and nothing beeping at you. This means you can actually work. You get your projects done and it's now 10:30 a.m. You open your door and wait for emergencies. There aren't any, because the people who would have interrupted you earlier in your day figured out a way to handle their problems themselves. Their issues are not urgent anymore. It's funny how once others have to take responsibility for their own hiccups and you aren't available, they can figure out how to get them done. They don't actually need you; you just happened to be there.

If there is indeed an urgent request, your brain is now calm enough to be able to delegate and complete the task. It is now 11:00 a.m. What will you do for the next hour? Work! Get old projects done and plan new ones. If everything is done, guess what? You have free time to plan dinner or check in on Facebook. After heading to lunch and spending the afternoon as planned, with a set time for interruptions and e-mails, you are done early and head out of the office at 4:00 p.m. There is nothing left pending. Once you arrive at home, you're able to enjoy your family. You turn off your phone and do not check your messages again until the next day at the scheduled time.

Just imagine a life where people have to leave you messages rather than being able to reach you at every moment. The younger generation cannot remember this time. I remember having an answering machine with a tape in it that told callers when I was not home. I would check my messages and return all social phone calls when I got back. I had the time to do that in the evenings because I was not bothered all day, so I got my work done. There was no e-mail to check, no cell phone, no Facebook. Remember that simplicity? How stressed were you then, compared to now? How scattered was your brain? Did you always feel like you could not keep up? Or did you accept that you would not reach people right away? I am making this point because people don't realize how stressed they actually are. You get floored when you reach someone's voicemail, or if someone doesn't respond to your text quickly. Let's be real. We have technology and it has its purpose. I am not intending to be hypocritical as I sit here in a coffee shop, writing on my Mac. But I encourage you to schedule your time. Schedule time for home, work, and play. Make keeping a schedule a priority. Tell people no. Your work will be so much more efficient and your body will not progress to illness because it's suffering from the stress of trying to do everything for everyone at a moment's notice.

When you make this time for yourself, you will find that you have more time to enjoy life. Suddenly, taking 30 minutes to play Legos with your kids is not such an imposition on your housecleaning time. Your day goes by more slowly, as you can fill it with multiple activities, instead of rushing everywhere. Can you commit to yourself like this? Committing to a lifestyle that allows you to find time and space for yourself will help heal your adrenal fatigue. It will also prevent adrenal fatigue from happening again in the future. You have to schedule time to enjoy yourself and to connect with your mind and body. And here's the great part: You only need 10 to 15 minutes of mindful meditation each day to reconnect with yourself. If you put yourself on a schedule that allows time for this, you will reach optimal health much faster and prevent further disease development.

# THE ART OF MEDITATION

Meditation is an art. It is not easy. To take your mind away from real life and plant it in the metaphysical is hard work! But the benefits are so incredibly vast that I encourage you to start learning to meditate. A recent study of meditation and addiction evaluated two groups of smokers, one that meditated and one that just relaxed. It showed that those who committed to daily meditation for 2 weeks showed a 60 percent reduction in smoking tobacco, while the subjects who simply relaxed showed no change in their smoking habits. In addition, brain scans for the meditation group showed increased activity in the areas of the brain that regulate self-control.[1] This is extremely beneficial, as nicotine is highly addictive and requires immense self-control to remove from your system. People spend their lives trying to quit. Maybe if my father had not been such a heavy smoker, he could have saved his heart.

I have seen addiction throughout my life—whether it was addiction to nicotine or food—and listened to excuses about why someone can't control the addiction. But it is often the case that people simply do not want to quit. Learn the techniques to teach your brain what it does or does not need, and it will believe what you teach it. Can you imagine what success you could have with eating a better diet and committing to exercise if you used meditation as an aid? If you can improve your self-control by accessing that portion of your brain, you can do anything!

Researchers are also studying the effects of meditation on cardiovascular health. A study released in 2013 showed that meditation may have beneficial effects on your blood pressure and the stimulation of your heart. Meditation was shown to have a positive effect on reducing inflammation in the body.[2] Another study evaluated women undergoing radiation therapy for breast cancer. The test group was given 12 meditation sessions during a 6-week radiation period. During that time, fatigue, anxiety, quality of life, and emotional well-being were all evaluated. After the meditation therapy, the participants saw an improvement in anxiety, fatigue, and overall quality of life compared with those without meditation therapy.[3]

And if you're still not convinced of the benefits of meditation for your adrenal fatigue, recent research has shown that meditation not only improves thinking, but it also reduces stress! Researchers studied the effects of meditation on physiology, cognitive function, IQ, and EQ (emotional quotient) in 34 male student volunteers. On two separate occasions 1 month apart, each student came to the lab for testing and monitoring. During the first session, the students spent 10 minutes playing a computer game (as a stressor). Then they spent a month learning guided meditation with the help of an instructor and tapes. During the second session they spent 10 minutes playing the computer game again, and then they spent 15 minutes meditating. Stress changed specific physiological variables, including cortisol levels, and it reduced performance of certain cognitive tasks. A month of regular meditation increased IQ and EQ, reduced physiological stress responses, and improved cognitive function.[4]

## Learning to Meditate

So how should you begin? There are many ways to meditate, most of which start with breathing. As you read this, check your breath. Are you breathing? Really listen to yourself. When was your last breath? How deep was it? Did your chest expand fully?

Most of us do not expand our chests when we breathe. Instead, we typically take small, shallow breaths. But your rib cage was built to move, and if you don't take large breaths and move your rib cage, your thoracic spine (the section of spine in the middle of your back) locks up, making breathing deeply even more difficult. This then causes your neck and lower back to become more mobile, resulting in spinal rotations and pain. If you are always at the chiropractor for rotating cervical and lumbar manipulations, or for locked ribs, deeper breathing will

## PRACTICING MEDITATION IN EACH STAGE OF ADRENAL FATIGUE

Meditation is important during all stages of adrenal fatigue because of its capacity to connect your mind and body and to prevent disease development. The focus of your meditation will change to address the specific needs of each stage.

**STAGE 1:** Those in Stage 1 are commonly on the go, moving very quickly and rarely taking a moment for themselves. It is important to spend your meditative time reminding yourself of who you are. What do you enjoy? What is your purpose in life? Most people in Stage 1 cannot meditate effectively because they spend their time thinking about what they have to get done. Instead, I suggest you focus on your breath. Focus on your health. Focus on your purpose. Let go of the day and the worry. Enjoy the stillness as you acknowledge the importance of your health.

**STAGE 2:** During Stage 2, symptoms usually occur and many people begin experiencing self-doubt. They feel overwhelmed and may even hate their bodies. Meditation is important during this stage because it helps you focus on your beauty. What makes you beautiful and unique? Why do your friends enjoy your company? What is special about you? Listen to your pulse as you reconnect with who you are. Breathe. Imagine yourself in a deep sleep, surrounded by calm water. See a deer in the woods. Watch it glide through its space. The world is in harmony. Find your place within that harmony. End your meditation sessions by again reminding yourself of your beauty.

**STAGE 3:** Finally, during Stage 3, many people are surrounded by pain or significant illness. These conditions tend to consume their thoughts. Those in Stage 3 need to focus on finding good in the day. Imagine yourself well and without pain. Focus on finding the strength within yourself to fight—it's a strength you used to have but have disconnected from. Use this time to focus on energy. See yourself completing tasks. You have the power to heal yourself. Find that fighter within. Try to feel the adrenaline of success. Notice the changes in your heartbeat when you think about energy. Notice the feeling of confidence. Those in Stage 3 need to meditate to focus on their goals and get them done.

help you immensely. Simply put, meditation will help you relieve pain by moving what was meant to move.

A good way to prepare for meditation is to find a quiet spot and focus on your breathing. Remember, your goal is to have full, well-filled lungs. If your body is not used to this, it will be exhausting to take those deep breaths. It may cause some discomfort and you may want to quit. Don't. Lie down if you need to reduce any back pain. Try to meditate for 5 minutes every day. Focus on making your rib cage expand with each breath and letting every bit of air out when you exhale. If your mind wanders, focus it back on your breath.

After you get your breath in order, listen to your heartbeat. Focus on your pulse. Is it fast or slow? Does it change as you breathe more deeply? You can reach a meditative state simply by focusing on your parasympathetic system, or on automatic functions like breathing and heart rate.

## Your Restorative Meditation Routine

I interviewed Ruth Hartung, the director of 7 Centers Yoga Arts in Sedona, Arizona, who agreed that meditation is beneficial when healing adrenal fatigue, noting that "Meditation [benefits] our health by activating the parasympathetic nervous system and allowing the mind and body to rest for short periods within a day." She also shared some tips on learning to meditate, especially for those with adrenal fatigue.

Begin by sitting in a comfortable position—either in a chair or on a pillow on the floor where you can be still and sit with your spine straight. Now become aware of your breath. Follow your breath as it comes in and goes out. Become aware of the sensations you experience as your breath first enters your nose and then exits it.

You may notice qualities of warmth or coolness in your breath. Keep your breath consistent; don't make your inhalations longer or shorter. Thoughts will come to distract you. Perhaps you hear your stomach gurgling or your attention is pulled to sounds around you. When this happens, gently redirect your attention back to your breath. In this way,

# SEVEN TIPS FOR JOURNALING YOUR WAY TO ADRENAL RESTORATION

Journaling can be a fantastic way to not only reduce your stress, but also to stay on track with the steps of emotional, as well as physical, healing. A study published in the *Journal of the American Medical Association* found that patients struggling with a chronic illness who wrote down their thoughts about stressful situations experienced fewer physical symptoms than patients who did not journal. In addition, these patients showed a significant (50 percent) improvement in their diseases after 4 months of journaling.[5]

Daily journaling will serve as a reminder of your three steps: Love yourself, stop making excuses, and commit to your new lifestyle. Everyone journals differently, and there is no right or wrong way to complete this task. But however you choose to journal, it should always remind you of your goals and focus. Your journal entries should always end on a positive note, making you feel peaceful and instilling motivation to continue your journey to total health.

Here are some suggestions for effective journaling.

1. List 5 things that happened during your day that were negative in nature, and rewrite them as positive experiences.
2. Write an imaginative story that visualizes you accomplishing your goals.
3. Write down positive descriptive words about yourself.
4. Write down what you love about yourself.
5. Each night, write why you are committing to this total health turnaround. Write down why you are worth this makeover.
6. Write down your excuses for not getting well. Then rewrite them with a positive spin. For example, "I cannot commit to exercise because I am in pain" becomes "I am not in pain. My body is simply trying to communicate with me, asking me to get well. I will listen to my body and commit to making it well."
7. Keep a record of your daily activities, including your dietary choices, supplements taken, exercise habits, sleeping patterns, and health markers, such as blood work. Seeing a log of these efforts and improvements will help you maintain motivation as you restore your adrenal function.

you'll begin to train your mind, which has a habit of scattering and moving constantly. This lack of focus creates both physical and emotional exhaustion. By focusing on your breath, you'll anchor your awareness in your body by becoming aware of its sensations and movements, and you'll begin to train your mind to one-pointedness. This is a much more efficient and effective way to use your mind in all areas of life.

Now it may be harder to remain focused the first few times you try this, and that's normal. But try to meditate for at least 5 minutes each day to create a sense of calmness and serenity. If you still find yourself feeling stressed after meditating, try the Restorative Yoga routine on page 256.

## THE MIND-BODY CONNECTION

Your mind is connected to your body, and the signals from your brain control your body. Is it so hard to believe that by adjusting your brain you can change your body? If your stereo was not working, would you check the wires? Of course! I encourage you to commit to yourself and open up to the possibility of healing emotionally. Once you do, your adrenal fatigue will finally begin to reverse and you can enjoy true, total health.

# MY TURNAROUND
## KIRSTEN AIRD, AGE: 19

At just 19 years old, Kirsten Aird's stress was taking a toll on her health. "My stress level was very high since I have a heavy college work load. I was also worried and frustrated about my health," she admits. "I was diagnosed with hypothyroidism and dealt with migraines, food allergies, muscle and joint pain, sleep issues, and, on top of that, weight gain."

Kirsten went to see a naturopathic physician but didn't get the help she needed. "The doctor's advice was to get more and more restrictive with my diet, but when I did that and didn't see any results, it became very frustrating. The doctor also increased the dosage of my thyroid medication from time to time, and I ended up taking too high of a dose, which overtaxed my adrenal glands. While my experience with that doctor was not optimal, I still preferred the way naturopathic physicians look at the patient as a whole to find the root cause instead of simply masking symptoms with drugs," she says.

Determined to find help, Kirsten scheduled an appointment with Dr. Pingel. "Before being diagnosed, I had not heard of adrenal fatigue. I wasn't familiar with what the adrenals were or why their health impacted my health," she shares.

After a few months on Dr. Pingel's plan, Kirsten could notice a difference. "I have almost no muscle and joint pain," she shares. In addition, her sleep has improved, her energy has increased, and her headaches are lessening. "My weight has slowly but steadily decreased, and I went from a size 11 to a size 7. My blood work also shows improvements in my thyroid numbers. Before, I was so tired and overwhelmed, but now I have had friends at school ask me how I manage to balance everything so effectively."

Today, Kirsten's stress level is significantly better. "Nowadays, I think I have learned to manage my stress level more effectively, and even though my college work load hasn't changed, feeling stronger and healthier helps me manage things better," she says. "My experience has helped me to be compassionate with other individuals who are going through the same thing. It's important to not lose hope, hold on to your faith, and just keep looking for an answer and someone to listen and take you seriously. When you find a doctor who takes you and your concerns seriously and whom you can trust to help you gain your health back, then you will start to feel like there is hope to feel better."

# MY TURNAROUND
## SUSAN SEKAN, AGE: 53

Susan Sekan began experiencing health problems a few years ago. "My OB/GYN said I was perimenopausal and put me on birth control to regulate my periods. I was suffering from sleep deprivation, night sweats, and mood swings. I also had high blood pressure and high cholesterol," she reveals.

On top of her health concerns, Susan was also experiencing a lot of stress at work. "I was working for a contractor and had been there for 30 years. The owner passed away rather quickly and left the business to his sons, and they eventually wanted me out. So there was a period of 6 months when I knew they wanted me to leave and I was really stressed out."

Concerned about her health and stress level, Susan spoke to a friend who recommended she see Dr. Pingel. Shortly after, she was diagnosed with adrenal fatigue. "I had heard of adrenal fatigue before, but I didn't think my symptoms were caused by adrenal fatigue," she admits. "I started taking supplements and changed my diet. Before, I was eating a lot of junk food and lots of butter and cream cheese. I also wouldn't eat regularly. I would pig out at lunch and eat no dinner, or I would skip breakfast. Now, I try to stick with whole grains, fruits, and vegetables, and I stay away from processed food."

Soon after starting Dr. Pingel's plan, Susan noticed a difference in her quality of life. "I started feeling a big change within the first month. I was quite shocked at how quickly I started feeling better. Sleep was a huge issue before, and I started sleeping so much better. I also lost 15 pounds," she says. "I don't feel as stressed, and I feel like I can handle things better. Now, I'm no longer on birth control or any other medications."

Now that she knows she's healthy, Susan has some peace of mind. "My mom and my daughter have seen such a change in me, which feels great," she states. "My stress is pretty low now. I have been really busy at work these last few weeks, but I feel more busy than stressed. It feels great to have my life back."

# PART III

## RECIPES FOR ADRENAL RESTORATION

The following recipes were created to provide the perfect amount of nutrients to support your adrenal glands and reverse adrenal fatigue. Remember: This is not about calorie counting but about providing your body with the nutrients it needs to heal your particular stage of adrenal fatigue.

Each of the breakfast, lunch, and dinner recipes offers modifications for the different stages of adrenal fatigue, allowing you to enjoy all of the recipes in this book, regardless of your current state of adrenal fatigue. In addition, you'll find adrenal-friendly recipes for snacks and even desserts (to be enjoyed on occasion). While making these recipes, I want to encourage you to take the time to enjoy the aspect of cooking for your health. You are doing something good for yourself, and your adrenal glands will thank you. So dig in and enjoy!

## BREAKFASTS

Honeydew Cucumber Smoothie 303
Fruited Carrot-Veggie Salad 304
Sweet Potato Hash
   with Poached Eggs 305
Tofu Scramble with Peppers
   and Mushrooms 306
Mexican Breakfast Burrito 307
Eggs Pipérade 308
Smoky Lentil, Egg,
   and Mushroom Skillet 309
Quinoa and Butternut
   Breakfast Bowl 310
Spicy Vegetable and Grain
   Omelet 311
Open-Face Egg Sandwich 312
Savory Oatmeal 313
Brown Rice Bowl 314

## LUNCHES

Grilled Portobello
   and Hummus Stacks 315

Rustic Lentil Soup 316

Speedy Salmon Wrap 317

Zesty Pasta Salad 318

Asparagus and Tofu Stir-Fry 319

Colorful Curry Bowl 320

Moroccan Stuffed Peppers 321

Kicked-Up Bean Tostadas 322

Mediterranean Chopped Salad 323

Salmon Miso Soup 324

## DINNERS

Chicken Peanut Noodle Bowl 325

Quinoa Tabbouleh 326

Grilled Tuna and Mango Salad 327

Hearty Chili 328

Broccoli Rabe and Bean Sauté 329

Roasted Root Vegetables 330

Tomato-Watermelon Gazpacho 331

Black Bean Stew 332

Chicken Tortilla Soup 333

Steamed Vegetables
with Red Pepper Sauce 334

## SNACKS

Quick Bean Burrito 335

Guacamole Deviled Eggs 335

Cucumber Boats 335

Peach Blueberry Smoothie 336

Fresh Fruit Salad Cup 336

3-Layer Mexican Dip 336

Smoked Salmon on
Cucumber Slices 337

Chocolate Lover's Trail Mix 337

Nutty Celery Sticks 337

Stuffed Lettuce Cups 338

## DESSERTS

Almond and Mixed Berry
Muffins 339

Wholesome Oat Muffins 340

Blueberry Muffins 341

Glazed Pineapple Cupcakes 342

Oat-Almond Mixed Berry Crisp 343

Plum-Blueberry Cobbler 344

Almond-Cherry Clafoutis 345

Red Fruit Crumble 346

# BREAKFASTS

## Honeydew Cucumber Smoothie

Prep Time: 5 minutes          Total Time: 10 minutes          Makes 1 serving

- ½    cup frozen green peas
- 1    tablespoon water
- ½    cup unsweetened almond milk
- ¾    cup cubed honeydew melon
- ½    cup finely chopped English cucumber
- 1    cup finely chopped kale
- 1    tablespoon almond butter
- 3    ice cubes
- 3    tablespoons oatmeal
-      Honey (optional)

In a small microwave-safe bowl, combine the peas and water. Cover and microwave on high power for 2 minutes, or until the peas are cooked. Drain the peas and rinse with cold water.

In a blender, combine the peas, almond milk, melon, cucumber, kale, almond butter, ice cubes, oatmeal, and honey to taste, if using. Blend until smooth. Serve with the oatmeal.

| MAKE IT STAGE 2: | MAKE IT STAGE 3: |
|---|---|
| Reduce the melon to ½ cup. Use 1 whole cucumber. | Decrease the melon to ¼ cup. Use 1 whole cucumber. |

STAGE 1

# Fruited Carrot-Veggie Salad

Prep Time: 20 minutes          Total Time: 20 minutes          Makes 4 servings

½ cup raisins
2 tablespoons olive oil
3 tablespoons lime juice
2 tablespoons fresh squeezed orange juice
½ teaspoon sea salt
⅛ teaspoon ground red pepper
3 large carrots, shredded (3 cups)
2 cups coarsely chopped baby spinach
2 cups halved cherry tomatoes
1½ cups chopped fresh pineapple
1 can (15 ounces) chickpeas, drained
⅓ cup toasted pumpkin seeds
1 avocado, cubed
4 gluten-free corn muffins

Soak the raisins in boiling water to cover. Let stand for 6 minutes or until softened, then drain well.

In a large bowl, whisk together the olive oil, lime juice, orange juice, salt, and pepper until blended. Stir in the carrots, spinach, tomatoes, pineapple, chickpeas, and raisins. Top with the pumpkin seeds and avocado. Serve with the muffins.

**TIP:** If made ahead, add additional lime juice to taste.

| MAKE IT STAGE 2: | MAKE IT STAGE 3: |
|---|---|
| Decrease the beans to 1 cup. | Increase the carrots to 3½ cups. Decrease the pineapple to 1 cup. |

STAGE 1

# Sweet Potato Hash with Poached Eggs

Prep Time: 20 minutes        Total Time: 55 minutes        Makes 4 servings

| | |
|---|---|
| 1 | tablespoon olive oil |
| ½ | large red onion, chopped |
| 2 | sweet potatoes (1 pound), peeled and chopped |
| ⅓ | cup water |
| 1 | large red bell pepper, chopped |
| ½ | teaspoon chopped fresh rosemary |
| ½ | teaspoon chopped fresh thyme |
| ½ | teaspoon sea salt |
| ¼ | teaspoon ground black pepper |
| ⅛ | teaspoon ground nutmeg |
| 3 | cups coarsely chopped mustard or turnip greens |
| 4 | eggs |
| 4 | pieces gluten-free bread |
| 2 | large peaches, cut into wedges |

In a large, heavy skillet, heat the oil over medium-high heat. Add the onion and cook, covered, for 4 minutes, stirring occasionally. Stir in the potatoes and water. Cook, stirring occasionally, for 6 minutes.

Add the bell pepper, rosemary, thyme, salt, black pepper, and nutmeg. Reduce the heat to medium. Cover and cook, stirring occasionally, for 4 minutes. Stir in the greens and cook for 4 minutes, or until tender.

Fill a small skillet with water and bring to a boil over high heat. Reduce the heat to medium-low. Break 1 egg into the skillet. Cook for 3 to 4 minutes, or until the white is set and the yolk is soft-cooked. Repeat with the remaining eggs.

Meanwhile, toast the bread. Serve the poached eggs on top of the hash with the toast and peaches.

| **MAKE IT STAGE 2:** | **MAKE IT STAGE 3:** |
|---|---|
| Decrease the bread to 2 pieces, sausage to 1½ links, and use 2 medium peaches. | Use 2½ sweet potatoes (1¼ pounds), and decrease the bread to 2 pieces, sausage to 1½ links, and use 1 large peach. |

# Tofu Scramble with Peppers and Mushrooms

Prep Time: 15 minutes        Total Time: 35 minutes        Makes 4 servings

| | |
|---|---|
| 1 | carton (14 ounces) soft tofu, drained |
| ⅜ | cup brown rice |
| 2 | tablespoons olive oil, divided |
| 1 | large onion, chopped |
| 2 | bell peppers, finely chopped |
| 10 | ounces cremini mushrooms, quartered |
| ½ | teaspoon sea salt, divided |
| 1 | egg, lightly beaten |
| ¼ | cup chopped fresh basil |
| 1 | tablespoon nutritional yeast |
| 1 | avocado, sliced |
| 2 | pieces gluten-free bread |
| 2 | cups mixed berries |

Line a plate with a double layer of paper towels. Coarsely crumble the tofu onto the plate and set it aside. Cook the rice according to package directions.

In a large nonstick skillet, heat 1 tablespoon of the oil over medium heat. Add the onion, bell peppers, mushrooms, and ¼ teaspoon of the salt. Increase the heat to medium-high and cook, stirring frequently, for 8 minutes, or until the liquid evaporates and the vegetables are tender. Remove from the skillet and set aside.

Wipe out the skillet. Add the remaining 1 tablespoon oil and heat over medium heat. Add the tofu and cook, stirring frequently, for 5 minutes, or until hot. Stir in the brown rice, egg, and remaining ¼ teaspoon salt. Cook, stirring frequently, for 2 minutes, or until the egg is set. Stir in the basil, yeast, and reserved vegetables. Continue to cook, stirring frequently, for 1 minute, or until the vegetables are hot. Top with the avocado. Meanwhile, toast the bread. Serve the scramble with the toast and berries.

| MAKE IT STAGE 2: | MAKE IT STAGE 3: |
|---|---|
| Decrease the tofu by half. Omit the egg and the bread. | Decrease the tofu by half, the brown rice to ¼ cup, and the berries to 1 cup. Omit the bread. |

STAGE 2

# Mexican Breakfast Burrito

Prep Time: 10 minutes        Total Time: 25 minutes        Makes 4 servings

- 10  ounces extra-firm tofu, drained and cut into ¾" cubes
- ½  cup brown rice
- 8  leaves collard greens, stems removed
- 2  tablespoons water
- 2  tablespoons olive oil
- 1  red onion, halved and sliced
- 1  large tomato, coarsely chopped
- ½  teaspoon sea salt
- 2  Hass avocados, pitted, peeled, and sliced
- 1½  cups fresh cilantro
- ¼  cup toasted pumpkin seeds
    Hot sauce
- 2  cups sliced fresh fruit

Place the tofu on a plate between layers of paper toweling; press lightly and let stand 10 minutes. Cook the rice according to package directions.

Meanwhile, place 4 collard leaves on a microwaveable plate and add 1 tablespoon of the water. Cover and microwave on high power for 1 minute, or until the leaves soften slightly. Repeat with the remaining leaves and water.

In a large nonstick skillet, heat 1 tablespoon of the oil over medium heat. Add the tofu. Increase the heat to medium-high and cook, turning the tofu frequently, for 5 minutes, or until lightly browned. Set aside.

Add the remaining 1 tablespoon oil to the skillet and set it over medium heat. Add the onion and cook, stirring frequently, for 5 to 6 minutes, or until lightly browned. Stir in the rice, tomato, and salt. Cook, stirring frequently, for 4 to 5 minutes, or until the rice is hot. Stir in the reserved tofu.

To assemble the burritos, divide the rice mixture evenly among the collard leaves. Top with the avocado, cilantro, pumpkin seeds, and hot sauce to taste. Roll to enclose the filling. Serve with the fruit.

| **MAKE IT STAGE 1:** | **MAKE IT STAGE 3:** |
| --- | --- |
| Serve with 1 glass of fresh-pressed juice of choice. | Decrease the fruit to 1 cup. |

STAGE 2

# Eggs Pipérade

Prep Time: 10 minutes          Total Time: 30 minutes          Makes 4 servings

½  cup quinoa, rinsed and drained
2  teaspoons olive oil
1  onion, sliced
1  small red bell pepper, sliced
1  small green bell pepper, sliced
1  jalapeño chile pepper, seeded and chopped
   (wear plastic gloves when handling)
1  small tomato, diced
½  teaspoon chopped fresh thyme
1  teaspoon ancho chili powder
4  eggs
1  grapefruit, cut into 8 wedges

Cook the quinoa according to package directions. In a large ovenproof skillet, heat the oil. Add the onion, bell peppers, and jalapeño chile pepper. Cook, stirring occasionally, for 6 minutes or until softened. Stir in the tomatoes, thyme, and chili powder. Bring to a simmer, cover, and cook for 6 minutes, or until the vegetables are almost tender.

Make 4 indentations in the vegetable mixture with the back of a large spoon. One at a time, break an egg and drop it into each indentation. Simmer, covered, for 6 to 8 minutes, or until the eggs are set and cooked to desired doneness.

Place the quinoa in shallow bowls and top with the pipérade-egg mixture. Serve with the grapefruit.

| MAKE IT STAGE 1: | MAKE IT STAGE 3: |
|---|---|
| Use 2 small grapefruits. Top dish with ½ avocado, sliced. Serve with 1 cup of green juice (1 cucumber, 1" ginger root, handful of kale, and 1 apple). | Omit the grapefruit. |

STAGE 2

# Smoky Lentil, Egg, and Mushroom Skillet

Prep Time: 10 minutes     Total Time: 30 minutes     Makes 4 servings

| | |
|---|---|
| 1 | cup lentils, rinsed and drained |
| 2 | tablespoons olive oil |
| 1 | onion, chopped |
| 8 | ounces cremini mushrooms, sliced |
| ½ | teaspoon sea salt |
| 1½ | cups packaged, matchstick-cut carrots |
| 1 | cup halved grape tomatoes |
| 1 | jalapeño chile pepper, seeded and finely chopped (wear plastic gloves when handling) |
| ¾ | teaspoon smoked paprika |
| ½ | cup reduced-sodium vegetable broth |
| ¼ | cup chopped flat-leaf parsley + additional for garnish |
| 4 | eggs |
| 1 | avocado, sliced |

Cook the lentils according to package directions. In a large skillet, heat 1 tablespoon of the oil over medium heat. Add the onion and cook, stirring frequently, for 5 minutes, or until it begins to brown. Add the mushrooms and salt. Cook for 6 minutes, stirring frequently, or until lightly browned.

Add the carrots, tomatoes, jalapeño chile pepper, and paprika. Cook for 3 minutes, stirring occasionally, or until the vegetables soften. Add the lentils and broth. Simmer for 2 minutes, or until the lentils are hot. Stir in the ¼ cup parsley. Remove the skillet from the heat and cover to keep warm.

Fill a small skillet with water and bring to a boil over high heat. Reduce the heat to medium-low. Break 1 egg into the skillet. Cook for 3 to 4 minutes, or until the white is set and the yolk is soft-cooked. Repeat with the remaining eggs.

Spoon the lentil mixture onto 4 plates and top each with a poached egg. Sprinkle with additional parsley. Top with the avocado.

| **MAKE IT STAGE 1:** | **MAKE IT STAGE 3:** |
|---|---|
| Use 8 eggs (2 per serving). Serve with ½ cup of berries. | No changes necessary. |

STAGE 2

# Quinoa and Butternut Breakfast Bowl

Prep Time: 10 minutes          Total Time: 25 minutes          Makes 4 servings

| | |
|---|---|
| 1 | cup quinoa, rinsed and drained |
| 1⅓ | cups coconut milk beverage |
| 2 | cups peeled, chopped butternut squash |
| 1 | cup shredded carrots |
| 4 | teaspoons ground flaxseeds |
| 3 | tablespoons maple syrup |
| 1 | teaspoon ground cinnamon |
| ⅛ | teaspoon ground allspice |
| ½ | cup chopped dried plums |
| | Stevia |
| ¼ | cup toasted walnuts |
| 1½ | cups fresh blueberries |

In a medium saucepan, combine the quinoa, coconut milk, squash, carrots, flaxseeds, maple syrup, cinnamon, and allspice. Bring to a simmer and cook, covered, for 20 minutes. Add the plums during the last 5 minutes of cooking. Stir in stevia to taste and top with the walnuts. Serve with the blueberries.

| MAKE IT STAGE 1: | MAKE IT STAGE 3: |
|---|---|
| Serve with 2 pieces of gluten-free toast. Increase the blueberries to 2 cups. | Increase the amount of carrots to 1⅓ cups and decrease the blueberries to 1 cup. |

STAGE 3

# Spicy Vegetable and Grain Omelet

Prep Time: 15 minutes          Total Time: 25 minutes          Makes 4 servings

⅓   cup amaranth
2   teaspoons olive oil, divided
1   onion, chopped
1½  cups coarsely chopped mushrooms
1   cup fresh kale
½   teaspoon chile pepper
¼   teaspoon sea salt, divided
1   tablespoon nutritional yeast
4   eggs
½   teaspoon dried tarragon or dill
¾   cup shredded Cheddar-style soy cheese
1   cup raw cashews
1   cup water
1   teaspoon Dijon mustard
1   teaspoon lemon juice
    Salt and pepper

Cook the amaranth according to package directions. In a large nonstick skillet, heat 1 teaspoon of the oil over medium-high heat. Add the onion and cook for 4 minutes, stirring. Add the mushrooms, kale, chile pepper, and ⅛ teaspoon of the salt. Cook for 6 minutes, or until tender. Place the vegetable mixture in a bowl and stir in the nutritional yeast and half of the amaranth.

In a separate bowl, whisk together the eggs, tarragon or dill, remaining ⅛ teaspoon salt, and remaining amaranth. Wash and dry the skillet, place it over medium heat, and heat the remaining 1 teaspoon oil. Add the whisked egg mixture and cook for 9 minutes, gently lifting the edges with a rubber spatula to allow uncooked egg to flow underneath. Cook until the eggs are set. Meanwhile, in a blender, combine the cashews, water, mustard, and lemon juice. Blend until smooth. Season with salt and pepper to taste. In a small saucepan, heat the cashew hollandaise until warm. Spoon the vegetable mixture on top of the eggs and gently fold the untopped half of the eggs over the filling. Cut the omelet into 4 wedges and serve topped with the hollandaise sauce.

| **MAKE IT STAGE 1:** | **MAKE IT STAGE 2:** |
|---|---|
| Use 6 eggs (1½ eggs per serving) and serve with 2 navel oranges, cut into wedges. | Serve with 1 navel orange, cut into wedges. |

STAGE 3

# Open-Face Egg Sandwich

Prep Time: 5 minutes        Total Time: 10 minutes        Makes 1 serving

- 1   small navel orange, peel and white pith removed
- 1   tablespoon nutritional yeast
- 1½  teaspoons olive oil
- ⅛   teaspoon sea salt
- 1   cup baby arugula
- 1   cup baby spinach
- ⅓   cup halved grape or cherry tomatoes
- 1   egg
- 1   corn tortilla, warmed
    Handful of pumpkin seeds

Section the orange over a small bowl. Squeeze the membrane to yield 1 table-spoon juice; discard the membrane. Add the yeast, oil, and salt and whisk until blended.

In a large bowl, combine the arugula, spinach, and tomatoes.

Fill a small skillet with water and bring to a boil over high heat. Reduce the heat to medium-low. Break the egg into the skillet. Cook for 3 to 4 minutes, or until the white is set and the yolk is soft cooked.

While the egg cooks, add the dressing to the greens and toss. Top the warm tortilla with the greens and poached egg. Sprinkle with the pumpkin seeds.

| MAKE IT STAGE 1: | MAKE IT STAGE 2: |
|---|---|
| Add ¼ cup cooked soybeans to the greens. Use 2 oranges. Replace the tortilla with 1 slice of gluten-free toast. | Use 2 oranges. |

STAGE 3

# Savory Oatmeal

Prep Time: 5 minutes          Total Time: 15 minutes          Makes 1 serving

½   cup coconut water
¼   cup old-fashioned oats
1   cup packed baby spinach
½   cup sugar snap peas, strings removed, sliced
¼   cup shredded carrot
1   tablespoon nutritional yeast
2   teaspoons chia seeds
¼   cup unsweetened almond milk
2   tablespoons chopped almonds or walnuts
¼   cup blueberries

In a small saucepan, bring the coconut water to a boil. Stir in the oats. Reduce the heat to medium and simmer for 3 minutes. Stir in the spinach, peas, and carrot. Simmer for 3 minutes, stirring occasionally, until the water is absorbed. Remove the saucepan from the heat and stir in the yeast and chia seeds. Turn into a bowl, add the milk, and sprinkle with the almonds. Serve with the blueberries.

| MAKE IT STAGE 1: | MAKE IT STAGE 2: |
|---|---|
| Serve with 1 scrambled egg. Increase the blueberries to ½ cup. | Increase the blueberries to ½ cup. |

STAGE 3

# Brown Rice Bowl

Prep Time: 15 minutes        Total Time: 20 minutes        Makes 4 servings

⅓  cup short-grain brown rice
2  teaspoons olive oil
8  ounces baby bok choy, quartered
3  cups coarsely chopped turnip or mustard greens
2  cups snow peas, halved crosswise
8  ounces firm tofu, finely chopped
1  tablespoon nutritional yeast
2  tablespoons reduced-sodium soy sauce
1  tablespoon orange juice concentrate

Cook the rice according to package directions. In a large skillet, heat the oil over medium-high heat. Add the bok choy and cook, stirring, for 3 minutes. Stir in the greens and snow peas and cook for 2 minutes.

Stir in the rice, tofu, nutritional yeast, soy sauce, and orange juice concentrate. Cook, stirring, for 2 minutes, or until heated through. Serve with the grapefruit.

| MAKE IT STAGE 1: | MAKE IT STAGE 2: |
|---|---|
| Increase the rice to ¾ cup, the tofu to 16 ounces, and serve with 1 plum. | Serve with 1 plum. |

# LUNCHES

STAGE 1

## Grilled Portobello and Hummus Stacks

Prep Time: 25 minutes        Total Time: 35 minutes        Makes 4 servings

- 2    tablespoons olive oil
- 5    tablespoons balsamic vinegar
- 2    tablespoons honey mustard
- 1    teaspoon chopped fresh rosemary
- 2    cloves garlic, finely chopped
- ¼    teaspoon sea salt
- 3    large red bell peppers
- 4    portobello mushrooms (24 ounces)
- 2    gluten-free whole grain hamburger buns, split
- 3    cups arugula
- ¾    cup lemon-flavored hummus
- 4    small peaches

In a large bowl, whisk together the olive oil, vinegar, mustard, rosemary, garlic and salt until blended. Remove ¼ cup and set aside for grilling.

Preheat a grill or grill pan on medium high heat. Cut the peppers into slabs and place in a pie plate. Microwave on high power for 4 minutes, or until beginning to soften. Grill the peppers and mushrooms for 4 minutes per side or just until tender, brushing with the reserved dressing. Grill the bun halves for 2 minutes, or until toasted.

Add the arugula to the bowl with the dressing and toss until combined. Spread half of the hummus on the buns. Top with the mushrooms and spoon on the remaining hummus. Top with the grilled red peppers and arugula salad. Serve with the peaches and a small mixed-greens salad.

| MAKE IT STAGE 2: | MAKE IT STAGE 3: |
|---|---|
| Omit the peaches. | Omit the peaches. |

STAGE 1

# Rustic Lentil Soup

Prep Time: 15 minutes        Total Time: 1 hour 10 minutes        Makes 4 servings

- 1    tablespoon olive oil
- 1    large onion, chopped
- 3    cloves garlic, minced
- 2    carrots, sliced
- 2    ribs celery, coarsely chopped
- 1    large sweet potato, peeled and cut into ¾" pieces
- ½    cup brown lentils, sorted and rinsed
- 2    cups reduced-sodium vegetable broth
- 1½   cups water
- 1    small tomato, chopped
- ½    teaspoon dried thyme
- ½    cup brown rice
- 2    cups chopped kale
- ¼    teaspoon sea salt

In a Dutch oven, heat the oil over medium heat. Add the onion and cook, stirring frequently, for 4 minutes, or until softened. Stir in the garlic and cook, stirring frequently, for 1 minute. Add the carrots, celery, sweet potato, lentils, broth, water, tomatoes, and thyme. Bring to a boil over high heat. Reduce the heat to low, cover, and simmer for 30 minutes. Meanwhile, cook the rice according to package directions.

Add the kale and salt to the lentil soup. Bring to a boil. Reduce the heat, cover, and simmer for 20 minutes, or until the lentils and vegetables are tender. Serve the soup over the rice. Serve with the plums and a small mixed-greens salad.

| MAKE IT STAGE 2: | MAKE IT STAGE 3: |
|---|---|
| Replace the sweet potato with 2 cups peeled and finely chopped butternut squash. | Decrease the amount of brown rice to ¼ cup. |

STAGE 1

# Speedy Salmon Wrap

Prep Time: 20 minutes        Total Time: 25 minutes        Makes 4 servings

- ¾   cup short-grain brown rice
- 8   large leaves collard greens, stems removed
- 2   tablespoons water
- 3   tablespoons olive oil
- 2   tablespoons balsamic vinegar
- 2   teaspoons Dijon mustard
- 2   red bell peppers, cut into thin lengthwise strips
- 2   cups finely chopped English cucumber
- 2   pink or red grapefruits, peel and white pith removed, cut into segments
- 1   Hass avocado, pitted, peeled, and sliced
- 4   ounces cooked wild salmon, flaked

Cook the rice according to package directions. On a microwaveable plate, stack 4 of the collard leaves. Add 1 tablespoon of the water. Cover with a damp paper towel and microwave on high power for 1 minute, or until slightly softened. Repeat with the remaining collard leaves and water.

In a small bowl, whisk the oil, vinegar, and mustard until blended.

On a clean work surface, lay the collard leaves with a long side facing you. Spoon the rice in a strip along a long side, about 1" from the edge and ends, dividing evenly. Top with the bell pepper strips and cucumber, dividing evenly. Drizzle with the dressing. Top with the grapefruit, avocado, and salmon, dividing evenly. Roll up tightly from the filled side. Cut in half before serving.

| MAKE IT STAGE 2: | MAKE IT STAGE 3: |
|---|---|
| Decrease the amount of rice to ¼ cup and replace the salmon with 1 cup cooked soybeans or chickpeas. Spread 1 tablespoon almond butter on each collard green leaf. | Decrease the amount of rice to ¼ cup and use 1 grapefruit. |

**STAGE 1**

# Zesty Pasta Salad

Prep Time: 20 minutes          Total Time: 30 minutes          Makes 4 servings

|     |     |
| --- | --- |
| 6 | ounces gluten-free rotini pasta |
| 1¼ | cups fresh or frozen shelled edamame |
| 2 | ribs celery, chopped |
| 1 | pint cherry tomatoes, halved |
| 2 | cups baby spinach leaves |
| 1 | can (28 ounces) no-salt-added kidney beans, drained |
| 3 | tablespoons olive oil |
| ¼ | cup white wine vinegar |
| ½ | teaspoon sea salt |
| ½ | teaspoon ground black pepper |
| ½ | cup chopped fresh basil leaves |
|   | Rind of 1 lemon |
| 4 | large kiwifruit, peeled and sliced |

Bring a large pot of water to a boil. Add the pasta and cook according to package directions, adding the edamame during the last 4 minutes of cooking. Drain and rinse under cold running water. Place in a large bowl. Toss in the celery, tomatoes, spinach, and kidney beans. Refrigerate until ready to use.

In a medium bowl, whisk together the olive oil, vinegar, salt and pepper until blended. Add the dressing and basil to the pasta mixture. Toss until combined. Top with the lemon rind. Serve with the kiwifruit.

| **MAKE IT STAGE 2:** | **MAKE IT STAGE 3:** |
| --- | --- |
| Decrease the amount of pasta to 5 ounces. | Decrease the amount of pasta to 5 ounces and use 1½ cups edamame and 2½ cups spinach. Omit the kiwifruit and serve with a small side salad. |

STAGE 2

# Asparagus and Tofu Stir-Fry

Prep Time: 15 minutes　　　Total Time: 25 minutes　　　Makes 4 servings

| | |
|---|---|
| ½ | cup short-grain brown rice |
| 2 | tablespoons hoisin sauce |
| 1 | tablespoon balsamic vinegar |
| 1½ | teaspoons Sriracha |
| 2 | teaspoons chopped fresh ginger |
| 1 | clove garlic, finely chopped |
| 1 | teaspoon cornstarch |
| 3 | tablespoons cold water |
| 1 | tablespoon olive oil |
| ¾ | pound asparagus, cut into 1" pieces |
| 1 | large red bell pepper, sliced |
| 3 | cups sliced napa cabbage |
| 4 | scallions, sliced diagonally |
| 4 | ounces tofu, grilled |
| 2 | oranges, peeled and coarsely chopped |

Cook the rice according to package directions. In a small dish, stir together the hoisin sauce, vinegar, Sriracha, ginger, garlic, cornstarch, and water until combined.

In a wok or Dutch oven, heat the oil over medium-high heat. Add the asparagus and red bell pepper and cook, stirring constantly, for 3 minutes. Add the cabbage and scallions and cook, stirring constantly, for 2 minutes.

Stir in the tofu and continue to cook, stirring constantly, for 1 minute. Stir in the hoisin mixture. Cook for 1 minute, stirring, or until the sauce is thickened. Serve over the rice and top with the oranges.

| **MAKE IT STAGE 1:** | **MAKE IT STAGE 3:** |
|---|---|
| Increase the amount of rice to ¾ cup. Use 4 ounces large peeled and deveined split shrimp in place of tofu. | Use 2 red bell peppers and 1 pound asparagus. Use rind of ½ orange in place of whole orange. |

STAGE 2

# Colorful Curry Bowl

Prep Time: 15 minutes        Total Time: 55 minutes        Makes 4 servings

| | |
|---|---|
| 1 | tablespoon olive oil |
| 1 | onion, coarsely chopped |
| 3 | cloves garlic, minced |
| 2 | teaspoons curry powder |
| 1 | teaspoon garam masala |
| ½ | pound butternut squash, peeled, seeded, and cut into 1" chunks |
| 1 | can (15 ounces) chickpeas, rinsed and drained |
| 1 | small tomato, diced |
| 1¼ | cups reduced-sodium vegetable broth or coconut water |
| ¾ | cup quinoa |
| 4 | cups cauliflower florets |
| ½ | teaspoon sea salt |
| 2 | cups broccoli florets |
| ¾ | cup coconut milk |
| 1 | cup chopped fresh cilantro |
| 2 | cups cubed mango |

In a Dutch oven, heat the oil over medium heat. Add the onion and cook, stirring frequently, for 5 minutes, or until the onion begins to brown. Stir in the garlic, curry powder, and garam masala. Add the squash, chickpeas, tomatoes, and vegetable broth. Bring to a boil over high heat. Reduce the heat to medium-low, cover, and simmer for 20 minutes, stirring occasionally, or until the squash is just tender. Meanwhile, cook the quinoa according to package directions.

Stir in the cauliflower and salt. Return to a boil; reduce the heat to medium-low, cover, and simmer for 5 minutes. Stir in the broccoli and coconut milk. Simmer, covered, for 10 minutes, or until the vegetables are tender. Serve over the quinoa and sprinkle with the cilantro. Serve with the mango.

| **MAKE IT STAGE 1:** | **MAKE IT STAGE 3:** |
|---|---|
| Use 3 cups broccoli florets. | Decrease the amount of quinoa to ¼ cup and use 1 cup cubed mango. |

STAGE 2

# Moroccan Stuffed Peppers

Prep Time: 20 minutes         Total Time: 1 hour 15 minutes         Makes 4 servings

| | |
|---|---|
| ½ | cup millet |
| 4 | small bell peppers, halved lengthwise (any colors, preferably a variety) |
| 1½ | cups vegetable broth |
| 1 | tablespoon olive oil |
| 1 | small onion, chopped |
| 1 | can (15 ounces) chickpeas, rinsed and drained |
| 2 | cloves garlic, minced |
| 1 | teaspoon ground cumin |
| 1 | teaspoon curry powder |
| ¼ | teaspoon sea salt |
| 4 | cups coarsely chopped kale |
| 1 | small tomato, diced |
| ¼ | cup finely chopped dried apricots |
| ½ | pear |

Cook the millet according to package directions. Preheat the oven to 350°F. In a 13" x 9" baking dish, place the pepper halves cut sides down. Pour in ½ cup of the vegetable broth. Cover and microwave on high power for 10 minutes, or until the peppers soften. Turn the peppers over. Set aside.

In a large nonstick skillet, heat the oil over medium heat. Add the onion and chickpeas. Cook for 8 minutes, stirring frequently. Add the garlic, cumin, curry powder, and salt. Cook, stirring, for 1 minute. Add the kale and remaining 1 cup vegetable broth. Bring to a boil over high heat. Reduce the heat to medium and simmer for 2 minutes, or until the kale is wilted. Stir in the millet, tomatoes, and apricots. Simmer for 2 minutes.

Spoon the filling into the pepper halves. Bake for 25 to 30 minutes, or until the peppers are tender. Serve with the pear and a small mixed-greens salad.

| **MAKE IT STAGE 1:** | **MAKE IT STAGE 3:** |
|---|---|
| Increase the millet to ⅔ cup. Use 1 pear. | Replace the broth with coconut water, decrease the millet to ⅓ cup, and omit the pear. |

STAGE 3

# Kicked-Up Bean Tostadas

Prep Time: 20 minutes          Total Time: 30 minutes          Makes 4 servings

      4   (7") gluten-free tortillas
      1   teaspoon olive oil
      1   poblano chile pepper, finely chopped
          (wear plastic gloves when handling)
      1   can (15 ounces) no-salt-added adzuki beans, rinsed and drained
      ½   cup medium salsa
      4   scallions, sliced
      1   teaspoon ancho chili powder
      ½   teaspoon ground cumin
      3   tablespoons chopped fresh cilantro
      2   cups sliced baby spinach
      2   vine-ripened tomatoes, chopped
      1   avocado, finely chopped
          Shredded Cheddar-style dairy-free blend

Preheat the oven to 350°F. Brush the tops of the tortillas with the olive oil. Place them in a single layer directly on the middle oven rack. Bake until golden and crisped, 10 to 14 minutes. (If the tortillas puff, flatten them by pressing down on them with a spatula.) Place on 4 plates and set aside.

Heat a nonstick skillet over medium heat. Add the chile pepper and beans. Cook for 5 minutes, stirring and breaking up with a spoon. Stir in the salsa, scallions, chili powder, cumin, and cilantro. Cook for 2 minutes, or until the flavors have blended. Spoon onto the tortilla shells and top with the spinach, tomatoes, avocado, and a sprinkle of the dairy-free blend.

| MAKE IT STAGE 1: | MAKE IT STAGE 2: |
| --- | --- |
| Add organic, grass-fed beef to the skillet. Serve with 2 cups cherries. | No changes necessary. |

STAGE 3

# Mediterranean Chopped Salad

Prep Time: 20 minutes     Total Time: 20 minutes     Makes 4 servings

| | |
|---|---|
| 2 | tablespoons lemon juice |
| 2 | tablespoons extra-virgin olive oil |
| ½ | teaspoon sea salt |
| 4 | cups very thinly sliced kale |
| ⅓ | cup hummus |
| 1 | large tomato, finely chopped |
| 1 | cup cubed seedless watermelon |
| ½ | English cucumber, finely chopped |
| ½ | green bell pepper, finely chopped |
| ½ | small red onion, chopped |
| ⅓ | cup coarsely chopped flat-leaf parsley |

In a small bowl, whisk together the lemon juice, oil, and salt. Place the kale in a large bowl and add 1 tablespoon of the lemon dressing. Toss the kale with your hands, rubbing until wilted. Add ⅓ cup of the hummus to the remaining lemon dressing and whisk to combine.

Add the tomato, watermelon, cucumber, bell pepper, onion, and parsley to the kale and toss to combine. Serve the salad with the dressing on the side to drizzle over the top.

| MAKE IT STAGE 1: | MAKE IT STAGE 2: |
|---|---|
| Increase the amount of cubed watermelon to 2 cups. Serve with extra hummus and gluten-free crackers on the side. | Use 1 whole green bell pepper. |

STAGE 3

# Salmon Miso Soup

Prep Time: 15 minutes  Total Time: 25 minutes  Makes 4 servings

- 4 ounces uncooked soba noodles or gluten-free linguine
- 1 can (14.5 ounces) reduced-sodium vegetable broth
- 4 cups coconut water
- 2 tablespoons peeled, slivered fresh ginger
- 2 cups small broccoli florets (quartered or halved, if large)
- 1 cup watercress, large stems removed
- 4 scallions, sliced
- 3 tablespoons white or yellow miso (soybean paste)
- 4 ounces wild salmon, thinly sliced
- 1 teaspoon toasted sesame oil
- ¼ cup chopped fresh cilantro

Fill a large saucepan with water and bring to a boil. Add the noodles and cook according to package directions; drain well.

Meanwhile, in a large saucepan over medium-high heat, bring the broth, coconut water, and ginger to a simmer. Add the broccoli and simmer for 3 minutes. Add the watercress and scallions and simmer for 1 minute. Stir in the miso until dissolved. Add the salmon and sesame oil. Cook for 1 minute longer, or just until the salmon is cooked through.

Place the noodles in 4 soup bowls and top with the soup mixture. Sprinkle with the cilantro. Serve with a mixed-greens salad.

| MAKE IT STAGE 1: | MAKE IT STAGE 2: |
|---|---|
| Decrease the amount of broccoli to 1¾ cups. Replace the salmon with cubed, firm tofu. Add nuts and avocado to the salad. | Decrease the amount of broccoli to 1¾ cups. Add a handful of pumpkin seeds to the salad. |

# DINNERS

## Chicken Peanut Noodle Bowl

Prep Time: 15 minutes        Total Time: 35 minutes        Makes 4 servings

| | |
|---|---|
| 18 | ounces rice noodles |
| 1 | tablespoon olive oil, divided |
| 6 | ounces boneless, skinless chicken breast, cut into thin strips |
| 2 | large red bell peppers, cut into 1" strips |
| 3 | carrots, halved and thinly sliced |
| 4 | scallions, sliced diagonally |
| 1 | tablespoon slivered fresh ginger |
| 12 | ounces baby bok choy, quartered lengthwise |
| 1 | can (15 ounces) reduced-sodium vegetable broth |
| 3 | tablespoons peanut butter |
| 2 | tablespoons reduced-sodium soy sauce |
| 1 | teaspoon Sriracha sauce |
| | Lime wedges |
| 3 | cups fresh strawberries |

Cook the rice noodles according to package directions. In a large, deep skillet over medium-high heat, heat ½ tablespoon of the oil. Add the chicken and cook, stirring, for 3 minutes or until cooked through. Transfer to a plate.

Heat the remaining ½ tablespoon oil in the pan. Add the red peppers, carrots, scallions, and ginger. Cook, stirring, for 4 minutes. Stir in the bok choy and cook for 4 minutes, stirring until the vegetables are tender-crisp. Add the broth, peanut butter, soy sauce, and Sriracha. Bring to a simmer, and stir until the sauce is blended. Stir in the chicken and remove from the heat.

Place the noodles in 4 soup bowls and top with the vegetable-broth mixture. Serve with the lime wedges and strawberries.

| **MAKE IT STAGE 2:** | **MAKE IT STAGE 3:** |
|---|---|
| Decrease the amount of noodles to 12 ounces. Substitute tofu for the chicken. Add 2 cups kale and 1 head cauliflower cut into florets. Omit the strawberries. | Decrease the amount of noodles to 12 ounces. Decrease the amount of strawberries to 1 cup. |

STAGE 1

# Quinoa Tabbouleh

Prep Time: 15 minutes          Total Time: 30 minutes          Makes 4 servings

1¾  cups water
 4   cups coarsely chopped collard greens
 ¾   cup quinoa, rinsed and drained
 ½   teaspoon sea salt, divided
 3   tablespoons lemon juice
 2   tablespoons olive oil
 1   cucumber, peeled, seeded, and finely chopped
 2   tomatoes, finely chopped
 1   rib celery, chopped
 2   scallions, thinly sliced
 1   cup chopped flat-leaf parsley
 ½   cup chopped fresh mint
 ½   cup chopped walnuts
 2   cups fresh cherries

In a large saucepan, bring the water to a boil. Stir in the collard greens, quinoa, and ¼ teaspoon of the salt. Bring to a boil. Reduce the heat to low, cover, and simmer for 15 minutes, or until the quinoa is tender. Turn the mixture into a large bowl and let cool.

In a small bowl, whisk the remaining ¼ teaspoon salt, lemon juice, and olive oil. Add to the quinoa mixture. Add the cucumber, tomatoes, celery, scallions, parsley, and mint. Stir to combine. Let stand 15 minutes to allow flavors to blend. Sprinkle with the walnuts. Serve with the cherries.

| MAKE IT STAGE 2: | MAKE IT STAGE 3: |
| --- | --- |
| Decrease the quinoa by 3 tablespoons. | Decrease the amount of cherries to 1 cup. |

STAGE 1

# Grilled Tuna and Mango Salad

Prep Time: 25 minutes        Total Time: 35 minutes        Makes 4 servings

- ½  **pound green beans**
- ½  **cup red quinoa**
- 2  **mangos, peeled, finely chopped, and divided**
- 3  **tablespoons lime juice**
- 2  **tablespoons freshly squeezed orange juice**
- 2  **teaspoons honey or agave**
- 5  **teaspoons olive oil, divided**
- ½  **teaspoon sea salt, divided**
- 3  **cups chopped romaine lettuce**
- 3  **cups chopped escarole**
- 1  **red bell pepper, cut into 1" strips**
- 1  **piece (½ pound) yellowfin tuna steak, about 1" thick**
- ¼  **teaspoon coarse ground black pepper**
- 4  **lime wedges**

Cook the green beans. Cook the quinoa according to package directions.

In a mini food processor or blender, blend ¼ cup of the mango with all of the lime juice, orange juice, and honey or agave, 4 teaspoons of the olive oil, and ¼ teaspoon of the salt.

In a large bowl, toss together the romaine and escarole. Arrange the greens on 4 plates. Arrange the green beans, red pepper, quinoa, and remaining mango in mounds on top of the greens. (This step can be prepared up to 12 hours in advance. Just cover with plastic and refrigerate.)

Heat a grill pan over medium-high heat. Rub the remaining 1 teaspoon olive oil over the tuna. Sprinkle the tuna evenly with the remaining ¼ teaspoon salt and the black pepper. Add the tuna to the pan and grill for 5 minutes on each side, or until the fish is just opaque. Let stand for 10 minutes before slicing. Place fish slices on top of the salad and serve alongside the dressing and lime wedges.

| MAKE IT STAGE 2: | MAKE IT STAGE 3: |
|---|---|
| No changes necessary. | Use a large red bell pepper and 1 mango, and decrease the amount of quinoa to ⅓ cup. |

STAGE 1

# Hearty Chili

Prep Time: 15 minutes     Total Time: 50 minutes     Makes 4 servings

½   cup pearl barley
1   tablespoon olive oil
1   onion, chopped
1   red bell pepper, finely chopped
2   cloves garlic, minced
4   teaspoons chili powder
1½  teaspoons ground cumin
2   cups reduced-sodium vegetable broth
1   small tomato, diced
1   pound butternut squash, peeled, seeded, and finely chopped
1   can (15 ounces) kidney beans
1   large zucchini, finely chopped
½   teaspoon sea salt
¼   cup plain or coconut yogurt
2   tablespoons chopped fresh cilantro
1   nectarine, halved

Cook the barley according to package directions. In a Dutch oven, heat the oil over medium heat. Add the onion and bell pepper and cook, stirring frequently, for 5 minutes, or until the vegetables soften. Stir in the garlic, chili powder, and cumin and cook, stirring frequently, for 1 minute, until fragrant. Add the vegetable broth, tomato, and butternut squash. Bring to a boil over high heat. Reduce the heat to low, cover, and simmer for 15 minutes.

Add the kidney beans and zucchini. Bring to a boil. Reduce the heat, cover, and simmer for 10 minutes. Stir in the barley and salt. Simmer for 10 minutes, or until the vegetables are tender. Serve the chili topped with the yogurt and cilantro. Serve with a small mixed-greens salad.

| MAKE IT STAGE 2: | MAKE IT STAGE 3: |
| --- | --- |
| Substitute 1 cup coconut water for the vegetable broth. Omit the nectarine. | Decrease the barley to ¼ cup and substitute 1 cup coconut water for the vegetable broth. |

STAGE 2

# Broccoli Rabe and Bean Sauté

Prep Time: 15 minutes          Total Time: 50 minutes          Makes 4 servings

- 3 teaspoons olive oil, divided
- 1 onion, chopped
- 1 red bell pepper, chopped
- 8 ounces broccoli rabe, trimmed and coarsely chopped
- 2 cloves garlic, thinly slivered
- 3 tablespoons balsamic vinegar
- 1 can (15 ounces) no-salt-added white beans, drained
- 1 package (8 ounces) prepared polenta, cut into 8 slices
  Handful of slivered almonds

In a large skillet, heat 2 teaspoons oil over medium-high heat. Add the onion and pepper. Cook, stirring occasionally, for 6 minutes. Stir in the broccoli rabe, garlic, and vinegar. Cover and cook for 5 minutes, stirring occasionally, or until the vegetables are just tender. Stir in the white beans and cook for 2 minutes longer.

In a large skillet, heat the remaining oil over medium-high heat. Cook each polenta slice for 6 minutes, turning once. Spoon the broccoli rabe mixture on top. Sprinkle with the almonds and serve.

| MAKE IT STAGE 1: | MAKE IT STAGE 3: |
|---|---|
| No changes necessary. | Decrease the polenta to ¾ package (6 ounces) and omit the plums. |

# Roasted Root Vegetables

Prep Time: 20 minutes        Total Time: 50 minutes        Makes 4 servings

½    cup teff or other grain
8    carrots (about 1 pound), cut into 3" x ½" matchsticks
3    large parsnips (about 1 pound), cut into 3" x ½" matchsticks
1    red onion, halved and cut into ½" wedges through root ends
1    small pear, diced
1    sweet potato, diced
3    tablespoons olive oil, divided
½    teaspoon sea salt, divided
1    pound Brussels sprouts, halved
¼    cup tahini
3    tablespoons water
2    tablespoons lemon juice
1    cup flat-leaf parsley (whole leaves, not chopped)
½    cup chopped toasted almonds or hazelnuts

Cook the teff according to package directions. Preheat the oven to 375°F. In a large, shallow roasting pan, toss the carrots, parsnips, onion, pear, sweet potato, 2 tablespoons of the oil, and ¼ teaspoon of the salt. Spread the vegetables out. Roast, stirring once, for 15 minutes. Stir in the Brussels sprouts. Roast for 15 minutes longer, or until the vegetables are tender and lightly browned.

Meanwhile, in a small bowl, whisk together the remaining 1 tablespoon oil, ¼ teaspoon salt, tahini, water, and lemon juice.

Stir the parsley into the roasted vegetables. Serve the vegetables over the teff. Drizzle with the dressing and sprinkle with the almonds.

| MAKE IT STAGE 1: | MAKE IT STAGE 3: |
|---|---|
| Increase the amount of teff to ¾ cup. | Decrease the amount of teff to ¼ cup and use ½ pear. |

STAGE 2

# Tomato-Watermelon Gazpacho

Prep Time: 15 minutes          Total Time: 15 minutes          Makes 4 servings

½  cup red quinoa
1½  pounds vine-ripened tomatoes
 2  scallions, green ends only, chopped
½  jalapeño chile pepper, seeded (wear plastic gloves when handling)
 2  tablespoons chopped fresh mint
 2  cups cubed fresh watermelon, divided
 1  small cucumber, peeled, seeded, and cut into ¾" chunks
 1  small red bell pepper, cored and cut into ¾" chunks
 1  tablespoon olive oil
 2  tablespoons wine balsamic vinegar
½  teaspoon sea salt

Cook the quinoa according to package directions. In a blender, puree the tomatoes, scallions, jalapeño chile pepper, mint, and 1 cup of the watermelon. Add the cucumber, red pepper, oil, vinegar, and salt. Pulse until medium-fine.

Add the remaining watermelon and the quinoa and pulse until coarsely chopped. Pour into 4 bowls and serve with a mixed-greens salad.

| MAKE IT STAGE 1: | MAKE IT STAGE 3: |
| --- | --- |
| Top soup with 4 ounces lump crabmeat or cooked chopped shrimp. Add 1 diced avocado, 2 chopped beets, and a handful of walnuts to the salad. | Use 2 pounds tomatoes, and decrease the cubed watermelon to 1 cup and the quinoa to ⅓ cup. Add ¼ diced avocado and 1 chopped beet to the salad. |

STAGE 3

# Black Bean Stew

Prep Time: 15 minutes        Total Time: 55 minutes        Makes 4 servings

¾   cup brown rice
1    tablespoon olive oil
1    red onion, coarsely chopped
1    green bell pepper, finely chopped
2    cloves garlic, minced
1    teaspoon ground cumin
1    teaspoon paprika
1½  cups vegetable broth
1    pound butternut squash, peeled, seeded, and cut into 1" chunks
1    cup halved grape tomatoes
1    cup canned black beans, rinsed and drained
1    cup frozen corn kernels
¼   teaspoon sea salt
½   cup chopped fresh cilantro
     Hot sauce (optional)
½   cup cubed pineapple

Cook the rice according to package directions. In a Dutch oven, heat the oil over medium heat. Add the onion and bell pepper. Cook for 5 minutes, stirring occasionally, or until softened. Add the garlic, cumin, and paprika. Cook for 1 minute, stirring constantly, or until fragrant. Add the broth, squash, tomatoes, and beans. Bring to a boil over high heat. Reduce the heat to low, cover, and simmer for 20 minutes.

Add the corn and salt. Cover and simmer for 10 minutes, or until the vegetables are tender. Spoon the stew over the brown rice and sprinkle it with the cilantro. Serve with the hot sauce, if using, and the pineapple.

| MAKE IT STAGE 1: | MAKE IT STAGE 2: |
| --- | --- |
| Increase the amount of cubed pineapple to 1 cup. Serve with a mixed-greens salad. | Substitute 1 cup coconut water for the vegetable broth. |

STAGE 3

# Chicken Tortilla Soup

Prep Time: 10 minutes          Total Time: 20 minutes          Makes 4 servings

- **4** cups reduced-sodium vegetable broth
- **2** large sweet potatoes, peeled and cut into ½" chunks
- **1** cup canned black beans, rinsed and drained
- **1** cup frozen corn kernels
- **1** cup medium salsa
- **1** teaspoon ground cumin
- **1** container (5 ounces) baby spinach
- **2** ounces cooked chicken breast, chopped
- **2** ounces multigrain, gluten-free tortilla chips, broken into small pieces
- **1** avocado, pitted, peeled, and finely chopped
- **¼** cup chopped fresh cilantro
     Lime wedges
- **1** cup fresh fruit

In a large saucepan over high heat, combine the broth and sweet potatoes. Bring to a boil. Reduce the heat to low, cover, and simmer for 8 minutes, or until the sweet potatoes are tender. Add the beans, corn, salsa, and cumin. Bring to a boil. Reduce the heat to low and simmer for 5 minutes, or until the corn is cooked. Stir in the spinach and chicken and cook for 2 minutes, or until the spinach wilts.

Ladle the soup into bowls and top with the tortilla chips, avocado, and cilantro. Serve with the lime wedges to squeeze into the soup. Serve alongside the fruit.

| **MAKE IT STAGE 1:** | **MAKE IT STAGE 2:** |
| --- | --- |
| Serve with a mixed-greens salad topped with nuts. | Substitute 4 ounces finely chopped tofu for the chicken. Serve with a mixed-greens salad topped with nuts. |

STAGE 3

# Steamed Vegetables with Red Pepper Sauce

Prep Time: 15 minutes      Total Time: 20 minutes      Makes 4 servings

½  cup amaranth
¼  cup sliced almonds, toasted
¼  cup pumpkin seeds, toasted
¾  cup roasted red peppers
1  small tomato, chopped
3  cloves roasted garlic
1½  tablespoons extra-virgin olive oil
½  teaspoon ancho chili powder
1½  teaspoons sherry or red wine vinegar
¼  teaspoon sea salt
⅛  teaspoon ground red pepper
1  cup frozen shelled edamame
2  cups broccoli florets
2  zucchini, diagonally sliced
1  cup quartered strawberries

Cook the amaranth according to package directions. In a mini food processor, blend the almonds and pumpkin seeds until finely ground. Add the red peppers, tomatoes, garlic, olive oil, chili powder, sherry or vinegar, salt, and ground red pepper. Blend until smooth. (The sauce can be refrigerated for up to 3 days.)

Bring a large saucepan filled with a steamer basket and 1" of water to a simmer. Add the edamame, broccoli, and zucchini. Steam for 4 minutes or until the vegetables are just tender. Spoon the amaranth into shallow bowls and top with the steamed vegetables and Romesco sauce. Serve with the strawberries either on the side or on top of a mixed-greens salad.

| MAKE IT STAGE 1: | MAKE IT STAGE 2: |
|---|---|
| Use 1 zucchini, 2 cups of strawberries, and 1 cup of amaranth. | Increase the amount of amaranth to 1 cup. |

# SNACKS

## Quick Bean Burrito

Prep Time: 4 minutes        Total Time: 5 minutes        Makes 1 serving

- ¼   cup canned black beans, rinsed and drained
- 2   tablespoons finely chopped tomato
- 1   gluten-free tortilla

In a small bowl, mash the beans and tomato. Microwave the tortilla on high power for 15 seconds. Lay the tortilla on a flat surface and spread the bean mixture down the center. Fold the sides in toward the center and serve.

## Guacamole Deviled Eggs

Prep Time: 3 minutes        Total Time: 3 minutes        Makes 1 serving

- 1   hard-cooked egg, peeled
- 2   tablespoons packaged guacamole
    Dash of hot-pepper sauce

Halve the egg lengthwise, removing the egg yolk. In a small bowl, mash the yolk. Add the guacamole and hot-pepper sauce and stir to combine.

Fill each egg white half with the egg yolk mixture.

## Cucumber Boats

Prep Time: 5 minutes        Total Time: 5 minutes        Makes 2 servings

- 1   tablespoon quinoa pilaf mix
- 1   English cucumber, halved lengthwise and seeded

Prepare the quinoa pilaf according to package directions.

Fill each cucumber half with pilaf. Slice each half crosswise into 3 pieces and serve.

## Peach Blueberry Smoothie

Prep Time: 2 minutes          Total Time: 3 minutes          Makes 1 serving

- 1   cup almond or vanilla soy milk, chilled
- 4   slices fresh or frozen peaches (about ½ cup)
- ¼   cup blueberries
     Handful of kale
- ¼   teaspoon ground cinnamon

In a blender, combine the soy milk, peaches, kale, blueberries, and cinnamon. Blend until smooth.

## Fresh Fruit Salad Cup

Prep Time: 2 minutes          Total Time: 2 minutes          Makes 2 servings

- 1   cup chopped fresh fruit
- 2   tablespoons plain or vanilla soy yogurt
- 1   tablespoon chopped almonds or cashews

In a small dessert dish, place the fruit. Dollop with the yogurt and top with the chopped nuts.

## 3-Layer Mexican Dip

Prep Time: 2 minutes          Total Time: 2 minutes          Makes 1 serving

- ½   cup fresh tomato salsa
- ¼   cup finely chopped avocado
- ¼   cup canned black beans, rinsed and drained
     Gluten-free tortilla chips

In a small bowl, place the salsa. Top with the avocado and black beans. Serve with the chips.

# Smoked Salmon on Cucumber Slices

Prep Time: 5 minutes        Total Time: 5 minutes        Makes 2 servings

- 1     Japanese cucumber, cut into ½" rounds
- 2–3  tablespoons dairy-free sour cream
- 3     ounces smoked salmon slices
        Sprigs dill
        Rice crackers

Place the cucumber slices on a platter. Put a small dollop of the sour cream on each. Top with a bit of the salmon and a dill sprig. Serve with the rice crackers.

# Chocolate Lover's Trail Mix

Prep Time: 3 minutes        Total Time: 3 minutes        Makes 2 servings

- 2     tablespoons unsalted cashews, almonds, or walnuts
- ¼    cup unsweetened cranberries or goji berries
- 2     tablespoons hemp or pumpkin seed kernels
- 2     tablespoons dark chocolate chips
- ¼    cup gluten-free toasted oat cereal

In a small bowl, mix together the nuts, berries, seed kernels, chocolate chips, and cereal.

# Nutty Celery Sticks

Prep Time: 5 minutes        Total Time: 5 minutes        Makes 2 servings

- 4     ribs celery
- 2     tablespoons almond butter or cashew butter
- 1     teaspoon chopped unsalted nuts

Fill the celery ribs with the nut butter or tahini. Top with the chopped nuts.

# Stuffed Lettuce Cups

Prep Time: 5 minutes          Total Time: 10 minutes          Makes 4 servings

- ⅛   cup brown rice
- 1   teaspoon coconut oil
- 1   cup seasoned tofu cubes
- ¼   cup finely chopped avocado
- 4   leaves butterhead or Bibb lettuce

Cook the rice according to package directions.

In a small skillet over medium-high heat, warm the oil. When hot enough, add the tofu cubes and lightly brown them on all sides. Remove the cubes to a small bowl and add the rice and avocado. Fill the lettuce leaves with this mixture, and serve.

# DESSERTS

## Almond and Mixed Berry Muffins

Prep Time: 15 minutes        Total Time: 40 minutes        Makes 12 muffins

  2   cups almond flour
  ¾   cup coconut flour
  4   teaspoons baking powder
  ¼   cup ground flaxseeds
  ½   teaspoon salt
  ⅔   cup fresh blueberries
  ⅔   cup fresh raspberries
  1   cup almond milk
  1   egg
  ¼   cup applesauce
  ½   cup raw (turbinado) sugar
  ⅓   cup coconut oil
  1   teaspoon almond extract

Preheat the oven to 400°F. Line a 12-cup muffin pan with paper liners.

In a large bowl, combine the almond flour, coconut flour, baking powder, flaxseeds, and salt. Whisk to mix. Add the blueberries and raspberries and stir to coat.

In another bowl, combine the almond milk, egg, applesauce, sugar, oil, and almond extract. With a fork, beat until smooth.

Pour the egg mixture into the berry mixture and gently mix with a fork to moisten the dry ingredients. Don't overmix (a few lumps in the batter are normal). Dollop the batter into the prepared muffin cups.

Bake for 20 to 24 minutes, or until a wooden pick inserted into the center of a muffin comes out clean. Cool in the pan on a rack for 5 minutes. Remove to the rack and cool completely.

# Wholesome Oat Muffins

Prep Time: 1 hour          Total Time: 1 hour 20 minutes          Makes 12 muffins

| | |
|---|---|
| 1 | cup almond milk |
| 1 | teaspoon cider vinegar |
| 1 | cup + 2 tablespoons oats |
| 1 | cup gluten-free flour |
| 1½ | teaspoons baking powder |
| ½ | teaspoon baking soda |
| ¼ | teaspoon ground cinnamon |
| ¼ | teaspoon salt |
| ⅓ | cup coconut oil |
| 1 | egg |
| ⅓ | cup raw (turbinado) sugar |
| 1 | teaspoon vanilla extract |

Preheat the oven to 425°F. Grease a 12-cup muffin pan.

In a small bowl, mix the almond milk and vinegar. Let stand in a warm place for 20 minutes. Add 1 cup of the oats to the milk mixture. Let soak for 30 minutes.

In a medium bowl, combine the flour, baking powder, baking soda, cinnamon, and salt.

In a large bowl, stir together the oil, egg, sugar, and vanilla until well blended. Stir in the oat mixture. Stir in the flour mixture until just combined. Do not overmix.

Divide the batter evenly among the prepared muffin cups, filling them about two-thirds full. Sprinkle the remaining 2 tablespoons oats over the muffins. Bake for 11 to 15 minutes, or until a wooden pick inserted in the center of a muffin comes out clean. Cool in the pan on a rack for 5 minutes. Remove to the rack and cool completely.

**NOTE:** Ingredients for a changed serving size are based on a calculation and are not reviewed by the author or tested. Please also consider scaling up or down cooking containers as needed.

# Blueberry Muffins

Prep Time: 15 minutes          Total Time: 35 minutes          Makes 12 muffins

- 1½   cups almond flour
- ¼   cup coconut flour
- 2   teaspoons baking powder
- ½   teaspoon salt
- ½   teaspoon cinnamon
- ½   cup almond milk
- ¼   cup coconut oil
- 1   egg
- ⅓   cup raw (turbinado) sugar
- 1   teaspoon vanilla extract
- 1½   cups blueberries

Preheat the oven to 400°F. Grease a 12-cup muffin pan.

In a medium bowl, combine the almond flour, coconut flour, baking powder, salt, and cinnamon.

In a large bowl, stir together the almond milk, oil, egg, sugar, and vanilla until well blended. Stir in the flour mixture until just combined. Do not overmix. Gently fold in the blueberries.

Divide the batter evenly among the prepared muffin cups, filling them about two-thirds full. Bake for 17 to 20 minutes, or until a wooden pick inserted in the center of a muffin comes out clean. Cool in the pan on a rack for 5 minutes. Remove to the rack and cool completely.

# Glazed Pineapple Cupcakes

Prep Time: 20 minutes          Total Time: 40 minutes          Makes 12 cupcakes

¼   cup + 5 tablespoons raw (turbinado) sugar
1   cup canned pineapple chunks packed in juice, drained
     (reserve 3 tablespoons juice)
½   cup almond flour
½   cup soy flour
¾   teaspoon baking powder
½   teaspoon baking soda
2   eggs
     Dash of salt
½   cup plain or vanilla soy yogurt
¼   cup coconut oil
2   teaspoons vanilla extract

Preheat the oven to 350°F. Coat a nonstick 12-cup muffin pan with cooking spray. Scatter 1 packed teaspoon of the sugar into the bottom of each cup. Cut each pineapple chunk in half. Place 4 pieces in a single layer in each cup.

On a sheet of waxed paper, combine the almond flour, soy flour, baking powder, and baking soda. Blend with a fork.

Separate the eggs, putting the whites in the bowl of an electric mixer and the yolks into a large mixing bowl. Add the salt to the whites and beat on low speed for 1 minute to loosen. Increase the speed to high. Beat for 2 to 3 minutes, gradually adding 1 tablespoon of the sugar until the whites hold soft peaks. Set aside.

To the yolks, add the yogurt, oil, reserved pineapple juice, vanilla, and remaining 4 tablespoons sugar. With a fork, beat until smooth. Stir in the dry ingredients. Carefully fold the reserved whites into the batter. Dollop the batter into the muffin cups. Smooth the tops.

Bake for 15 minutes, or until the cupcakes are browned and spring back when pressed with a fingertip. Remove from the oven. Cool in the pan on a rack for 5 minutes. Place a heatproof tray over the pan. Using oven mitts, flip the pan over on the tray. Tap the cup bottoms to aid release. Serve warm.

# Oat-Almond Mixed Berry Crisp

Prep Time: 15 minutes        Total Time: 1 hour        Makes 6 servings

- 4  tablespoons raw (turbinado) sugar
- 1½  tablespoons tapioca starch
- 2  cups sliced fresh strawberries
- 2  cups fresh blueberries
- 1½  teaspoons almond extract
- ¾  cup old-fashioned oats
- 3  tablespoons sliced almonds
- 1  tablespoon coconut oil

Preheat the oven to 350°F. Coat an 8" × 8" baking dish with cooking spray.

In a medium bowl, combine 3 tablespoons of sugar and the tapioca starch. Stir to mix. Add the strawberries, blueberries, and almond extract. Toss to coat the berries thoroughly. Transfer to the baking dish.

In the same bowl, combine the oats, almonds, 1 tablespoon sugar, and oil. Toss to coat thoroughly. Scatter evenly over the berry mixture.

Bake for 45 minutes, or until the berriy juices bubble and are no longer opaque. Remove to a rack and let stand at room temperature for 5 minutes.

# Plum-Blueberry Cobbler

Prep Time: 15 minutes        Total Time: 1 hour 5 minutes        Makes 8 servings

  8   plums, pitted and quartered
  2   cups blueberries
  ⅓   cup + 4 teaspoons raw (turbinado) sugar
  ⅓   cup quinoa flour, divided
  ¾   cup almond flour
  ¾   teaspoon baking powder
  ⅛   teaspoon salt
  ½   cup almond milk
  1   egg
  1½  tablespoons coconut oil

Preheat the oven to 375°F. Coat a 9" × 9" baking dish with cooking spray.

In a large bowl, mix the plums, blueberries, ⅓ cup of the sugar, and 2 table-spoons of the quinoa flour. Place in the prepared baking dish.

In a medium bowl, mix 3 teaspoons of the remaining sugar, the remaining quinoa flour, and the almond flour, baking powder, and salt.

In a small bowl, mix the almond milk, egg, and oil. Pour into the flour mix-ture. Stir until a thick batter forms. Drop tablespoons of the batter on top of the fruit. Sprinkle with the remaining 1 teaspoon sugar.

Bake for 35 to 40 minutes, or until golden and bubbly. Cool on a rack for at least 10 minutes before serving.

# Almond-Cherry Clafoutis

Prep Time: 15 minutes    Total Time: 50 minutes    Makes 4 servings

| | |
|---|---|
| 12 | ounces pitted large fresh or frozen, drained, and thawed cherries |
| 4 | tablespoons raw (turbinado) sugar, divided |
| 3 | tablespoons sliced almonds |
| 3 | tablespoons quinoa flour |
| 3 | eggs |
| 1 | egg yolk |
| ¾ | cup almond milk |
| ¼ | teaspoon almond extract |
| | Pinch of salt |

Preheat the oven to 375°F. Coat four 8-ounce ramekins or custard cups lightly with cooking spray. In a medium bowl, toss the cherries with 2 tablespoons of the sugar. Divide the cherries among the ramekins.

In a food processor, combine the almonds, flour, eggs, egg yolk, almond milk, almond extract, salt, and the remaining 2 tablespoons of the sugar. Pulse for 30 seconds, or until the almonds are ground and the mixture forms a smooth batter.

Evenly divide the batter over the cherries. Bake for 35 minutes or until puffed and brown. Let cool until warm (the clafoutis will sink slightly). Serve warm.

# Red Fruit Crumble

Prep Time: 15 minutes          Total Time: 1 hour 20 minutes          Makes 8 servings

### Fruit

- 1 pound strawberries, hulled and thickly sliced
- 3 ripe plums, cut into 1" pieces (¾ pound)
- 1 cup fresh or frozen raspberries
- ¼ cup all-fruit raspberry or strawberry preserves, stirred smooth

### Topping

- 1 cup oats
- ⅓ cup almond flour
- ⅓ cup raw (turbinado) sugar
- ½ teaspoon ground cinnamon
- ⅛ teaspoon salt
- 3 tablespoons Earth Balance omega-3 buttery spread, cut into small pieces
- ¾ cup chopped walnuts

Preheat the oven to 375°F.

**TO MAKE THE FRUIT:** In an 8" × 8" glass baking dish, combine the strawberries, plums, raspberries, and fruit preserves and mix gently with a spatula.

**TO MAKE THE TOPPING:** In a medium bowl, mix the oats, flour, sugar, cinnamon, and salt. Crumble in the Earth Balance until well incorporated. Stir in the walnuts. Sprinkle the oat mixture over the fruit.

Bake, uncovered, for 35 to 40 minutes or until the fruit is tender and bubbly and the topping is lightly browned. Cool the baking dish on a rack for at least 30 minutes before serving.

# ENDNOTES

## CHAPTER 1

1  J. L. Wilson, *Adrenal Fatigue: The 21st Century Stress Syndrome* (Petaluma, CA: Smart Publications, 2001), 6.

2  B. Bleicken et al., "Delayed Diagnosis of Adrenal Insufficiency Is Common: A Cross-Sectional Study in 216 Patients," *American Journal of Medical Science* 339, no. 6 (June 2010): 525–31, doi:10.1097/MAJ.0b013e3181db6b7a.

3  N. Pranji, et al., "Is Adrenal Exhaustion Synonym of Syndrome Burnout at Workplace?" *Collegium Antropologicum* 36, no. 3 (September 2012): 911–9.

4  D. S. Goldstein, "Adrenal Responses to Stress," *Cellular and Molecular Neurobiology* 30, no. 8 (November 2010): 1433–40.

5  D. J. Powell and W. Schlotz, "Daily Life Stress and the Cortisol Awakening Response: Testing the Anticipation Hypothesis," *PLOS ONE* 7, no. 12 (2012): e52067, doi:10.1371/journal.pone.0052067.

6  F. Ye et al., "Hormones Other Than Aldosterone May Contribute to Hypertension in 3 Different Subtypes of Primary Aldosteronism," *Journal of Clinical Hypertension* (Greenwich) 15, no. 4 (April 2013): 264–9, doi:10.1111/jch.12070.

7  L. Ceccoli et al., "Bone Health and Aldosterone Excess," *Osteoporosis International* 24, no. 11 (November 2014): 2801–07, doi:10.1007/s00198-013-2399-1.

8  P. J. Fitzgerald, "Elevated Norepinephrine May Be an Etiological Factor in a Wide Range of Diseases: Age-Related Macular Degeneration, Systemic Lupus Erythematosus, Atrial Fibrillation, Metabolic Syndrome," *Medical Hypotheses* 80, no. 5 (May 2013): 558–63, doi:10.1016/j.mehy.2013.01.018.

9  J. Vafaeimanesh, M. Bagherzadeh, and M. Parham, "Adrenal Insufficiency As a Cause of Acute Liver Failure: A Case Report," Case Rep Endocrinol 2013 (published electronically February 25, 2013): 487189, doi:10.1155/2013/487189.

10  M. A. Demitrack et al., "Evidence for Impaired Activation of the Hypothalamic-Pituitary-Adrenal Axis in Patients with Chronic Fatigue Syndrome," *Journal of Clinical Endocrinology & Metabolism* 73 (1991): 1224–34.

11  R. Riva et al., "Fibromyalgia Syndrome Is Associated with Hypocortisolism," *International Journal of Behavioral Medicine* 17, no. 3 (September 2010): 223–33, doi:10.1007/s12529-010-9097-6.

## CHAPTER 2

1  CDC; www.diabetes.org/diabetes-basics/statistics/.

2  J. Li, X. Sun, and Y. Yu, "The Prevalence of Impaired Glucose Regulation in Psychiatric Patients with Sleep Disorders and Its Relationship with Altered Hypothalamopituitary-Adrenal and Hypothalamopituitary-Thyroid Axis Activity," *Sleep Medicine* 14, no. 7 (July 14, 2013): 662–67, doi:10.1016/j.sleep.2013.04.004.

3  Ibid.

4  B. Viollet et al., "Cellular and Molecular Mechanisms of Metformin: An Overview," *Clinical Science (London)* 122, no. 6 (March 2012): 253–70, doi:10.1042/CS20110386.

5  S. K. Musani et al., "Aldosterone, C-Reactive Protein, and Plasma B-Type Natriuretic Peptide Are Associated with the Development of Metabolic Syndrome and Longitudinal Changes

in Metabolic Syndrome Components: Findings from the Jackson Heart Study," *Diabetes Care* 36, no. 10 (October 2013): 3084–92.

6   www.diabetes.org/diabetes-basics/statistics/; "Economic Costs of Diabetes in the U.S. in 2012," American Diabetes Association, March 6, 2013, http://professional.diabetes.org/News_Display.aspx?TYP=9&CID=91943&loc=ContentPage-statistics.

7   www.lerner.ccf.org/qhs/risk_calculator/.

8   Mayo Clinic. www.mayoclinic.org.

9   "Glycemic Index," *Self* Nutrition Data, http://nutritiondata.self.com/topics/glycemic-index.

## CHAPTER 3

1   K. Reding et al., "Social Status Modifies Estradiol Activation of Sociosexual Behavior in Female Rhesus Monkeys," *Hormones and Behavior* 62, no. 5 (November 2012): 612–20, doi:10.1016/j.yhbeh.2012.09.010.

2   K. L. Felmingham, W. C. Fong, and R. A. Bryant, "The Impact of Progesterone on Memory Consolidation of Threatening Images in Women," *Psychoneuroendocrinology* 37, no. 11 (November 2012): 1896–900, doi:10.1016/j.psyneuen.2012.03.026.

3   S. Conova, "Estrogen's Role in Cancer," *in Vivo* 2, no. 10 (May 26, 2003): http://www.cumc.columbia.edu/publications/in-vivo/Vol2_Iss10_may26_03/; "Endometriosis," Mayo Clinic, April 2, 2013, http://www.mayoclinic.com/health/endometriosis/DS00289/DSECTION=treatments-and-drugs; "Uterine Fibroids," MedlinePlus, July 25, 2011, http://www.nlm.nih.gov/medlineplus/ency/article/000914.htm.

4   T. M. Barber and S. Franks, "The Link between Polycystic Ovary Syndrome and Both Type 1 and Type 2 Diabetes Mellitus: What Do We Know Today?" *Women's Health* 8, no. 2 (March 2012): 147–54, doi:10.2217/whe.11.94.

5   A. J. Plechner, "Cortisol Abnormality As a Cause of Elevated Estrogen and Immune Destabilization: Insights for Human Medicine from a Veterinary Perspective," *Medical Hypotheses* 62, no. 4 (2004): 575–81.

6   S. Bellanger, "Saturated Fatty Acid Exposure Induces Androgen Overproduction in Bovine Adrenal Cells," *Steroids* 77, no. 4 (March 10, 2012): 347–53, doi:10.1016/j.steroids.2011.12.017.

7   S. Benson et al., "Disturbed Stress Responses in Women with Polycystic Ovary Syndrome," *Psychoneuroendocrinology* 34, no. 5 (June 2009): 727–35, doi:10.1016/j.psyneuen.2008.12.001.

8   R. A. Lobo et al., "Psychological Stress and Increases in Urinary Norepinephrine Metabolites, Platelet Serotonin, and Adrenal Androgens in Women with Polycystic Ovary Syndrome," American Journal of Obstetrics and Gynecology 145, no. 4 (February 15, 1983): 496–503.

## CHAPTER 4

1   S. Cohen et al., "Chronic Stress, Glucocorticoid Receptor Resistance, Inflammation, and Disease Risk," *Proceedings of the National Academy of Sciences of the United States of America* 109, no. 16 (2012): 5995–99, doi:10.1073/pnas.1118355109.

2   T. Pudrovska et al., "Higher-Status Occupations and Breast Cancer: A Life-Course Stress Approach," *Social Science and Medicine* 89 (July 2013): 53–61, doi:10.1016/j.socscimed.2013.04.013.

3   J. Vuyyuri et al., "Ascorbic Acid and a Cytostatic Inhibitor of Glycolysis Synergistically Induce Apoptosis in Non-Small Cell Lung Cancer Cells," *PLOS ONE* 8, no. 6 (June 11, 2013): e67081.

4   A. T. Masi et al., "Lower Serum Androstenedione Levels in Pre-Rheumatoid Arthritis versus Normal Control Women: Correlations with Lower Serum Cortisol Levels," *Autoimmune Diseases* (published electronically May 22, 2013): 593493, doi:10.1155/2013/593493.

5   E. Haus, L. Sackett-Lundeen, and M. H. Smolensky, "Rheumatoid Arthritis: Circadian Rhythms in Disease Activity, Signs and Symptoms, and Rationale for Chronotherapy with

Corticosteroids and Other Medications," *Bulletin of the NYU Hospital for Joint Diseases* 70, sup. 1 (2012): 3–10; V. P. Kouri et al., "Circadian Timekeeping is Disturbed in Rheumatoid Arthritis at Molecular Level," *PLOS ONE* 8, no. 1 (published electronically January 15, 2013): e54049, doi:10.1371/journal.pone.0054049.

## CHAPTER 5

1   www.cdc.gov/cholesterol/facts.htm.

2   "Detection, Evaluation, and Treatment of High Blood Cholesterol in Adults (Adult Treatment Panel III): Final Report," National Institutes of Health, September 2002, http://www.nhlbi.nih.gov/guidelines/cholesterol/atp3full.pdf.

3   D. Il'yasova et al., "Circulating Levels of Inflammatory Markers and Cancer Risk in the Health Aging and Body Composition Cohort," *Cancer Epidemiology, Biomarkers, and Prevention* 14, no. 10 (October 2005): 2413–8; M. D. Barber, J. A. Ross, and K. C. Fearon, "Changes in Nutritional, Functional, and Inflammatory Markers in Advanced Pancreatic Cancer," *Nutrition and Cancer* 35, no. 2 (1999): 106–10; J. A. Smigielski et al., "Application of Biochemical Markers CA 19-9, CEA and C-Reactive Protein in Diagnosis of Malicious and Benign Pancreatic Tumors," *Archives of Medical Science* 9, no. 4 (August 30, 2013): 677–83; M. Y. Donath and S. E. Shoelson, "Type 2 Diabetes as an Inflammatory Disease," *Nature Reviews Immunology* 11, no. 2 (February 2011): 98–107, doi:10.1038/nri2925; G. L. King, "The Role of Inflammatory Cytokines in Diabetes and Its Complications," *Journal of Periodontology* 79, sup. 8 (August 2008): 1527–34, doi:10.1902/jop.2008.080246.

4   I. Kawachi et al., "Symptoms of Anxiety and Risk of Coronary Heart Disease. The Normative Aging Study," *Circulation* 90 (1994): 2225–29.

5   W. S. Jones et al., *Treatment Strategies for Patients with Peripheral Artery Disease* (Agency for Healthcare Research and Quality: Rockville, MD, May 2013).

6   A. Matsusima et al., "Acute and Chronic Flow-Mediated Dilation and Blood Pressure Responses to Daily Intake of Boysenberry Juice: A Preliminary Study," *International Journal of Food Sciences and Nutrition* (published electronically July 12, 2013).

7   "DASH Diet: Healthy Eating to Lower Your Blood Pressure," Mayo Clinic, May 15, 2013, http://www.mayoclinic.com/health/dash-diet/HI00047.

8   G. A. Spiller and B. Bruce, "Vegan Diets and Cardiovascular Health," *Journal of the American College of Nutrition* 17, no. 5 (October 1998): 407–8.

9   F. L. Crowe et al., "Risk of Hospitalization or Death from Ischemic Heart Disease among British Vegetarians and Nonvegetarians: Results from the EPIC-Oxford Cohort Study," *American Journal of Clinical Nutrition* 97, no. 3 (March 2013): 597–603, doi:10.3945/ajcn.112.044073; N. I. Alrabadi, "The Effect of Lifestyle Food on Chronic Diseases: A Comparison between Vegetarians and Non-Vegetarians in Jordan," *Global Journal of Health Science* 5, no. 1 (November 4, 2012): 65–9, doi:10.5539/gjhs.v5n1p65; C. T. McEvoy, N. Temple, and J. V. Woodside, "Vegetarian Diets, Low-Meat Diets, and Health: A Review," *Public Health Nutrition* 15, no. 12 (December 2012): 2287–94, doi:10.1017/S1368980012000936; S. Y. Yang et al., "Chinese Lacto-Vegetarian Diet Exerts Favorable Effects on Metabolic Parameters, Intima-Media Thickness, and Cardiovascular Risks in Healthy Men," *Nutrition in Clinical Practice* 27, no. 3 (June 2012): 392–8, doi:10.1177/0884533611436173; B. J. Pettersen et al., "Vegetarian Diets and Blood Pressure among White Subjects: Results from the Adventist Health Study-2 (AHS-2)," *Public Health Nutrition* 15, no. 10 (October 2012): 1909–16, doi:10.1017/S1368980011003454; M. Krajcovicova-Kudlackova et al., "Selected Biomarkers of Age-Related Diseases in Older Subjects with Different Nutrition," *Bratislava Medical Journal* 112, no. 11 (2011): 610–3; S. Y. Yang et al., "Relationship of Carotid Intima-Media Thickness and Duration of Vegetarian Diet in Chinese Male Vegetarians," *Nutrition and Metabolism* 8, no. 1 (September 19, 2011): 63, doi:10.1186/1743-7075-8-63.

10  Y. Ingenbleek and K. S. McCully, "Vegetarianism Produces Subclinical Malnutrition, Hyperhomocysteinemia, and Atherogenesis," *Nutrition* 28, no. 2 (February 2012): 148–53, doi:10.1016/j.nut.2011.04.009.

11  N. D. Powell et al., "Social Stress Up-Regulates Inflammatory Gene Expression in the Leukocyte Transcriptome via O-Adrenergic Induction of Myelopoiesis," Proceedings of the National Academy of Sciences 110, no. 41 (October 8, 2013): 16574–79, doi:10.1073/pnas.1310655110.

12 S. Cohena et al., "Chronic Stress, Glucocorticoid Receptor Resistance, Inflammation, and Disease Risk," Proceedings of the National Academy of Sciences 109, no. 16 (2012): 5995–99, doi:10.1073/pnas.1118355109.

## CHAPTER 6

1 K. N. et al., "Elevated Thyroid Stimulating Hormone Is Associated with Elevated Cortisol in Healthy Young Men and Women," *Thyroid Research* 5, no. 1 (October 2012 13), doi:10.1186/1756-6614-5-13; A. C. Hackney and J. D. Dobridge, "Thyroid Hormones and the Interrelationship of Cortisol and Prolactin: Influence of Prolonged, Exhaustive Exercise," *Polish Journal of Endocrinology* 60, no. 4 (July–August 2009): 252–7; W. Seeling et al., "Blood Glucose, ACTH, Cortisol, T4, T3 and rT3 after Cholecystectomy. Comparative Studies of Continuous Peridural Anesthesia and Neuroleptanalgesia," *Regional-Anaesthesie* 7, no. 1 (January 1984): 1–10.

2 Centers for Disease Control and Prevention. www.cdc.gov.

3 P. N. Taylor et al., "A Review of the Clinical Consequences of Variation in Thyroid Function within the Reference Range," Journal of Clinical Endocrinology and Metabolism 98, no. 9 (September 2013): 3562–71, doi:10.1210/jc.2013-1315.

4 K. N. Walter et al., "Elevated Thyroid Stimulating Hormone Is Associated with Elevated Cortisol in Healthy Young Men and Women," *Thyroid Research* 5, no. 1 (October 30, 2012): 13, doi:10.1186/1756-6614-5-13.

5 EmedicineHealth – Hashimotos. www.emedicinehealth.com/hashimotos_disease/article_em.htm.

6 A. Dizdarevic-Bostandic et al., "Inflammatory Markers in Patients with Hypothyroidism and Diabetes Mellitus Type 1," *Medicinski Arhiv* 67, no. 3 (2013): 160–1; Y. T. Yu et al., "Subclinical Hypothyroidism is Associated with Elevated High-Sensitive C-Reactive Protein among Adult Taiwanese," *Endocrine* 44, no. 3 (December 2013): 716–22; R. Krysiak and B. Okopien, "Coexistence of Primary Aldosteronism and Hashimoto's Thyroiditis," *Rheumatology International* 32, no. 8 (August 2012): 2561–3, doi:10.1007/s00296-011-2032-6.

7 D. Armanini et al., "Microalbuminuria and Hypertension in Pregnancy: Role of Aldosterone and Inflammation," *Journal of Clinical Hypertension* 15, no. 9 (September 2013): 612–4.

8 K. Kusche-Vihrog et al., "C-Reactive Protein Makes Human Endothelium Stiff and Tight," *Hypertension* 57, no. 2 (February 2011): 231–7; D. Menicucci et al., "Minimal Changes of Thyroid Axis Activity Influence Brain Functions in Young Females Affected by Subclinical Hypothyroidism," *Archives Italiennes de Biologie* 151, no. 1 (March 2013): 1474; D. S. Greco, "Endocrine Causes of Calcium Disorders," *Topics in Companion Animal Medicine* 27, no. 4 (November 2012): 150–5.

9 M. Kozai, "Thyroid Hormones Decrease Plasma 10,25-dihydroxyvitamin D Levels through Transcriptional Repression of the Renal 25-Hydroxyvitamin D3 10-Hydroxylase Gene (CYP27B1)," *Endocrinology* 154, no. 2 (February 2013): 609–22.

10 N. J. Aljohani et al., "Differences and Associations of Metabolic and Vitamin D Status among Patients with and without Sub-Clinical Hypothyroid Dysfunction," *BMC Endocrine Disorders* 13, no. 1 (August 20, 2013): 31, doi:10.1186/1472-6823-13-31.

11 Kozai M, Yamamoto H, Ishiguro M, et al. "Thyroid Hormones Decrease Plasma 1a,25-dihydroxyvitamin D Levels through Transcriptional Repression of the Renal 25-hydroxyvitamin D3 1a-hydroxylase Gene (CYP27B1)," *Endocrinology* 154, no. 2 (February 2013): 609–22.

12 Aljohani et al. "Differences and Associations," . . .

## CHAPTER 7

1 B. Bleicken et al., "Delayed Diagnosis of Adrenal Insufficiency Is Common: A Cross-Sectional Study in 216 Patients," *American Journal of Medical Sciences* 339, no. 6 (June 2010): 525–31.

2 J. S. Prendiville and L. N. Manfredi, "Skin Signs of Nutritional Disorders," *Seminars in Dermatology* 11, no. 1 (March 1992): 88–97; M. L. Heath and R. Sidbury, "Cutaneous Manifestations of Nutritional Deficiency," *Current Opinion in Pediatrics* 18, no. 4 (August 2006): 417–22; N. Scheinfeld, M. J. Dahdah, and R. Scher, "Vitamins and Minerals: Their Role

in Nail Health and Disease," *Journal of Drugs in Dermatology* 6, no. 8 (August 2007): 782–7; "Micronutrients and Skin Health," Linus Pauling Institute, September 2011, http://lpi.oregonstate.edu/infocenter/skin.html.

3   N. Sugaya et al., "Adrenal Hormone Response and Psychophysiological Correlates under Psychosocial Stress in Individuals with Irritable Bowel Syndrome," *International Journal of Psychophysiology* 84, no. 1 (April 2012): 39–44.

4   B. Björkstén et al., "Allergy Development and the Intestinal Microflora during the First Year of Life," *Journal of Allergy and Clinical Immunology* 108, no. 4 (October 2001): 516–20.

5   E. J. Woodmansey, "Intestinal Bacteria and Ageing," *Journal of Applied Microbiology* 102, no. 5 (May 2007): 1178–86.

6   J. B. Adams et al., "Gastrointestinal Flora and Gastrointestinal Status in Children with Autism—Comparisons to Typical Children and Correlation with Autism Severity," *BMC Gastroenterology* 11, no. 22 (March 16, 2011).

7   http://www.greatplainslaboratory.com/home, Great Plains Laboratory.

8   V. M. Bondarenko and E. V. Riabichenko, "Intestinal-Brain Axis. Neuronal and Immune-Inflammatory Mechanisms of Brain and Intestine Pathology," *Zhurnal mikrobiologii, epidemiologii, i immunobiologii* 2 (March–April 2013): 112–20.

9   M. El-Salhy, "Irritable Bowel Syndrome: Diagnosis and Pathogenesis," *World Journal of Gastroenterology* 18, no. 37 (October 7, 2012): 5151–63.

10  W. H. Wilson et al., "Intestinal Microbial Metabolism of Phosphatidylcholine and Cardiovascular Risk," *New England Journal of Medicine* 368, no. 17 (2013): 1575.

11  D. Grady, "Studies Focus on Gut Bacteria's Role in Weight," *New York Times,* March 27, 2013, http://www.nytimes.com/2013/03/28/health/studies-focus-on-gut-bacteria-in-weight-loss.html?_r=0.

12  A. Duseja and Y. K. Chawla, "Obesity and NAFLD: The Role of Bacteria and Microbiota," *Clinics in Liver Disease* 18, no. 1 (February 2014): 59–71.

13  Y. T. Tsai, P. C. Cheng, and T. M. Pan, "Anti-Obesity Effects of Gut Microbiota Are Associated with Lactic Acid Bacteria," *Applied Microbiology and Biotechnology* (published electronically November 14, 2013); R. Luoto et al., "Reshaping the Gut Microbiota at an Early Age: Functional Impact on Obesity Risk?" *Annals of Nutrition and Metabolism* 63, sup. 2 (2013): 17–26.

14  S. M. Finegold, "Intestinal Bacteria—The Role They Play in Normal Physiology, Pathologic Physiology, and Infection," *California Medicine* 110, no. 6 (June 1969): 455–59.

15  X. Li et al., "Combat-Training Increases Intestinal Permeability, Immune Activation, and Gastrointestinal Symptoms in Soldiers," *Alimentary Pharmacology and Therapeutics* 37, no. 8 (April 2013): 799–809.

16  G. S. Kelly, "Hydrochloric Acid: Physiological Functions and Clinical Implications," *Alternative Medicine Review* 2, no. 2 (1997): 116–27, http://www.thorne.com/media/alternative_medicine_review/1997/volume_2/Number_2/Hydrochloric_Acid.pdf; J. English, "Gastric Balance: Heartburn Not Always Caused by Excess Acid," *Nutrition Review,* http://nutritionreview.org/2013/04/gastric-balance-heartburn-caused-excess-acid/.

17  R. J. Laheij et al., "Risk of Community-Acquired Pneumonia and Use of Gastric Acid-Suppressive Drugs," *Journal of the American Medical Association* 292, no. 16 (October 27, 2004): 1955–60.

18  V. Plourde, "Stress-Induced Changes in the Gastrointestinal Motor System," *Canadian Journal of Gastroenterology* 13, suppl. A (March 1999): 26A–31A.

19  R. L. Earley, L. S. Blumer, and M. S. Grober, "The Gall of Subordination: Changes in Gall Bladder Function Associated with Social Stress," *Proceedings of the Royal Society B: Biological Sciences* 271, no. 1534 (January 7, 2004): 7–13.

20  D. Nellesen et al., "Comorbidities in Patients with Irritable Bowel Syndrome with Constipation or Chronic Idiopathic Constipation: A Review of the Literature from the Past Decade," *Postgraduate Medicine* 125, no. 2 (March 2013): 40–50.

21  C. C. Vere et al., "Psychosocial Stress and Liver Disease Status," *World Journal of Gastroenterology* 15, no. 24 (June 28, 2009): 2980–86.

## CHAPTER 8

1 *Morbidity and Mortality Weekly Report,* Centers for Disease Control and Prevention, 60, no. 8, March 4, 2011, http://www.cdc.gov/mmwr/PDF/wk/mm6008.pdf.

2 D. F. Kripke, R. D. Langer, and L. E. Kline, "Hypnotics' Association with Mortality or Cancer: A Matched Cohort Study," *BMJ Open* (February 2012): 2: e000850, doi:10.1136/bmjopen-2012-000850.

3 G. Terán-Pérez et al., "Steroid Hormones and Sleep Regulation," *Mini Reviews in Medicinal Chemistry* 12, no. 11 (October 2012): 1040–8.

4 A. N. Vgontzas et al., "Chronic Insomnia Is Associated with Nyctohemeral Activation of the Hypothalamic-Pituitary-Adrenal Axis: Clinical Implications," *Journal of Clinical Endocrinology and Metabolism* 86, no. 8 (August 2001): 3787–94.

5 G. Cizza et al., "Chronic Sleep Deprivation and Seasonality: Implications for the Obesity Epidemic," *Journal of Endocrinological Investigation* 34, no. 10 (November 2011): 793–800, doi:10.3275/7808.

6 A. Liu, C. A Kushida, and G. M. Reaven, "Habitual Shortened Sleep and Insulin Resistance: An Independent Relationship in Obese Individuals," *Metabolism* 62, no. 11 (November 2013): 1553–56, doi:10.1016/j.metabol.2013.06.003.

7 S. R. Iyer, "Sleep and Type 2 Diabetes Mellitus—Clinical Implications," *Journal of the Association of Physicians of India* 60 (October 2012): 42–7.

8 R. H. Farkas, E. F. Unger, and R. Temple, "Zolpidem and Driving Impairment—Identifying Persons at Risk," *New England Journal of Medicine* 369, no. 8 (August 22, 2013): 689–91, doi:10.1056/NEJMp1307972; M. Mitka, "Zolpidem-Related Surge in Emergency Department Visits," *Journal of the American Medical Association* 309, no. 21 (June 5, 2013): 2203, doi:10.1001/jama.2013.6289; A. G. Bach et al., "51-Year-Old-Man Found Somnolent on the Street," *Deutsche Medizinische Wochenschrift* 138, no. 9 (March 2013): 421–2, doi:10.1055/s-0032-1327373.

9 I. C. Amiháesei and O. C. Mungiu, "Main Neuroendocrine Features and Therapy in Primary Sleep Troubles," *Revista Medico-Chiruricala A Societatii de Medici si Naturalisti Din Iasi* 116, no. 3 (July–September 2012): 862–66.

10 C. Cummings, "Melatonin for the Management of Sleep Disorders in Children and Adolescents," *Paediatrics and Child Health* 17, no. 6 (June 2012): 331–36; E. Holvoet et al., "Disturbed Sleep in Children with ADHD: Is There a Place for Melatonin as a Treatment Option?" *Tijdschrift voor Psychiatrie* 55, no. 5 (2013): 349–57.

11 B. Claustrat, J. Brun, and G. Chazot, "The Basic Physiology and Pathophysiology of Melatonin," *Sleep Medicine Reviews* 9, no. 1 (February 2005): 11–24.

12 C. Campino et al., "Melatonin Reduces Cortisol Response to ACTH in Humans," *Revista Medica de Chile* 136, no. 11 (November 2008): 1390–97.

13 G. Rizzo et al., "Low Brain Iron Content in Idiopathic Restless Legs Syndrome Patients Detected by Phase Imaging," *Movement Disorders* 28, no. 13 (November 2013): 1886–90, doi:10.1002/mds.25576.

14 R. Gupta, V. Lahan, D. Goel, "A Study Examining Depression in Restless Legs Syndrome," *Asian Journal of Psychiatry* 6, no. 4 (August 2013): 308–12, doi:10.1016/j.ajp.2013.01.011.

15 S. Brand et al., "Patients Suffering from Restless Legs Syndrome Have Low Internal Locus of Control and Poor Psychological Functioning Compared to Healthy Controls," *Neuropsychobiology* 68, no. 1 (2013): 51–58, doi:10.1159/000350957.

## CHAPTER 9

1 A. Brito et al., "Folate, Vitamin $B_{12}$, and Human Health," *Revista Médica de Chile* 140, no. 11 (November 2012): 1464–75.

2 C. F. Hughes et al., "Vitamin $B_{12}$ and Ageing: Current Issues and Interaction with Folate," *Annals of Clinical Biochemistry* 50, pt. 4 (July 2013): 315–29, doi:10.1177/0004563212473279.

3 S. Hashimoto et al., "Vitamin $B_{12}$ Enhances the Phase-Response of Circadian Melatonin Rhythm to a Single Bright Light Exposure in Humans," *Neuroscience Letters* 220 (1996): 129–32.

4   K. Honma et al., "Effects of Vitamin $B_{12}$ on Plasma Melatonin Rhythm in Humans: Increased Light Sensitivity Phase-Advances the Circadian Clock?" *Experientia* 48 (1992): 716–20.

5   C. R. Robinson et al., "The Effects of Nicotinamide upon Sleep in Humans," *Biological Psychiatry* 12 (1977): 139–43.

6   "Vitamin $B_6$ Dietary Supplement Fact Sheet," National Institutes of Health, September 15, 2011, http://ods.od.nih.gov/factsheets/VitaminB6-HealthProfessional/.

7   J. A. Rumberger et al., "Pantethine, a Derivative of Vitamin B(5) Used as a Nutritional Supplement, Favorably Alters Low-Density Lipoprotein Cholesterol Metabolism in Low- to Moderate-Cardiovascular Risk North American Subjects: A Triple-Blinded Placebo and Diet-Controlled Investigation," *Nutrition Research* 31, no. 8 (August 2011): 608–15, doi:10.1016/j.nutres.2011.08.001.

8   K. Head and G. Kelly, "Nutrients and Botanicals for Treatment of Stress: Adrenal Fatigue, Neurotransmitter Imbalance, Anxiety and Restless Sleep," *Alternative Medicine Review* 14, no. 2 (June 2009): 114–40.

9   L. H. Leung, "Pantothenic Acid Deficiency as the Pathogenesis of Acne Vulgaris," *Medical Hypotheses* 44, no. 6 (June 1995): 490–92.

10  www.hammernutrition.com/knowledge/humans-lack-the-ability-to-make-vitamin-c.278.html

11  S. Brody et al., "A Randomized Controlled Trial of High Dose Ascorbic Acid for Reduction of Blood Pressure, Cortisol, and Subjective Responses to Psychological Stress," *Psychopharmacology* 159, no. 3 (January 2002): 319–24.

12  S. J. Padayatty and M. Levine, "New Insights into the Physiology and Pharmacology of Vitamin C," *Canadian Medical Association Journal* 164, no. 3 (February 6, 2001): 353–55.

13  C. S. Johnston and L. L. Thompson, "Vitamin C Status of an Outpatient Population," *Journal of the American College of Nutrition* 17, no. 4 (August 1998): 366–70.

14  B.D. Vallance and R. Hume, "Vitamin C, Disease, and Surgical Trauma," *British Medical Journal* 1, no. 6168 (April 7, 1979): 955–56.

15  O. Fain, "Vitamin C," *Revue du Praticien* 63, no. 8 (October 2013): 1091–96; Medline.

16  J. A. Simon and E. S. Hudes, "Serum Ascorbic Acid and Gallbladder Disease Prevalence Among US Adults: The Third National Health and Nutrition Examination Survey (NHANES III)," *Archives of Internal Medicine* 160, no. 7 (April 10, 2000): 931–36.

17  S. M. Fishman, P. Christian, and K. P. West, "The Role of Vitamins in the Prevention and Control of Anaemia," *Public Health Nutrition* 3, no. 2 (June 2000): 125–50.

18  Age-Related Eye Disease Study Research Group, "A Randomized, Placebo-Controlled, Clinical Trial of High-Dose Supplementation with Vitamins C and E, Beta Carotene, and Zinc for Age-Related Macular Degeneration and Vision Loss: AREDS Report no. 8," *Archives of Ophthalmology* 119, no. 10 (October 2001): 1417–36.

19  M. Langlois et al., "Serum Vitamin C Concentration is Low in Peripheral Arterial Disease and Is Associated with Inflammation and Severity of Atherosclerosis," *Circulation* 103, no. 14 (April 10, 2001): 1863–68.

20  The Natural Database. naturaldatabase.therapeuticresearch.com.

21  A. R. Gaby, "Intravenous Nutrient Therapy: The Meyers' Cocktail," *Alternative Medicine Review* 7, no. 5 (2002): 389–403, http://www.thorne.com/altmedrev/.fulltext/7/5/389.pdf.

22  http://articles.mercola.com/sites/articles/archive/2012/01/30/calcium-supplement-on-heart-attack.aspx.

23  M. J. Bolland et al., "Effect of Calcium Supplements on Risk of Myocardial Infarction and Cardiovascular Events: Meta-Analysis," *BMJ* 341 (July 29, 2010: c3691, doi:10.1136/bmj.c3691.

24  S. Afzal, S. E. Bojesen, and B. G. Nordestgaard, "Reduced 25-Hydroxyvitamin D and Risk of Alzheimer's Disease and Vascular Dementia," *Alzheimer's and Dementia* (published electronically July 18, 2013): pii: S1552-5260(13)02425-4, doi:10.1016/j.jalz.2013.05.1765; A. Hossein-Nezhad and M. F. Holick, "Vitamin D for Health: A Global Perspective," *Mayo Clinic Proceedings* 88, no. 7 (July 2013): 720–55, doi:10.1016/j.mayocp.2013.05.011.

25  W. González et al., "Magnesium: The Forgotten Electrolyte," *Boletín de la Asociación Médica de Puerto Rico* 105, no. 3 (2013): 17–20.

26 I. M. Cox, M. J. Campbell, and D. Dowson, "Red Blood Cell Magnesium and Chronic Fatigue Syndrome," *Lancet* 337, no. 8744 (March 30, 1991): 757–60; M. Hornyak et al., "Magnesium Therapy for Periodic Leg Movements-Related Insomnia and Restless Legs Syndrome: An Open Pilot Study," *Sleep* 21, no. 5 (August 1, 1998): 501–5; S. L. Volpe, "Magnesium in Disease Prevention and Overall Health," *Advances in Nutrition* 4, no. 3 (May 1, 2013): 378S-83S, doi:10.3945/an.112.003483.

27 P. Schenk et al., "Intravenous Magnesium Sulfate for Bronchial Hyperreactivity: A Randomized, Controlled, Double-Blind Study," *Clinical Pharmacology and Therapeutics* 69, no. 5 (May 2001): 365–71.

28 M. A. Belfort et al., "A Comparison of Magnesium Sulfate and Nimodipine for the Prevention of Eclampsia," *New England Journal of Medicine* 348, no. 4 (January 23, 2003): 304–11; D. Altman et al., "Do Women with Pre-Eclampsia, and Their Babies, Benefit from Magnesium Sulphate? The Magpie Trial: A Randomised Placebo-Controlled Trial," *Lancet* 359, no. 9321 (June 1, 2002): 1877–90.

29 L. Ceremuzyński et al., "Hypomagnesemia in Heart Failure with Ventricular Arrhythmias. Beneficial Effects of Magnesium Supplementation," *Journal of Internal Medicine* 247, no. 1 (January 2000): 78–86.

30 W. J. Fawcett, E. J. Haxby, and D. A. Male, "Magnesium: Physiology and Pharmacology," *British Journal of Anaesthesia* 83, no. 2 (1999): 302–20, http://bja.oxfordjournals.org/content/83/2/302.full.pdf; T. Shimosawa et al., "Magnesium Inhibits Norepinephrine Release by Blocking N-Type Calcium Channels at Peripheral Sympathetic Nerve Endings," *Hypertension* 44, no. 6 (December 2004): 897–902.

31 W. W. Douglas and R. P. Rubin, "The Mechanism of Catecholamine Release from the Adrenal Medulla and the Role of Calcium in Stimulus-Secretion Coupling," *Journal of Physiology* 167, no. 2 (July 1963): 288–310. PMCID: PMC1359395.

32 R. Gärtner et al., "Selenium Supplementation in Patients with Autoimmune Thyroiditis Decreases Thyroid Peroxidase Antibodies Concentrations," *Journal of Clinical Endocrinology and Metabolism* 87, no. 4 (April 2002): 1687–91; L. H. Duntas, E. Mantzou, and D. A. Koutras, "Effects of a Six Month Treatment with Selenomethionine in Patients with Autoimmune Thyroiditis," *European Journal of Endocrinology* 148, no. 4 (April 2003): 389–93; F. Gärtner and B. C. Gasnier, "Selenium in the Treatment of Autoimmune Thyroiditis," *Biofactors* 19, no. 3-4 (2003): 165–70; E. E. Mazokopakis et al., "Effects of 12 Months Treatment with L-Selenomethionine on Serum Anti-TPO Levels in Patients with Hashimoto's Thyroiditis," *Thyroid* 17, no. 7 (July 2007): 609–12.

33 B. E. Hurwitz et al., "Suppression of Human Immunodeficiency Virus Type 1 Viral Load with Selenium Supplementation: A Randomized Controlled Trial," *Archives of Internal Medicine* 167, no. 2 (January 22, 2007): 148–54.

34 M. P. Rayman, "The Importance of Selenium to Human Health," *Lancet* 356, no. 9225 (July 15, 2000): 233–41.

35 M. P. Rayman et al., "Effect of Supplementation with High-Selenium Yeast on Plasma Lipids: A Randomized Trial," *Annals of Internal Medicine* 154, no. 10 (May 17, 2011): 656–65, doi:10.7326/0003-4819-154-10-201105170-00005.

36 M. Sakamoto et al., "Selenomethionine Protects against Neuronal Degeneration by Methylmercury in the Developing Rat Cerebrum," *Environmental Science and Technology* 47, no. 6 (March 19, 2013): 2862–68, doi:10.1021/es304226h.

37 "What are the Signs and Symptoms of Iron-Deficiency Anemia?" National Heart, Lung, and Blood Institute, April 1, 2011, http://www.nhlbi.nih.gov/health/health-topics/topics/ida/signs.html.

38 M. Muñoz, I. Villar, and J. A. García-Erce, "An Update on Iron Physiology," *World Journal of Gastroenterology* 15, no. 37 (October 7, 2009): 4617–26, doi:10.3748/wjg.15.4617PMCID: PMC2754509.

39 "Anemia or Iron Deficiency," Centers for Disease Control and Prevention, May 30, 2013, http://www.cdc.gov/nchs/fastats/anemia.htm.

40 C. Niederau, "Diabetes Mellitus in Hemochromatosis," *Zeitschrift für Gastroenterologie* suppl. (June 1999): 22–32.

41  H. Haase and L. Rink, "Functional Significance of Zinc-Related Signaling Pathways in Immune Cells," *Annual Review of Nutrition* 29 (August 2009): 133–52.

42  D. N. Marreiro et al., "Role of Zinc in Insulin Resistance," *Arquivos Brasileiros de Endocrinologia & Metabologia* 48, no. 2 (April 2004): 234–39.

43  M. Ruz et al., "Zinc as a Potential Coadjuvant in Therapy for Type 2 Diabetes," *Food and Nutrition Bulletin* 34, no. 2 (June 2013): 215–21.

44  A. Betsy, M. Binitha, and S. Sarita, "Zinc Deficiency Associated with Hypothyroidism: An Overlooked Cause of Severe Alopecia," *International Journal of Trichology* 5, no. 1 (January 2013): 40–42, doi:10.4103/0974-7753.114714.

45  R. Nazanin et al., "Zinc and Its Importance for Human Health: An Integrative Review," *Journal of Research in Medical Sciences* 18, no. 2 (February 2013): 144–157.

46  C. N. Kuratko et al., "The Relationship of Docosahexaenoic Acid (DHA) with Learning and Behavior in Healthy Children: A Review," *Nutrients* 5, no. 7 (July 2013): 2777–810, doi:10.3390/nu5072777.

47  A. R. Patten et al., "Omega-3 Fatty Acids Can Reverse the Long-Term Deficits in Hippocampal Synaptic Plasticity Caused by Prenatal Ethanol Exposure," *Neuroscience Letters* 551 (September 13, 2013): 7–11, doi:10.1016/j.neulet.2013.05.051.

48  S. Peter, S. Chopra, and J. J. Jacob, "A Fish a Day, Keeps the Cardiologist Away!—A Review of the Effect of Omega-3 Fatty Acids in the Cardiovascular System," *Indian Journal of Endocrinology and Metabolism* 17, no. 3 (May 2013): 422–29, doi:10.4103/2230-8210.111630.

49  D. Mozaffarian and J. H. Wu, "Omega-3 Fatty Acids and Cardiovascular Disease: Effects on Risk Factors, Molecular Pathways, and Clinical Events," *Journal of the American College of Cardiology* 58 (2011): 2047–67.

50  A. K. Papazafiropoulou, M. S. Kardara, and S. I. Pappas, "Pleiotropic Effects of Omega-3 Fatty Acids," *Recent Patents on Endocrine, Metabolic, and Immune Drug Discovery* 6 (2012): 40–46.

## CHAPTER 10

1  "Nearly 7 in 10 Americans Take Prescription Drugs, Mayo Clinic, Olmsted Medical Center Find," Mayo Clinic, June 19, 2013, http://www.mayoclinic.org/news2013-rst/7543.html.

2  "Top Therapeutic Classes by Dispensed Prescriptions (U.S.)," IMS Health, March 22, 2013, http://www.imshealth.com/deployedfiles/imshealth/Global/Content/Corporate/Press%20 Room/2012_U.S/Top_Therapeutic_Classes_Dispensed_Prescriptions_2012.pdf.

3  http://www.imshealth.com/deployedfiles/imshealth/Global/Content/Corporate/Press%20 Room/2012_U.S/Top_25_Medicines_Dispensed_Prescriptions_U.S.pdf.

4  N. Abdoli et al., "Mechanisms of the Statins Cytotoxicity in Freshly Isolated Rat Hepatocytes," *Journal of Biochemical and Molecular Toxicology* 27, no. 6 (June 2013): 287–94.

5  V. M. Alla et al., "A Reappraisal of the Risks and Benefits of Treating to Target with Cholesterol Lowering Drugs," *Drugs* 73, no .10 (July 2013): 1025–54.

6  R. C. Parish and L. J. Miller, "Adverse Effects of Angiotensin Converting Enzyme (ACE) Inhibitors. An Update," *Drug Safety* 7, no. 1 (January–February 1992): 14–31.

7  R. J. Lehane, "Lisinopril-Induced Angioedema of the Lip," *New York State Dental Journal* 79, no. 3 (April 2013): 25–7.

8  A. J. Barron et al., "Systematic Review of Genuine Versus Spurious Side-Effects of Beta-Blockers in Heart Failure Using Placebo Control: Recommendations for Patient Information," *International Journal of Cardiology* (June 21, 2013): pii: S0167-5273(13)00996-0.

9  M. F. Conrad et al., "Progression of Asymptomatic Carotid Stenosis Despite Optimal Medical Therapy," *Journal of Vascular Surgery* 58, no. 1 (July 2013): 128–35.e1, doi:10.1016/j. jvs.2013.04.002.

10  "CDC Grand Rounds: Prescription Drug Overdoses—a U.S. Epidemic," *Morbidity and Mortality Weekly Report* 61, no. 1 (January 13, 2012): 10–13, http://www.cdc.gov/mmwr/ preview/mmwrhtml/mm6101a3.htm.

11  Ibid.

12 S. Purkayastha and D. Cai, "Neuroinflammatory Basis of Metabolic Syndrome," *Molecular Metabolism* 2, no. 4 (October 5, 2013): 356–63; D. Nuzzo et al., "Inflammatory Mediators as Biomarkers in Brain Disorders," *Inflammation* (published electronically December 1, 2013); H. Baba et al., "C-reactive Protein as a Significant Prognostic Factor for Stage IV Gastric Cancer Patients," *Anticancer Research* 33, no. 12 (December 2013): 5591–95.

13 R. Zhang et al., "Mechanisms of Acupuncture-Electroacupuncture on Persistent Pain," *Anesthesiology* 120, no. 2 (February 2014): 428–503.

14 A. L. Cavalcante et al., "Role of NMDA Receptors in the Trigeminal Pathway, and the Modulatory Effect of Magnesium in a Model of Rat Temporomandibular Joint Arthritis" *European Journal of Oral Sciences* 121, no. 6 (December 2013): 573–83.

15 E. Gertsch et al. "Intravenous Magnesium as Acute Treatment for Headaches: A Pediatric Case Series," *Journal of Emergency Medicine* 46, no. 2 (February 2014): 308–12, doi:10.1016/j.jemermed.2013.08.049.

16 "Antibiotics: Will They Work When You Really Need Them?" Centers for Disease Control and Prevention, November 5, 2013, http://www.cdc.gov/getsmart/healthcare/learn-from-others/factsheets/antibiotics.html.

17 "Sharp Rise in Emergency Department Visits Involving the Sleep Medication Zolpidem," Substance Abuse and Mental Health Services Administration, May 1, 2013, http://www.samhsa.gov/newsroom/advisories/1304303131.aspx.

18 J. S. Poceta, "Zolpidem ingestion, automatisms, and sleep driving: a clinical and legal case series," *Journal of Clinical Sleep Medicine* 7, no. 6 (December 15, 2011): 632–8.

19 R. Giordano et al., "Acute Administration of Alprazolam, a Benzodiazepine Activating GABA Receptors, Inhibits Cortisol Secretion in Patients with Subclinical but Not Overt Cushing's Syndrome," *Pituitary* 26, no. 3 (September 2013): 363–9.

20 R. Giordano et al., "Alprazolam (a Benzodiazepine Activating GABA Receptor) Reduces the Neuroendocrine Responses to Insulin-Induced Hypoglycaemia in Humans," *Clinical Endocrinology* 59, no. 3 (September 2003): 314–20.

21 S. M. Wilhelm et al., "Perils and Pitfalls of Long-Term Effects of Proton Pump Inhibitors," Expert Review of Clinical Pharmacology 6, no. 4 (July 2013): 443–51; S. Abraham, "Proton Pump Inhibitors: Potential Adverse Effects," *Current Opinion in Gastroenterology* 28, no. 6 (2012): 615–20.

22 "Proton Pump Inhibitors (PPI): Class Labeling Change," U.S. Food and Drug Administration, March 23, 2011, http://www.fda.gov/safety/medwatch/safetyinformation/safetyalertsfor humanmedicalproducts/ucm213321.htm.

## CHAPTER 11

1  G. S. Kelly, "Nutritional and Botanical Interventions to Assist with the Adaptation to Stress," *Alternative Medicine Review* 4, no. 4 (1999): 249–65.

2  A. J. Tomiyama et al., "Low Calorie Dieting Increases Cortisol," *Psychosomatic Medicine* 72, no. 4 (May 2010): 357–64.

## CHAPTER 12

1  Natural Database. naturaldatabase.therapeuticresearch.com.

2  K. Lu et al., "The Acute Effects of L-theanine in Comparison with Alprazolam on Anticipatory Anxiety in Humans," *Humam Psychopharmacology* 19, no. 7 (October 2004): 457–65.

3  S. Kasper, "An Orally Administered Lavandula Oil Preparation (Silexan) for Anxiety Disorder and Related Conditions: An Evidence Based Review," *International Journal of Psychiatry in Clinical Practice* 17, sup. 1 (November 2013): 15–22; P. Sasannejad et al., "Lavender Essential Oil in the Treatment of Migraine Headache: A Placebo-Controlled Clinical Trial," *European Neurology* 67, no. 5 (2012): 288–91; J. A. Hawrelak, T. Cattley, and S. P. Myers, "Essential Oils in the Treatment of Intestinal Dysbiosis: A Preliminary in Vitro Study," *Alternative Medicine Review* 14, no. 4 (December 2009): 380–4; J. Baker et al., "Medicinal Lavender Modulates the Enteric Microbiota to Protect against *Citrobacter rodentium*–Induced Colitis," *American*

*Journal of Physiology—Gastrointestinal and Liver Physiology* 303, no. 7 (October 2012): G825-36, doi:10.1152/ajpgi.00327.2011.

4   P. Sasannejad et al., "Lavender Essential Oil in the Treatment of Migraine Headache: A Placebo-Controlled Clinical Trial," *European Neurology* 67, no. 5 (2012): 288–91.

5   P. W. Lin et al., "Efficacy of Aromatherapy (*Lavandula angustifolia*) as an Intervention for Agitated Behaviours in Chinese Older Persons with Dementia: A Cross-Over Randomized Trial," *International Journal of Geriatric Psychiatry* 22, no. 5 (May 2007): 405–10.

6   K. Hirokawa, T. Nishimoto, and T. Taniguchi, "Effects of Lavender Aroma on Sleep Quality in Healthy Japanese Students," *Perceptual and Motor Skills* 114, no. 1 (February 2012): 111–22.

7   G. T. Lewith, A. D. Godfrey, and P. Prescott, "A Single-Blinded, Randomized Pilot Study Evaluating the Aroma of *Lavandula augustifolia* as a Treatment for Mild Insomnia," *Journal of Alternative and Complementary Medicine* 11, no. 4 (August 2005): 631–7.

8   N. Morris, "The Effects of Lavender (*Lavendula angustifolium*) Baths on Psychological Well-Being: Two Exploratory Randomised Control Trials," *Complementary Therapies in Medicine* 10, no. 4 (December 2002): 223–28.

9   S. Kasper et al., "Efficacy and Safety of Silexan, a New, Orally Administered Lavender Oil Preparation, in Subthreshold Anxiety Disorder—Evidence from Clinical Trials," *Wiener Medizinische Wochenschrift* 160, no. 21–22 (December 2010): 547–56.

10  P. Aslanargun et al., "Passiflora incarnata Linneaus as an Anxiolytic before Spinal Anesthesia," Journal of Anesthesia 26, no. 1 (February 2012): 39–44, doi:10.1007/s00540-011-1265-6; E. M. Konta et al., "Evaluation of the Antihypertensive Properties of Yellow Passion Fruit Pulp (Passiflora edulis Sims f. flavicarpa Deg.) in Spontaneously Hypertensive Rats," *Phytotherapy Research* 28, no. 1 (January 2014): 28–32, doi:10.1002/ptr.4949; S. Akhondzadeh et al., "Passionflower in the Treatment of Opiates Withdrawal: A Double-Blind Randomized Controlled Trial," Journal of Clinical Pharmacy and Therapeutics 26, no. 5 (October 2001): 369–73.

11  S. Akhondzadeh et al., "Passionflower in the Treatment of Generalized Anxiety: A Pilot Double-Blind Randomized Controlled Trial with Oxazepam," *Journal of Clinical Pharmacy and Therapeutics* 26, no. 5 (October 2001): 363–67.

12  A. Mori et al., "Clinical Evaluation of Passiflamin (Passiflora Extract) on Neurosis—Multicenter Double Blind Study in Comparison with Mexazolam," *Rinsho Hyouka (Clinical Evaluation)* 21 (1993): 383–440.

13  Natural Database. naturaldatabase.therapeuticresearch.com.

14  Natural Database. Ibid.

15  Natural Database. Ibid.

16  K. De Bock K et al., "Acute Rhodiola rosea intake can improve endurance exercise performance," *International Journal of Sport Nutrition and Exercise Metabolism* 14 (2004): 298–307; A. A. Spasov et al., "A Double-Blind, Placebo-Controlled Pilot Study of the Stimulating and Adaptogenic Effect of *Rhodiola rosea* SHR-5 Extract on the Fatigue of Students Caused by Stress During an Examination Period with a Repeated Low-Dose Regimen," *Phytomedicine* 7 (2000): 85–89.

17  A. Bystritsky, L. Kerwin, and J. D. Feusner, "A Pilot Study of *Rhodiola rosea* (Rhodax) for Generalized Anxiety Disorder (GAD)," *Journal of Alternative and Complementary Medicine* 14 (2008): 175–80.

18  G. Darbinyan, G. Aslanyan, and E. Amroyan, "Clinical Trial of *Rhodiola rosea* L. Extract SHR-5 in the Treatment of Mild to Moderate Depression," *Nordic Journal of Psychiatry* 61 (2007): 343–48; "Rhodiola," Natural Medicines Comprehensive Database, http://naturaldatabase.therapeuticresearch.com/nd/Search.aspx?cs=NONMP&s=ND&pt=100&id=883&ds=.

19  A. Panossian, G. Wikman, and J. Sarris, "Rosenroot (*Rhodiola rosea*): Traditional Use, Chemical Composition, Pharmacology and Clinical Efficacy," *Phytomedicine* 17, no. 7 (June 2010): 481–93, doi:10.1016/j.phymed.2010.02.002.

20  S. Ishaque et al., "Rhodiola rosea for Physical and Mental Fatigue: A Systematic Review," *BMC Complementary and Alternative Medicine* 12 (May 29, 2012): 70, doi:10.1186/1472-6882-12-70.

21  E. M. Olsson„ B. von Scheele, and A. G. Panossian, "A Randomised, Double-Blind, Placebo-Controlled, Parallel Group Study of the Standardised Extract SHR-5 of the Roots of Rhodiola rosea in the Treatment of Subjects with Stress-Related Fatigue," *Planta Medica* 75 (2009): 105–112.

22  L. Zhang et al., "Protective Effects of Salidroside on Hydrogen Peroxide–Induced Apoptosis in SH-SY5Y Human Neuroblastoma Cells," *European Journal of Pharmacology* 564, no. 1–3 (June 14, 2007): 18–25.

23  C. Cifani et al., "Effect of Salidroside, Active Principle of *Rhodiola rosea* Extract, on Binge Eating," *Physiology and Behavior* 101, no. 5 (December 2, 2010): 555–62, doi:10.1016/j.physbeh.2010.09.006.

24  S. W. Chan, "*Panax ginseng, Rhodiola rosea,* and *Schisandra chinensis,*" *International Journal of Food Sciences and Nutrition* 63, sup. 1 (March 2012): 75–81.

25  K. M. Ko and P. Y. Chiu, "Biochemical Basis of the "Qi-Invigorating" Action of Schisandra Berry (wu-wei-zi) in Chinese Medicine," *American Journal of Chinese Medicine* 34, no. 2 (2006): 171–6; A. Panossian et al., "Synergy and Antagonism of Active Constituents of ADAPT-232 on Transcriptional Level of Metabolic Regulation of Isolated Neuroglial Cells," *Frontiers and Neuroscience* 7 (February 20, 2013): 16; H. J. Pu et al., "Correlation between Antistress and Hepatoprotective Effects of Schisandra Lignans Was Related with Its Antioxidative Actions in Liver Cells," *Evidence Based Complementary and Alternative Medicine* (2012): 161062; K. M. Ko et al., "Long-Term Schisandrin B Treatment Mitigates Age-Related Impairments in Mitochondrial Antioxidant Status and Functional Ability in Various Tissues, and Improves the Survival of Aging C57BL/6J Mice," *Biofactors* 34, no. 4 (2008): 331–42, doi:10.3233/BIO-2009-1086; T. Zhao et al., "Antitumor and Immunomodulatory Activity of a Water-Soluble Low Molecular Weight Polysaccharide from *Schisandra chinensis* (Turcz.) Baill," *Food and Chemical Toxicology* 55 (May 2013): 609–16; S. Takeda et al., "Effects of TJN-101, a Lignan Compound Isolated from Schisandra Fruits, on Liver Fibrosis and on Liver Regeneration after Partial Hepatectomy in Rats with Chronic Liver Injury Induced by CCl4," *Nihon Yakurigaku Zasshi* 90, no. 1 (July 1987): 51–65; P. Xia, L. J. Sun, and J. Wang, "Effects of *fructus schisandrae* on the Function of the Pituitary-Testis Axis and Carbohydrate Metabolism in Rats Undergoing Experimental Navigation and High-Intensity Exercise," *Zhonghua Nan Ke Xue* 17, no. 5 (May 2011): 472–76; S. Park et al., "Huang-Lian-Jie-Du-Tang Supplemented with *Schisandra chinensis* Baill. and *Polygonatum odoratum* Druce Improved Glucose Tolerance by Potentiating Insulinotropic Actions in Islets in 90% Pancreatectomized Diabetic Rats," *Bioscience, Biotechnollgy, and Biochemistry* 73, no. 11 (November 2009): 2384–92; P. J. Young et al., "Antihypertensive Effect of Gomisin A from *Schisandra chinensis* on Angiotensin II-Induced Hypertension via Preservation of Nitric Oxide Bioavailability," *Hypertension Research* 35, no. 9 (September 2012): 928–34; V. S. Baranova et al., "The Antiradical Activity of Plant Extracts and Healthful Preventive Combinations of these Extracts with the Phospholipid Complex," *Biomeditsinskaya Khimiya* 58, no. 6 (November–December 2012): 712–26; S. Y. Pan et al., "Effective Kinetics of Schisandrin B on Serum/Hepatic Triglyceride and Total Cholesterol Levels in Mice with and without the Influence of Fenofibrate," *Naunyn-Schmiedeberg's Archives of Pharmacology* 383, no. 6 (June 2011): 585–91, doi:10.1007/s00210-011-0634-x; A. Panossian and G. Wikman, "Pharmacology of *Schisandra chinensis* Bail.: An Overview of Russian Research and Uses in Medicine," *Journal of Ethnopharmacology* 118, no. 2 (July 23, 2008): 183–212, doi:10.1016/j.jep.2008.04.020; "Schisandra," The Natural Medicines Comprehensive Database, February 14, 2014, http://naturaldatabase.therapeuticresearch.com/nd/Search.aspx?cs=NONMP&s=ND&pt=100&id=376&ds=&name=SCHISANDRA&searchid=42860175.

26  R. Upton, ed., *Schisandra Berry: Analytical, Quality Control, and Therapeutic Monograph* (Santa Cruz, CA: American Herbal Pharmacopoeia, 1999), 1–25.

27  H. D. Sun et al., "Nigranoic Acid, a Triterpenoid from *Schisandra sphaerandra* that Inhibits HIV-1 Reverse Transcriptase," *Journal of Natural Products* 59, no. 5 (May 1996): 525–27.

28  I. S. Lee et al., "Structure-Activity Relationships of Lignans from *Schisandra chinensis* as Platelet Activating Factor Antagonists," *Biological and Pharmaceutical Bulletin* 22, no. 3 (March 1999): 265–67.

29 J. Gnabre et al., "Isolation of Lignans from *Schisandra chinensis* with Anti-Proliferative Activity in Human Colorectal Carcinoma: Structure-Activity Relationships," *Journal of Chromatography B Sci* 878, 28 (October 15, 2010): 2693–700.

30 Natural Database. naturaldatabase.therapeuticresearch.com.

31 P. D. Leathwood et al., "Aqueous Extract of Valerian Root (*Valeriana officinalis* L.) Improves Sleep Quality in Man," *Pharmacology Biochemistry and Behavior* 17, no. 1 (July 1982): 65–71; F. Donath et al., "Critical Evaluation of the Effect of Valerian Extract on Sleep Structure and Sleep Quality," *Pharmacopsychiatry* 33, no. 2 (March 2000): 47–53.

32 P. J. Houghton, "The Scientific Basis for the Reputed Activity of Valerian," *Journal of Pharmacy and Pharmacology* 51, no. 5 (May 1999): 505–12; B. M. Dietz et al., "Valerian Extract and Valerenic Acid are Partial Agonists of the 5-HT5a Receptor in Vitro," *Molecular Brain Research* 138, no. 2 (August 18, 2005): 191–97.

33 C. S. Yuan et al., "The Gamma-Aminobutyric Acidergic Effects of Valerian and Valerenic Acid on Rat Brainstem Neuronal Activity," *Anesthesia and Analgesia* 98, no. 2 (February 2004): 353–58.

34 Natural Database. naturaldatabase.therapeuticresearch.com.

35 T. Cenacchi et al., "Cognitive Decline in the Elderly: A Double-Blind, Placebo-Controlled Multicenter Study on Efficacy of Phosphatidylserine Administration," *Aging* 5, no. 2 (April 1993): 123–33.

36 T. H. Crook et al., "Effects of Phosphatidylserine in Age-Associated Memory Impairment," *Neurology* 41, no. 5 (May 1991): 644–49.

37 S. Schreiber et al., "An Open Trial of Plant-Source Derived Phosphatydilserine for Treatment of Age-Related Cognitive Decline," *Israel Journal of Psychiatry and Related Sciences* 37, no. 4 (2000): 302–7.

38 T. Crook, "Effects of Phosphatidylserine in Alzheimer's Disease," *Psychopharmacology Bulletin* 28, no. 1 (1992): 61–66.

39 D. Bentonet al., "The Influence of Phosphatidylserine Supplementation on Mood and Heart Rate When Faced with an Acute Stressor," *Nutritional Neuroscience* 4, no. 3 (2001): 169–78.

40 P. Monteleone et al., "Effects of Phosphatidylserine on the Neuroendocrine Response to Physical Stress in Humans," *Neuroendocrinology* 52, no. 3 (September 1990): 243–48.

41 P. Monteleone et al., "Blunting by Chronic Phosphatidylserine Administration of the Stress-Induced Activation of the Hypothalamo-Pituitary-Adrenal Axis in Healthy Men," *European Journal of Clinical Pharmacology* 42, no. 4 (1992): 385–88.

42 J. E. McElhaney et al., "A Placebo-Controlled Trial of a Proprietary Extract of North American Ginseng (CVT-E002) to Prevent Acute Respiratory Illness in Institutionalized Older Adults," *Journal of the American Geriatric Society* 52, no. 1 (January 2004): 13–19; G. N. Predy et al., "Efficacy of an Extract of North American Ginseng Containing Poly-Furanosyl-Pyranosyl-Saccharides for Preventing Upper Respiratory Tract Infections: A Randomized Controlled Trial," *Canadian Medical Association Journal* 173, no. 9 (October 25, 2005): 1043–48; J. E. McElhaney et al., "Efficacy of COLD-fX in the Prevention of Respiratory Symptoms in Community-Dwelling Adults: A Randomized, Double-Blinded, Placebo-Controlled Trial," *Journal of Alternative and Complementary Medicine* 12, no. 2 (March 2006): 153–57.

43 A. Caso Marasco et al., "Double-Blind Study of a Multivitamin Complex Supplemented with Ginseng Extract," *Drugs under Experimental and Clinical Research* 22 (1996): 323–29.

44 V. Vuksan et al., "Similar Postprandial Glycemic Reductions with Escalation of Dose and Administration Time of American Ginseng in Type 2 Diabetes," *Diabetes Care* 23, no. 9 (September 2000): 1221–26.

45 "Ginseng, American," Comprehensive Natural Database, February 14, 2014, http://naturaldatabase.therapeuticresearch.com/nd/Search.aspx?cs=NONMP&s=ND&pt=1 00&id=967&ds=&name=Ginseng+(GINSENG%2c+AMERICAN)&searchid=42911233.

46 A. G. Turpie, J. Runcie, and T. J. Thomson, "Clinical Trial of Geglydyrrhizinized Liquorice in Gastric Ulcer," *Gut* 10, no. 4 (April 1969): 299–302.

47 A. Madisch et al., "Treatment of Functional Dyspepsia with a Herbal Preparation. A Double-Blind, Randomized, Placebo-Controlled, Multicenter Trial," *Digestion* 69, no. 1 (2004): 45–52.

48 J. Melzer et al., "Meta-Analysis: Phytotherapy of Functional Dyspepsia with the Herbal Drug Preparation STW 5 (Iberogast)," *Alimentary Pharmacology and Therapeutics* 20, no. 11–12 (December 2004): 1279–87.

49 S. Tamir et al., "Estrogenic and Antiproliferative Properties of Glabridin from Licorice in Human Breast Cancer Cells," *Cancer Research* 60, no. 20 (October 15, 2000): 5704–709; D. Armanini, G. Bonanni, and M. Palermo, "Reduction of Serum Testosterone in Men by Licorice," *New England Journal of Medicine* 341, no. 15 (October 7, 1999): 1158.

50 H. A. Sigurjonsdottir et al., "Is Blood Pressure Commonly Raised by Moderate Consumption of Liquorice?" *Journal of Human Hypertension* 9, no .5 (May 1995): 345–48.

51 "Licorice," Natural Comprehensive Database, February 14, 2014,http://naturaldatabase. therapeuticresearch.com/nd/Search.aspx?cs=NONMP&s=ND&pt=100&id=881&fs=ND&sea rchid=42911233.

52 L. C. Mishra, B. B. Singh, and S. Dagenais, "Scientific Basis for the Therapeutic Use of *Withania somnifera* (Ashwagandha): A Review," *Alternative Medicine Review* 5, no. 4 (August 2000): 334–46.

53 Natural Database. naturaldatabase.therapeuticresearch.com.

54 R. Upton, ed., *Ashwagandha Root (Withania somnifera): Analytical, Quality Control, and Therapeutic Monograph* (Santa Cruz, CA: American Herbal Pharmacopoeia, 2000): 1–25; Mishra, "Scientific Basis for the Therapeutic Use of *Withania somnifera*," 334–46.

55 Upton, *Ashwagandha Root*, 1–25.

56 Mishra "Scientific Basis for the Therapeutic Use of *Withania somnifera*," 334–46.

57 Upton, *Ashwagandha Root*, 1–25.

58 "Ashwagandha," Natural Medicine Comprehensive Database, February 14, 2014, http:// naturaldatabase.therapeuticresearch.com/nd/Search.aspx?cs=NONMP&s=ND&pt=100&id= 953&ds=&name=Ashwaganda++(ASHWAGANDHA)&searchid=42860175

## CHAPTER 13

1 "Exercise or Phyiscal Activity," Centers for Disease Control and Prevention, February 28, 2014, http://www.cdc.gov/nchs/fastats/exercise.htm. [ed: page not available; please check/ replace source.]

2 Physical Activity and Health. www.cdc.gov/nccdphp/sgr/pdf/sgrfull.pdf.

3 M. Wilhelm et al., "Effect of Resistance Exercises on Function in Older Adults with Osteo-porosis or Osteopenia: A Systematic Review," *Physiotherapy Canada* 64, no. 4 (Fall 2012): 386–94, doi:10.3138/ptc.2011-31BH; M. Gray, R. Di Brezzo, and I. L. Fort, "The Effects of Power and Strength Training on Bone Mineral Density in Premenopausal Women," *Journal of Sports Medicine and Physical Fitness* 53, no. 4 (August 2013): 428–36.

4 V. Tomic et al., "The Effect of Maternal Exercise during Pregnancy on Abnormal Fetal Growth," *Croatian Medical Journal* 54, no. 4 (August 28, 2013): 362–68.

5 M. Hamer, K. L. Lavoie, and S. L. Bacon, "Taking Up Physical Activity in Later Life and Healthy Ageing: The English Longitudinal Study of Ageing," *British Journal of Sports Medicine* (published electronically November 25, 2013): doi:10.1136/bjsports-2013-092993.

6 A. W. Li and C. A. Goldsmith, "The Effects of Yoga on Anxiety and Stress," *Alternative Medicine Review* 17, no. 1 (March 2012): 21–35.

7 A. Michalsen et al., "Rapid Stress Reduction and Anxiolysis among Distressed Women as a Consequence of a Three-Month Intensive Yoga Program," *Medical Science Monitor* 11, no. 12 (December 2005): CR555–561.

8 H. Zouhal "Catecholamines and the Effects of Exercise, Training, and Gender," *Sports Medicine* 38, no. 5 (2008): 401–23.

9 J. A. Blumenthal et al., "Effects of Exercise Training on Older Patients with Major Depres-sion," *Archives of Internal Medicine* 159 (1999): 2349–56.

10 "Boost your Immune System and Shake Off Stress by Taking a Walk in the Woods," Loyola Medicine, October 2, 2013, http://loyolamedicine.org/newswire/news/boost-your-immune-system-and-shake-stress-taking-walk-woods.

## CHAPTER 14

1  Y. Y. Tang, R. Tang, and M. I. Posner, "Brief Meditation Training Induces Smoking Reduction," *Proceedings of the National Academy of Sciences* 110, no. 34 (August 20, 2013): 13971–75, doi:10.1073/pnas.1311887110.

2  S. Olex, A. Newberg, and V. M. Figueredo, "Meditation: Should a Cardiologist Care?" *International Journal of Cardiology* (published electronically July 24, 2013): pii: S0167-5273(13)01141-8, doi:10.1016/j.ijcard.2013.06.086.

3  Y. H. Kim et al., "Effects of Meditation on Anxiety, Depression, Fatigue, and Quality of Life of Women Undergoing Radiation Therapy for Breast Cancer," *Complementary Therapies in Medicine* 21, no. 4 (August 2013): 379–87, doi:10.1016/j.ctim.2013.06.005.

4  Y. Singh and A. Ratna, "Immediate and Long-Term Effects of Meditation on Acute Stress Reactivity, Cognitive Functions, and Intelligence," *Alternative Therapies in Health and Medicine* 18, no. 6 (2012): 46–53.

5  J. M. Smyth et al., "Effects of Writing about Stressful Experiences on Symptom Reduction in Patients with Asthma or Rheumatoid Arthritis: A Randomized Trial," *Journal of the American Medical Association* 281, no. 14 (April 14, 1999): 1304–49.

# INDEX

Underscored page references indicate boxed text.

## A

ACE inhibitors, 183
Acetylcholine, 233
Acid, 124–25
Acne, vitamin B₅ for, 154
ACTH, 66, 134
Adaptogen, 228, 234, 236–37
Addiction, 290
Addison's disease, 14
ADHD, 140–41, 231
Adrenal fatigue
  cardiovascular system and, 83–93
  diagnosis, 4–5
  exercise and, 242–79
    secrets to success, 251
    Stage 1, 243–44, 270–79
    Stage 2, 244–47, 260–69
    Stage 3, 247–48, 254–59
    workout program, 250–79
  GI issues as symptoms of, 116
  herbs for combating, 224–38
  hormones and, 52–67
  immune system and, 73–75
  low blood pressure and, 90–91
  nutrients affected by, 145–46
  polycystic ovarian syndrome link, 63, 66–67
  prevalence, 4
  sleep and, 132–43
  stages, 16–29
    exercise during, 243–79
    herbs beneficial for different stages, 230–37
    immune system and, 73–75
    journaling in, 294
    mediation during, 292
    nutrition plans, 213–22
    quiz for determining your stage, 17–20
    sex hormone balance, 61
    Stage 1, 21–22
    Stage 2, 22–26
    Stage 3, 26–28
  symptoms, 3–6
    list of common, 6
    Stage 1, 21
    Stage 2, 22–26
    Stage 3, 26–28
  thyroid gland and, 95–110

Adrenal glands
  Addison's disease, 14
  anatomy, 10–11
  blood pressure regulation, 40–41
  control of sleep by, 143
  Cushing's disease, 14, 15
  hormones released by, 8, 10–16, 54
  HPA axis, 8
  nutrients used by, 21–22
  roles in the body, 5–6
  as ruler of thyroid gland, 106–7
Adrenaline. *See* Epinephrine
Adrenal insufficiency, 4–5, 27
Adrenocorticotropic hormone (ACTH), 66
Aldosterone
  effects, 12–15, 50, 88
  link to
    metabolic syndrome, 41
    thyroid gland, 107
  targeted by ACE inhibitors, 183
Allergies, intestinal microflora link to, 117
Almonds
  Almond and Mixed Berry Muffins, 339
  Almond-Cherry Clafoutis, 345
  Oat-Almond Mixed Berry Crisp, 343
Alzheimer's disease, 232–33
Anemia, 36, 166–67
Angiotensin-converting enzyme (ACE) inhibitors, 183
Anise, 236
Antibiotics, 119, 122, 190–93
Antidepressants, 195–96
Antihistamines, 117
Antihypertensive drugs, 183–87
Anxiety
  conditions associated with
    Graves' disease, 109
    Stage 2 adrenal fatigue, 22–23
  dopamine increase in, 139
  improvement with
    ashwagandha, 236–37
    lavender, 226
    L-theanine, 225
    passiflora, 226
    rhodiola, 228–29

valerian, 231
  yoga, 244
  medication for, 194–95
Arrhythmia, 87, 142, 164
Ashwagandha, 236–37
Asparagus
  Asparagus and Tofu Stir-Fry, 319
Aspirin, 89, 90
Assisted Front Plank, 263
Assisted Side Plank, 263
Atherosclerosis, 87, 89
Attention deficit hyperactivity disorder
    (ADHD), 140–41, 231
Autism, 117–18
Autoimmune disease, 79–81
  Graves' disease, 109
  Hashimoto's thyroiditis, 98, 103–7
  IgA levels in, 122–23

# B

Bacteria, intestinal. *See* Flora, GI
Bacterial overgrowth, 118, 120, 125
Ball Eccentric Crunches, 274
Beans
  Black Bean Stew, 332
  Broccoli Rabe and Bean Sauté, 329
  Kicked-Up Bean Tostadas, 322
  Quick Bean Burrito, 335
  3-Layer Mexican Dip, 336
Benzodiazepines, 133, 138, 226–27, 237
Berries
  Almond and Mixed Berry Muffins,
    339
  Oat-Almond Mixed Berry Crisp, 343
  Red Fruit Crumble, 346
Beta-blockers, 183–85
Bile, 126
Binge eating, 229
Bioidentical hormone replacement therapy,
    6, 52, 58
Birth control pills, 54, 61
Blood pressure
  aldosterone effect on, 12–15, 50, 88
  high (*see* Hypertension)
  increase by glycyrrhiza, 235
  lowering with
    antihypertensive drugs, 183–87
    ashwagandha, 236–37
    meditation, 90–91, 290
  medication for, 41–42
  regulation by adrenal glands, 40–41
Blood sugar. *See also* Diabetes; Glucose
  diabetes diagnosis and, 43–44
  hormonal regulation, 32–34
  sleep linked to regulation of, 135
Blood thinners, 89, 90
Blood type, 213

Blueberries
  Blueberry Muffins, 341
  Peach Blueberry Smoothie, 336
  Plum-Blueberry Cobbler, 344
Bone health, aldosterone link to, 15
Boron, food sources of, 209
Breath holding as a coping response, 254
Breathing during meditation, 291–93, 295
Bridges (with March), 262
Broccoli
  Broccoli Rabe and Bean Sauté, 329
Burrito
  Mexican Breakfast Burrito, 307
  Quick Bean Burrito, 335
Butternut squash
  Quinoa and Butternut Cereal, 310
B vitamins, 92–93, 149–54, 153. *See also*
    *specific vitamins*

# C

Calcitonin, 108
Calcium
  diuretic effect on, 186–87
  effect on vitamin D level, 159–61
  food sources of, 161, 162, 209
  hormones affecting
    calcitonin, 108
    parathyroid hormone, 15
  kidney stones, 163
  magnesium balanced by, 164, 185–86
  overview of, 157–59
Calcium channel blockers, 185–86
Calorie counting, 204, 205
Calories
  burned in
    exercise, 241
    REM sleep, 135
  storage of, 245
Cancer
  author's mother's case, 69–70
  breast, 76, 291
  colorectal, 231
  herbs beneficial in
    ginseng, 234
    rhodiola, 228, 229
    schisandra berry, 231
  hormone-based, 52, 55
  immune system and, 70–71, 76–77
  in Stage 3 adrenal fatigue, 27
Candida, 120, 122, 213
Carbohydrate cravings, 48
Cardiovascular intervals, 264, 275
Cardiovascular system/health
  adrenal fatigue and, 83–93
  aldosterone effect on, 12–15, 50, 88
  arrhythmia, 87, 142, 164
  atherosclerosis, 87, 89

Cardiovascular system/health (*cont.*)
blood pressure (*see* Blood pressure;
Hypertension)
C-reactive protein as marker, 86
decline in diabetes, 35, 39, 42–43
dehydration effects, 87
diet impact on, 89–93, 90
heart attack, 88–89, 90, 184
improvement with
diet, 89–90, 90, 172–73
exercise, 89–90, 90
meditation, 289–90
probiotics link to, 118–19
in vitamin B₁₂ deficiency, 150
Carrots
Fruited Carrot-Veggie Salad, 304
Celery
Nutty Celery Sticks, 337
Chair Pose, 263
Cherries
Almond-Cherry Clafoutis, 345
Chicken
Chicken Peanut Noodle Bowl, 325
Chicken Tortilla Soup, 333
Children
autism in, 117–18
exercise by, 241
Chili
Hearty Chili, 328
Chocolate
Chocolate Lover's Trail Mix, 337
Cholesterol
deposition in arteries, 87
evaluating lab values, 84–86
inflammation and, 86–87
levels in
diabetes, 42–43, 50
Stage 2 adrenal fatigue, 22, 24
Stage 3 adrenal fatigue, 27
low-density lipoprotein (LDL), 84–86
lowering with
niacin, 151
omega-3 fatty acids, 172
statins, 181–82
vitamin B₅, 153
prevalence of high, 84
roles in body, 84
vitamin D production from, 84, 108
Chronic fatigue syndrome, 28
Cognitive function, improvement with
ashwagandha, 236
meditation, 291
phosphatidylserine, 232–33
Constipation, 127–28
Cooldown, 257, 265, 275
Core exercises
Stage 1 protocol, 273–74
Stage 2 protocol, 263–64

Cortisol
abnormality, 63, 66
decrease with
melatonin, 141
phosphatidylserine, 233
effects, 8, 11–12
blood sugar regulation, 33–35, 37–39
insulin release, 35–36, 47–48, 50
thyroid hormone storage, 101
increase with dieting, 206
levels in
Addison's disease, 14
Cushing's disease, 14
fibromyalgia, 28
insomnia, 134
rheumatoid arthritis, 80
Stage 1 adrenal fatigue, 21
Stage 2 adrenal fatigue, 22–24, 195
Stage 3 adrenal fatigue, 26–28
link to progesterone, 60
patterns in sleep, 136
Cortisol awakening response, 11–12
Cravings, sugar/carbohydrates, 38, 48
C-reactive protein, 86, 156
Cucumber
Cucumber Boats, 335
Honeydew Cucumber Smoothie, 303
Smoked Salmon on Cucumber Slices, 337
Curry
Colorful Curry Bowl, 320
Cushing's disease, 14, 15

**D**

Dairy products, eliminating, 208
DASH diet, 91–92
Dehydration, 47, 49, 87, 206, 216
Dementia
improvement with
lavender, 226
phosphatidylserine, 232–33
in vitamin B₁₂ deficiency, 150
Dependency, 193–97
Depression
in adrenal fatigue, 22, 25, 27, 242, 247–48
comorbid with restless leg syndrome, 142
improvement with rhodiola, 228, 229
medication for, 195
serotonin associated with, 139
DHEA, 24, 56–57, 59–61
Diabetes, 31–50
codiagnosed conditions, 32, 42–43
conventional approach to diagnosing, 43–45
cost of, 42–43
gestational, 241
malnutrition and, 47–49
polycystic ovarian syndrome (PCOS) link,
63, 66

prevalence, 31
problems with dietary guidelines, 45–47
reversing, 31–32, 43
side effects, 35
steps to becoming diabetes-free, 49–50
treating with medication, 35–43
  adrenal support *versus* medication, 37–38
  blood pressure medication, 41–42
  metformin, 35–36, 38–39, <u>48</u>
  vicious cycle of suppressive therapy,
    38–40
type 2, 31–33, 35, 43, 45, 48–49, 63, 66
Diet
  anti-inflammatory, 89, <u>90</u>, 92
  DASH, 91–92
  impact on
    cardiovascular health, 89–93, <u>90</u>
    type 2 diabetes, 45–50
  vegan/vegetarian, 92–93, 219
Dietary Approaches to Stop Hypertension
  (DASH) diet, 91–92
Diet foods/drinks, 91–92, 207, 245
Dieting
  stress from, <u>206</u>
  yo-yo, 9, 38, 245
Dip
  3-Layer Mexican Dip, 336
Diuretics, 186–87
Dopamine
  inverse relationship with serotonin,
    139–40, 143
  for restless leg syndrome treatment, 142–43
  rhodiola's effect on, 228
Downward Dog, 271–72

**E**

Eating
  more, not less, 207
  in predictable pattern, 207–8
Eccentric Crunches, 264
Eggs
  Eggs Pipérade, 308
  Guacamole Deviled Eggs, 335
  Open-Face Egg Sandwich, 312
  Smoky Lentil, Egg, and Mushroom Skillet,
    309
  Spicy Vegetable and Grain Omelet, 311
  Sweet Potato Hash with Poached Eggs, 305
  Tofu Scramble with Peppers and
    Mushrooms, 306
Emotions
  in adrenal fatigue, 246, 247
  emotional healing, steps to, 283–86
    committing to new lifestyle, 285–86
    complete love of yourself, 284
    no excuses for your ailments, 284–85
  thyroid gland function and, 107–8

Endocrine system, 10, 37, 54
Environment of health, 53–54
Epinephrine
  effects, 8, 16
  increase during exercise, 246
  tyrosine as precursor to, 147
Erectile dysfunction, 55
Estrogen
  adrenal gland production of, 15–16
  dominance, 60–61, <u>64</u>
  hormone imbalances, 58–62, <u>62</u>, <u>64–65</u>
  supplementation, 58, 59
  testosterone conversion to, 55, 56–57
Excuses for ailments, stop making, 284–85
Exercise(s). *See also specific exercises*
  achieving your goals, 249–50
  benefits of, 240–41, 243
    cardiovascular health, 89–90, <u>90</u>
  calories burned by, 241
  CDC minimum required amount, 240–41
  by children, 241
  choosing enjoyable, <u>251</u>
  consistency, 246, <u>251</u>
  frequency, <u>251</u>, 253
  getting started with routine, 249
  guidelines, 253–54
    breathing, 253–54
    movement, 254
    posture, 254
  overexercising, 243–44
  Stage 1 protocol, 270–75
  Stage 2 protocol, 260–64
  Stage 3 protocol, 255–57
  time of day for, <u>251</u>
  time required for, 252–53

**F**

Fat(s)
  absorption after gallbladder removal, 126
  for diabetes reversal, 49
  energy from, 32–33
  processed by liver, 41, 42
  storage of, 47, 207
Fatigue
  in adrenal fatigue stages, 22, 25, 247, 248
  reduced with rhodiola, 229
  SSRIs for treatment of, 196
  stress-related, 229
Fibromyalgia, 28, 236
Fight-or-flight reaction, 6–8, 14, 244
Fish oil, <u>90</u>, 126
Flora, GI. *See also* Probiotics
  colonization by, 117
  effect of antibiotics on, 191
  IBS link to, 118
  imbalance, 118, 121–23
  roles of, 119–20

Folate, 92, 149, 150, <u>153</u>
Food. *See also* Nutrition; *specific foods*
  evaluating, 204–5
  fast, 119
  processed, 119, 207
  sources for basic nutrients, <u>209–12</u>
Food intolerance, 121, 122
Front Plank, 273–74
Fruits, colorful, 219, 222
Furosemide, 187

## G

Gallbladder, 126–27
Gamma-aminobutyric acid (GABA), 138–40,
  225, 231, 237
Gastroesophageal reflux disease (GERD),
  113, 124–25, 196
Gastrointestinal system
  acid problem, 196–97
  apartment complex analogy, 120–21
  autism link to health of, 117–18
  constipation, 127–28
  gallbladder, 126–27
  gastroesophageal reflux disease, 113,
    124–25, 196
  glycyrrhiza for disorders of, 235
  interdependence with other systems,
    130
  irritable bowel syndrome, 113–14,
    118
  liver, 128–29
  normal functioning of, 114–15
  probiotics (*see* Probiotics)
  stress and, 112–30
  symptoms of adrenal fatigue, <u>116</u>
  ulcers, 124, 167, 235
GERD, 113, 124–25, 196
Gestational diabetes, 241
Ginseng, 234–35
Glucose. *See also* Blood sugar
  energy from, 32–33
  production by liver, 33, 36–38,
    44, 49
  2-hour postprandial glucose test, 44
Glutamate, 138, 139
Glutamine, 170–71
Glute/Hamstring Ball Curls, 272
Gluten, 216
Glycemic index, 46
Glycyrrhiza, 235–36
Goals, achieving fitness, 249–50
Grains
  alternative, 208, 219
  USDA guidelines, 203, 204
Graves' disease, 109–10
Guacamole
  Guacamole Deviled Eggs, 335

## H

Hashimoto's thyroiditis, 98, 103–7
HbA1c, 39, 43–45
Headaches, improvement with lavender,
  226
Heart attack, 88–89, 90, 184
Heartburn. *See* Gastroesophageal reflux
  disease
Heart health. *See* Cardiovascular system/
  health
Heart rate, during meditation, 293
*Helicobacter pylori,* 167
Hemochromatosis, 168
Hemoglobin A1c (HbA1c), 39, 43–45
Hemorrhoids, 227
Hepatitis, 129, 230, 235
Herbs, for combating adrenal fatigue
  ashwagandha, 236–37
  ginseng, 234–35
  glycyrrhiza, 235–36
  lavender, 226–27
  L-theanine, 225
  passiflora, 227
  phosphatidylserine, 232–34
  rhodiola, 224, 228–30
  schisandra berry, 230–31
  valerian, 231–32
High sensitivity C-reactive protein (HSCRP),
  86
HIV/AIDS
  immune system and, 77–78
  schisandra berry for, 230
Homocysteine, 92–93, 150
Honeydew
  Honeydew Cucumber Smoothie, 303
Horizontal Tai Chi Circles, 255
Hormone(s). *See also specific hormones*
  adrenal fatigue and, 52–67
  blood sugar regulation, 32–34
  feedback loop, 54
  imbalances, 52
    polycystic ovarian syndrome, 63
    in women, 58–67, <u>62</u>, <u>64–65</u>
  rhythms in women, 57–58
  stress and release of, 8
Hot flashes, 58, <u>65</u>, 196, 231
HPA axis, 8, 138
HSCRP, 86
Hummus
  Grilled Portobello and Hummus Stacks,
    315
Hydrochloric acid, stomach, 115, 196–97
Hydrochlorothiazide, 186–87
Hydrocodone, 187–88
Hypertension
  aldosterone effect on, 13–15
  antihypertensive drugs, 182–87

conditions related to
    dehydration, 87
    diabetes, 42
    Stage 2 adrenal fatigue, 24
    Stage 3 adrenal fatigue, 27
  DASH diet, 91–92
Hyperthyroidism, 103, 109–10
Hypnotic medications, 133–34
Hypoglycemia, 38, 48–49
Hypothalamic-pituitary-adrenocortical
    (HPA) axis, 8, 138
Hypothyroidism, 98, 99, 101–2, 107–8, 110

## I

IBS, 113–14, 118
IgA, 122–23
Immune system
  adrenal fatigue and, 73–75
  ashwagandha effect on, 237
  components, 72–73
  disease, 75–81
    autoimmune disease, 79–81
    cancer, 70–71, 76–77
    HIV/AIDS, 77–78
  IgA, 122–23
  role of, 71
Inflammation
  anti-inflammatory diet, 89, 90, 92
  anti-inflammatory herbs, 227, 236
  blood markers of, 39
  cholesterol and, 86–87
  high sensitivity C-reactive protein
    (HSCRP) as marker, 86
  liver, 39–40, 42
  from omega-6 fatty acids, 39
  reducing with meditation, 291
  related conditions
    cancer, 70
    diabetes, 35, 39–40
    stress, 93
Insomnia
  in adrenal fatigue stages, 22–25, 27
  dopamine increase in, 139
  drugs for, 133–34, 136–37, 193–94
  effects of, 136
  improvement with
    lavender, 226
    valerian, 231–32
  prevalence, 132
  rebound, 139
  stress hormone levels in, 134
  treatment, 28
Insulin
  blood sugar regulation, 32–35
  fasting insulin test, 45
  reduction with metformin, 36
  release with cortisol, 35–36, 47–48, 50

Insulin resistance, 27, 34–35, 39, 45, 66,
    135–36
Intervals, cardiovascular, 264, 275
Intestinal permeability, 121
Iodine, 100
Iron
  deficiency, 166–67
  overview of, 166–68
  role in restless leg syndrome development,
    142
  storage, elevated, 167–68
Irritable bowel syndrome (IBS), 113–14,
    118

## J

Journaling, 294

## K

Kidney disease, diabetes-related, 42
Kidney stones, 163

## L

Lactic acidosis, 36
Lavender, 226–27
LDL, 84–86
Leaky gut syndrome, 121, 122–23
Lentils
  Rustic Lentil Soup, 316
  Smoky Lentil, Egg, and Mushroom Skillet,
    309
Lettuce
  Stuffed Lettuce Cups, 338
Levothyroxine, 97, 98, 101–2, 106, 237
Libido, decreased, 9, 55, 64–65
Licorice, 235–36
Lifestyle, committing to new, 285–86
Limb amputation, diabetes-related, 42
Liver
  blood pressure medication and, 41–42
  damage from statins, 181–82
  functions, 41–42, 128–29
  glucose production, 33, 36–38, 44, 49
  herbs for health of
    glycyrrhiza, 235–36
    schisandra berry, 230
  inflammation, 39–40, 42
  in Stage 3 adrenal fatigue, 27
Love for yourself, developing, 284
Low-density lipoprotein (LDL), 84–86
Lower body exercises
  Stage 1 protocol, 272–73
  Stage 2 protocol, 262–63
L-theanine, 225
Lymph nodes, 72
Lymphocytes, 72–73

# M

Magnesium
  benefits/roles of, 162–64
  calcium balanced by, 164, 185–86
  food sources of, 209
Malnutrition and diabetes, 47–49
Manganese, food sources of, 209–10
Mango
  Grilled Tuna and Mango Salad, 327
Medications, 175–98
  anti-anxiety, 194–95
  antibiotics, 190–92
  business of prescription, 178–79
  dependency, 193–97
  eliminating, 197–98
  gastric acid suppressers, 196–97
  most commonly prescribed, 180
  nervous system and, 195–96
  pain management, 187–90
  side effects, 181 (see also specific drugs)
  sleep-inducing, 193–94
  treating symptoms not causes, 179–82
Meditation
  in adrenal fatigue stages, 244, 246, 247, 292
  benefits of, 290–91
  learning to meditate, 291–95
  restorative routine, 293, 295
Melatonin, 140–41, 143, 151
Memory loss, schisandra berry for, 230
Men, testosterone in, 54–57
Menopause, 64–65, 67, 91
Menstrual cycle
  herbs affecting
    ashwagandha, 236
    glycyrrhiza, 235
  hormones, 57–58, 60–62, 64–65
  irregularities in
    hyperthyroidism, 109
    Stage 2 adrenal fatigue, 22
Mental clarity, schisandra berry for, 230
Metabolic syndrome, 35, 41, 136
Metformin, 35–36, 38–39, 48, 63
Mind-body connection, 281–95
  commitment sacrifice, 282–83
  fat deposition, 246
  meditation, 290–95, 292
  steps to emotional healing, 283–86
  tools for success, 286–90
Mindfulness walking, 257
Minerals. See also specific minerals
  affected by adrenal fatigue, 157–59, 162–70, 163
  described, 146–47
  imbalances in restless leg syndrome, 141–42
Modified Pushups (Close Hands), 260
Modified Pushups (Neutral Hands), 260

Mood, improvement with
  lavender, 226
  L-theanine, 225
  phosphatidylserine, 233
  rhodiola, 228–30
  valerian, 231
Movement, exercise guidelines for, 254
Muffins
  Almond and Mixed Berry Muffins, 339
  Blueberry Muffins, 341
  Wholesome Oat Muffins, 340
Mushrooms
  Grilled Portobello and Hummus Stacks, 315
  Smoky Lentil, Egg, and Mushroom Skillet, 309
  Tofu Scramble with Peppers and Mushrooms, 306
Myers' cocktail, 156
My Turnaround profiles
  Aird, Kirsten, 296
  Debbie, 239
  Ennesser, Jennifer, 131
  Hartwell, Sheree, 94
  Jessica, 30
  Marcus, John, 68
  Matt, Tanya, 82
  Mulkins, Erin, 111
  Porter, Morgan, 174
  Predebon, Sheri, 280
  Sekan, Susan, 297
  Snell, Liz, 51
  Terrell, Teal, 223
  Wareham, Pat, 199
  Zimmerman, John, 144

# N

Natural medicine, principles of, 177–78
Naturopathic physician, oath of, 177–78
Negative feedback loop, 10
Nervous system disorders, treatment of, 179, 195–96
Neural tube defects, 149
Neurotransmitters, 118, 139–40, 143, 155. See also specific neurotransmitters
Niacin, 151–52, 153
Nicotine, 290
Non-Hodgkin's lymphoma, 69–70
Non-REM sleep, 134–35, 137
Norepinephrine
  effects, 8, 16
  increase during exercise, 246
  tyrosine as precursor to, 147
Nutrients
  fat-soluble and water-soluble, 147
  food sources for basic, 209–12
  synergy of, 148

Nutrition
adrenal restoration nutritional plan,
205–22
customizing, 213
guidelines, 206–8
Stage 2 plan, 216–19
Stage 3 plan, 213–16
balance of nutrients, 148
malnutrition and diabetes, 47–49
portion breakdown, 208
in Stage 1 adrenal fatigue, 21–22
USDA guidelines, 203–4
Nutritional deficiencies, 145–46, 148
Nuts
Nutty Celery Sticks, 337

**O**

Oatmeal
Savory Oatmeal, 313
Oats
Oat-Almond Mixed Berry Crisp, 343
Wholesome Oat Muffins, 340
Obesity
in children, 241
sleep decrease link to, 135
in Stage 3 adrenal fatigue, 247
Oblique Crunches, 274
Oils, 90
Omega-3 fatty acids, 49, 171–73, 210
Omega-6 fatty acids, 171
Opioids, 188–90
Osteopenia, 15, 108, 241
Osteoporosis, 108, 150, 241
Overweight children, 241
Oxycodone, 188–89

**P**

Pain management drugs, 187–90
Parasympathetic nervous system, 114, 121,
125, 253, 281, 293
Parathyroid hormone, 12, 14
Passiflora, 227
Pasta
Zesty Pasta Salad, 318
PCOS, 63, 66–67, 136
Peaches
Peach Blueberry Smoothie, 336
Peanut butter
Chicken Peanut Noodle Bowl, 325
Peppers
Moroccan Stuffed Peppers, 321
Steamed Vegetables with Red Pepper Sauce,
334
Tofu Scramble with Peppers and
Mushrooms, 306
Perimenopause, 64–65, 245

Phosphatidylserine, 232–34
Pilates, 252
Pineapple
Glazed Pineapple Cupcakes, 342
Plums
Plum-Blueberry Cobbler, 344
Red Fruit Crumble, 346
PMS, 57, 61–62
Polycystic ovarian syndrome (PCOS), 63,
66–67, 136
Posture, 253, 254
Potassium
aldosterone effect on, 12, 14, 15
diuretic effect on, 186–87
food sources of, 210
increase by
ACE inhibitors, 183
glycyrrhiza, 235
retention and low blood pressure, 91
role in restless leg syndrome, 141–42
PPI, 196–97
Prediabetes, 31, 38, 42–43, 136
Pregnancy
gestational diabetes, 241
in Stage 2 adrenal fatigue, 245
Pregnenolone, 24, 57, 60
Premenstrual syndrome (PMS), 57, 61–62
Probiotics
benefits of, 117
cardiovascular system link to, 118–19
described, 115
dosage, 191, 192
following antibiotic use, 191–93
weight loss and, 119
Progesterone
adrenal gland production of, 15–16
effects, 59–60
hormone imbalances, 58–62, 62, 64–65
link to cortisol, 60
Prone Multifidi, 263–64
Proteins
energy from, 32–33
liver role in building and breaking down, 41
sources of, 203, 208, 216, 219
USDA guidelines, 203–4
Proton pump inhibitor (PPI), 196–97
Psychiatric disorders, sleep and, 137–40
Pushups (Close Hands), 270
Pushups (Neutral Hands), 270

**Q**

Quarter Dog, 261
Quinoa
Quinoa and Butternut Cereal, 310
Quinoa Tabbouleh, 326
Quiz, to determine stage of adrenal fatigue,
17–20

## R

Rapid eye movement (REM) sleep, 134–37
Raspberries
    Red Fruit Crumble, 346
Recommended daily amount (RDA), 203–4
Recovery, slowed by extreme exercise, 243
REM sleep, 134–37
Restless leg syndrome, 12, 141–43
Reverse Bridge with March on Bench or Ball, 272
Reverse T3, 100–103, 105–8
Rheumatoid arthritis, 80–81
Rhodiola, 224, 228–30
Rice
    Brown Rice Bowl, 314
Rice noodles
    Chicken Peanut Noodle Bowl, 325

## S

Salads
    Fresh Fruit Salad Cup, 336
    Fruited Carrot-Veggie Salad, 304
    Grilled Tuna and Mango Salad, 327
    Mediterranean Chopped Salad, 323
    Zesty Pasta Salad, 318
Salmon
    Salmon Miso Soup, 324
    Smoked Salmon on Cucumber Slices, 337
    Speedy Salmon Wrap, 317
Sandwich
    Open-Face Egg Sandwich, 312
Scheduling your time, 289–90
Schisandra berry, 230–31
Scurvy, 155
Selective serotonin reuptake inhibitors (SSRIs), 195–96
Selenium
    benefits/roles of, 100, 102, 164–66
    food sources of, 210
Serotonin
    inverse relationship with dopamine, 139–40, 143
    precursors, 225, 231
    production in the intestine, 118
    rhodiola's effect on, 228
    selective serotonin reuptake inhibitors (SSRIs), 195–96
    vitamins needed for production, 146
Sex hormones. See also Estrogen;
        Progesterone; Testosterone
    adrenal gland production of, 15–16
    decrease in Stage 3 adrenal fatigue, 27
    hormone imbalances, 58–62, 62
Sexual desire, 9, 59. See also Libido
Side-Lying Leg Raise, 262
Side Plank, 274

Silicon, food sources of, 210
Single Leg Chair Lifts, 262
Single Leg Chair Pose, 273
Sleep, 132–43. See also Insomnia
    attention deficit hyperactivity disorder (ADHD) and, 140–41
    cortisol awakening response, 11–12
    daytime sleepiness, 27
    essential nature of, 132
    improvement with
        lavender, 226
        L-theanine, 225
        valerian, 231–32
        yoga, 244
    low testosterone effect on, 55
    normal cycle, 134–35
    prescription sleep aides, 133–34, 136–37, 193–94
    psychiatric disease and, 137–40
    rapid eye movement (REM), 134–37
    restless leg syndrome and, 141–43
    role of vitamin $B_6$ in, 151–52
Smoking, 176–77, 290
Smoothie
    Honeydew Cucumber Smoothie, 303
    Peach Blueberry Smoothie, 336
Sodium
    aldosterone effect on, 12, 14, 15
    diuretic effect on, 186–87
    dumping in low blood pressure, 91
Soups
    Chicken Tortilla Soup, 333
    Rustic Lentil Soup, 316
    Salmon Miso Soup, 324
    Tomato-Watermelon Gazpacho, 331
Spleen, 72
SSRIs, 195–96
Standing Lunges, 262
Standing Momentum Arm Raises (Front and Sides), 261
Standing Momentum Arm Raises (Front and Sides) with Weight, 271
Standing Terror Bands, 272
Statins, 84, 181–82
Steroids, therapeutic use of, 113, 117
Strawberries
    Red Fruit Crumble, 346
Strength training, CDC recommended amount, 240–41
Strep, 123–24
Stress
    adaptation to, 5–6, 11, 228–29
    in adrenal fatigue stages, 25, 27–28, 245–46
    author's stress-related illness, 78
    cortisol release in, 11, 33
    dieting as source of, 206
    digestive system and, 112–30

effect on
  blood sugar, 32–35
  cancer, 69–70, 76
  gallbladder function, 127
  heart health, 88–89
  liver health, 129
  polycystic ovarian syndrome, 66–67
  progesterone level, 62
  sex hormone balance, 61
  sexual desire, 59
  thyroid function, 110
effects of chronic on society, 7–8
fight-or-flight reaction to, 7
hormonal response to, 8
inflammation with, 93
reducing with
  ginseng, 234
  meditation, 291
  walking outside, 257
  yoga, 244
Stroke, diabetes-related, 42
Strontium, food sources of, 210
Sweet potato
  Sweet Potato Hash with Poached Eggs, 305
Sympathetic nervous system, 8, 14, 114, 183, 254

T

Tai chi, 252, 255
Testosterone
  adrenal gland production of, 15–16
  bioavailable, 54–55, 56
  conversion to estrogens, 55, 56–57
  supplementation, 55–57
  in women, 57–59, 64–65
Thymus, 72
Thyroid gland
  adrenal gland as ruler of, 106–7
  ashwagandha effect on, 237
  basics of, 99–100
  business analogy, 95–97
  calcitonin, 108
  constipation with low function, 128
  emotional side of, 107–8
  Hashimoto's thyroiditis, 98, 103–7
  hyperthyroidism, 103, 109–10
  low-functioning thyroid (hypothyroidism),
    98, 99, 101–2, 107–8, 110
  prevalence of malfunction, 98–99
  selenium for health of, 164–66
  stress effects on, 110
Thyroid hormones, 98, 100–103, 105–8
Thyroid stimulating hormone (TSH), 97,
    99–103, 105, 107–8
Tofu
  Asparagus and Tofu Stir-Fry, 319
  Tofu Scramble with Peppers and
    Mushrooms, 306

Tomatoes
  Tomato-Watermelon Gazpacho, 331
Toxin, removal by liver, 128–29
TPO antibodies, 103, 105
Trail mix
  Chocolate Lover's Trail Mix, 337
Tryptophan, 141
Ts, 261
TSH, 97, 99–103, 105, 107–8
Ts Over the Ball, 271
Tuna
  Grilled Tuna and Mango Salad, 327
2-hour postprandial glucose test, 44
Tyrosine, 147

U

Ulcers, 124, 167, 235
Upper body exercises
  Stage 1 protocol, 270–72
  Stage 2 protocol, 260–61
Upper respiratory infections, ginseng for, 234
USDA guidelines, 203–4

V

Valerian, 231–32
Vegan/vegetarian diets, 92–93, 219
Vegetables
  Fruited Carrot-Veggie Salad, 304
  in nutritional plan
    Stage 1, 222
    Stage 2, 216
    Stage 3, 216
  Roasted Root Vegetables, 330
  Spicy Vegetable and Grain Omelet, 311
  Steamed Vegetables with Red Pepper Sauce,
    334
  water-rich, 216
Vertical Tai Chi Circles, 255
Visualization exercise, 249
Vitamin(s)
  affected by adrenal fatigue, 149–57, 159–61
  B vitamins, 92–93, 149–54, 153
  fat-soluble and water-soluble, 147
  vitamin A, 100
  vitamin B₁, 153
  vitamin B₃, 153
  vitamin B₅, 92, 205
    benefits/roles of, 152–54, 153
    food sources of, 210–11
  vitamin B₆, 92, 138, 146
    benefits/roles of, 150–52, 153
    food sources of, 211
  vitamin B₇, 153
  vitamin B₁₂
    anemia, 36
    benefits/roles of, 146, 150, 153

Vitamin(s) (*cont.*)
  vitamin B$_{12}$ (*cont.*)
    deficiency, 92, 149, 150
    food sources of, <u>211</u>
  vitamin C, 78
    administration of, 156–57
    benefits/roles of, 146, 154–57
    food sources of, 155, <u>211</u>
  vitamin D
    cholesterol role in production, 84, 108
    deficiency with
      aldosterone excess, 15
      gallbladder removal, 126
      hypothyroidism, 108
    food sources of, 161, <u>162</u>, <u>211</u>
    overview of, 159–61
    parathyroid hormone effect on, 15
  vitamin K, food sources of, <u>211–12</u>

# W

Walking, 254–55, 257, 260, 270
Walking Lunges, 273
Warmup, 254–59, 260, 270
Water, daily recommended amount, 206
Watermelon
  Tomato-Watermelon Gazpacho, 331
Weight gain
  exercising to avoid, 242
  in Stage 2 adrenal fatigue, 246
Weight loss
  in adrenal fatigue
    Stage 1, 243
    Stage 2, 245–46, 247
    Stage 3, 248
  with exercise, 242
  failure to achieve goals, 9–10
  in hyperthyroidism, 109
  probiotics and, 119
*Withania somnifera*, 236–37
Women
  hormonal imbalances, 58–67, <u>62</u>, <u>64–65</u>
  hormonal rhythms, 57–58
  symptoms of unbalanced system, 58–61
  testosterone in, 57–59, <u>64–65</u>

Workout program, 250–79
  described, 250, 252
  secrets to success, <u>251</u>
  Stage 1 protocol, 270–79
    exercises, 270–75
    warmup, 270
    weeks 1 & 2, 276–77
    weeks 3 & 4, 277
    weeks 5 & 6, 278
    weeks 7 & 8, 279
  Stage 2 protocol, 260–69
    exercises, 260–64
    warmup, 260
    weeks 1 & 2, 266–67
    weeks 3 & 4, 267
    weeks 5 & 6, 268
    weeks 7 & 8, 269
  Stage 3 protocol, 254–59
    exercises, 255–57
    warmup, 254–59
    weeks 1 & 2, 258
    weeks 3 & 4, 258
    weeks 5 & 6, 259
    weeks 7 & 8, 259

# Y

Yoga
  in adrenal fatigue stages, 244, 247
  benefits of, 244
  restorative sequence, 256–57
    Assisted Bridge Pose, 256
    Legs Up on a Chair Pose, 256
    Supported Child's Pose, 256
    Supported Goddess Pose, 256–57
Ys, 261
Ys Over the Ball, 271

# Z

Zinc
  benefits/roles of, 100, 102, 168–69
  deficiency, 169–70
  food sources of, <u>212</u>
  supplementing, 170